J. H. Peter T. Podszus P. von Wichert (Eds.)

Sleep Related Disorders and Internal Diseases

Springer-Verlag
Berlin Heidelberg New York
London Paris Tokyo

PD Dr. med. Jörg Hermann Peter
Dr. med. Thomas Podszus
Prof. Dr. med. P. von Wichert
Zentrum für Innere Medizin
Med. Poliklinik
Baldinger Straße
3550 Marburg

ISBN-13: 978-3-642-72562-3 e-ISBN-13: 978-3-642-72560-9
DOI: 10.1007/978-3-642-72560-9

Library of Congress Cataloging-in-Publication Data.

Sleep related disorders and internal diseases. Based on a symposium held at the Philipps-Universität, Marburg/Lahn, FRG on May 26-28, 1986. 1. Sleep apnea syndromes - Congresses. 2. Sleep disorders - Congresses. I. Peter, J. H. (Jörg Hermann), 1945- . II. Podszus, Th. (Thomas), 1950- III. Wichert, P. von (Peter) [DNLM: 1. Sleep-physiology-congresses. 2. Sleep Apnea Syndromes-congresses. 3. Sleep Disorders-congresses.

Softcover reprint of the hardcover 1st edition 1987

Printed: E. Kieser, Augsburg
Binding: J. Schäffer, Grünstadt
2119-3140-543210

Preface

The normal function of the organism in various stages of activity can be seen as a process of mutual interaction of different regulation mechanisms building up the behaviour of the organism in changing situations and/or ages and/or levels of health or disease. Insights into these very complex relations which steer the action of the organism are particularly important for the study of internal medicine. They can be seen as directly related to the understanding of pathological conditions.

Recently, the medical community has focused its interest on the physiology and pathophysiology of events which happen during sleep. Although some information on pathological regulation during sleep was collected in the 1930s, the modern technology of registration methods is required to analyse the phenomena of sleep-related physiological and pathophysiological patterns. It is interesting that the modern research in this field developed from neuropsychiatry and is now expanding into other fields of medicine, although some problems, for instance the Pickwickian syndrome, were also for a long time considered part of the field of internal medicine. It becomes clearer that sleep is not only a neuropsychiatric phenomenon, but also has profound consequences for other physiological circuits, perhaps even an important role in pathogenesis.

Sleep also has profound consequences for internal diseases. This was shown very clearly recently by many groups, although their data have not yet received the attention which they deserve. It is now clear that the role of sleep is very important in relation to widespread problems such as arterial hypertension, respiratory insufficiency, and overweight, which are important for public health, including therefore also aspects of health costs, and social interaction.

We are now in the position to see the magnitude of the problem and how much work is still needed to gain a deeper knowledge of the mechanisms, epidemiology, pathogenesis, and therapy of sleep-related disorders as well as to develop better diagnostic tools. Internal medicine in particular is dependent on insights into physiological and pathophysiological regulation; it can be seen at least in part as applied pathophysiology. Therefore any information on, and insights into, the regulatory processes can lead directly to diagnostic and therapeutic measures.

As the amount of information which has been accumulated lately seems to us important for internal medicine, we organised this international symposium on sleep-related disorders and internal medicine at the Philipps-Universität, Marburg/Lahn, FRG. I would like to thank the many authors and participants at the symposium for their contributions, which are collected in this volume.

It was the aim of this symposium, organised by the working group "Disorders of regulation of breathing and circulation" of the Deutsche Gesellschaft für Pneumologie and the working group "Zeitreihenanalyse" (time series analysis) of the Medizinische Poliklinik der Philipps-Universität, Marburg, to review our present knowledge of the role of sleep-related alterations in internal diseases and to develop new ideas in this field as well as to stimulate future research. It was the first symposium on this subject. The work of Drs. Bonsignore, Hildebrandt, Kurtz, Martin, Matthys and Siegrist on the advisory committee of the Symposium is gratefully acknowledged.

This symposium was generously supported by the Deutsche Forschungsgemeinschaft, the Hessische Minister für Wissenschaft und Kunst, and the Philipps-Universität Marburg.

Many institutions and companies have contributed to our work in this field, thus making it possible to arrange this symposium. Among them are: Bayer AG, Bayropharm GmbH, Behringwerke AG, Boehringer Mannheim GmbH, Bristol Myers GmbH, Byk Gulden Lomberg Chem. Fabrik GmbH, Degussa Pharma Gruppe (Homburg), Hoechst AG, Hoffmann La Roche AG, Klinge Pharma GmbH, Knoll AG, Mundipharma GmbH, Pharma Schwarz GmbH, Röhm Pharma GmbH, Sandoz AG, Sanol Schwarz GmbH, Hellige GmbH, Intertechnique GmbH, Madaus Medizin Elektronik GmbH & Co. KG, Schubart Physik Elektronik Medizin, SEFAM, Stimotron Medizinische Geräte, and Paul-Martini-Stiftung der med. pharm. Studienges. e.V.

My particular thanks go to the administration of the University Hospital, to our secretaries and many colleagues. I am indebted also to Springer-Verlag Heidelberg, particularly Dr. Graf-Baumann, for publishing the results of the symposium in the present volume.

P. von Wichert

ACKNOWLEDGEMENT. The editors wish to thank Mr. M. Faust for the excellent planning and organization of the symposium. In addition, we are grateful to him for his contribution in reviewing the papers and in cooperating with Springer Press.

The contributors from the "Zeitreihenlabor", Marburg, would also like to thank Mr. T. S. Wohlfeil for translating their contributions, and for his help in shaping them.

Foreword

An international symposium is difficult to arrange, organise and complete. Thus, I highly commend Drs. von Wichert and Peter and their organising committee for the interesting and informative symposium on sleep-related disorders and internal diseases. The exchange of information and ideas at this conference was timely and stimulating. The symposium covered wide areas of pathology associated with the sleep cycle, thus reinforcing the concept that most diseases must be viewed with equal regard for sleeping and waking cycles. The importance of this view is that disease processes continue to act during sleep, many times in an exaggerated or different manner than during wakefulness.

The study of sleep itself, and associated diseases, has rapidly expanded in the past 15 years. Originally, this field was largely a basic science research effort, mostly limited to psychiatry. Today, as this symposium illustrates, there are applications throughout all areas of medicine. Many new specialties, both on a research and a clinical basis, have found the need to investigate the sleep cycle. To name a few, these disciplines include pulmonary medicine, cardiology, neurology, gastroenterology, urology and physiology. As the interest and knowledge of the importance of the sleep cycle continues to develop, virtually all areas of medicine will be involved in assessing diseases during sleep.

Although the written word cannot convey the verbal interaction at a symposium such as this, what is covered in this book brings forth both new information as well as concise summaries of various areas of sleep-related internal diseases. This book fills the need to disseminate pertinent information in this area, and make better understanding of it available to the reader. Research and therapeutic interventions will continue to develop rapidly here, and all of us will need continually to update our knowledge in this new and exciting area.

R. J. Martin
Director, Adult Special Care Unit
Director, Sleep Disorders Program
National Jewish Center for Immunology
and Respiratory Medicine, 1400 Jackson Street,
and
Associate Professor of Medicine,
University of Colorado Health Sciences Center, Denver, Colorado 80206, USA

Contents

Part 1: Sleep and Disordered Sleep

Sleep – Introductory Notes
P. Lavie 3

Chronobiological Aspects of Sleep Disorders
G. Hildebrandt 9

Critical Assessment Issues in Disordered Sleep and Wakefulness
K.-O. Liebmann 30

The Interaction of Drugs with Sleep
W. P. Koella 36

Part 2: Measurement

Measurement of Sleep Fragmentation
S. A. Rothenberg 63

Paroxysmal Awakenings from Sleep – A Model of Sleep Fragmentation Causing Excessive Daytime Sleepiness
R. Peled 75

Various Components of Respiratory Control During Sleep, Rest, and Strain
F. Raschke 83

Interindividual Differences in Sleep Patterns During Night and Shift Work
R. Moog 89

The Application of Time-Series Analysis to the Diagnosis of Complex Internal Disorders: Sleep Apnea
T. Penzel, and J. H. Peter 100

Techniques to Construct Respiratory Waveforms from VCG/ECG
F. Pinciroli, R. Rossi, and L. Vergani 110

Use of Tracheal Sound Recordings to Monitor Airflow During Sleep
N. MESLIER, and J. L. RACINEUX 121

Thoracoabdominal Motion in Health and Disease
M. J. TOBIN 125

Assessment of the Time Structure of Sleep Apneas
F. RASCHKE, J. MAYER, T. PENZEL, J. H. PETER, T. PODSZUS, and
P. VON WICHERT 135

An Apnea-Monitoring Device Based on Variation of Heart Rate and
Snoring
J. H. PETER, E. FUCHS, M. HÜGENS, U. KÖHLER, K. MEINZER,
U. MÜLLER, P. VON WICHERT, and M. ZAHORKA 140

Vigilance and Performance in Sleep Apnea Under Single-Dose
Theophylline Therapy
K. WEBER, B. EHRIG, E. FUCHS, T. PENZEL, and J. H. PETER 147

Computerization of Respiratory Parameters During Sleep
D. ROSE, P. AUBRY, T. VELEINE, and Z. RIDA 157

EEG-Analysis Among Patients with Sleep Apnea by Means
of a Microcomputer
H.-G. DAUN 161

Acquisition and Storage of Sleep-Related Biosignals
T. PENZEL, K. MEINZER, and J. H. PETER 166

Part 3: Epidemiology I

Sleep Disturbances and Cardiovascular Risk: A Biopsychosocial Approach
J. SIEGRIST 173

Sleep and Stress
T. ÅKERSTEDT 183

Prevalence of Sleep Complaints Among Swedish Men –
An Epidemiological Study
T. GISLASON 192

Part 4: Epidemiology II – Snoring

Clinical Approach to Heavy Snorers' Disease and Other Sleep-Related
Respiratory Disorders
E. LUGARESI, F. CIRIGNOTTA, and P. MONTAGNA 201

Snoring as a Risk Factor for Ischaemic Heart Disease and Stroke in Men
M. KOSKENVUO, J. KAPRIO, T. TELAKIVI, M. PARTINEN, K. HEIKKILÄ, and S. SARNA 211

Snoring, Sleep Apnea, and Hypertension in a Field Study
M. ZAHORKA, U. HESS, H. HIMMELMANN, U. KÖHLER, J. MAYER, J. H. PETER, T. PODSZUS, J. SIEGRIST and E. SOHN 219

Part 5: Epidemiology III - Sleep-Related Breathing Disorders

Rediscovering Sleepy Patients: The Sleep Apnea Syndrome
P. LAVIE 227

The Prevalence of Increased Pulmonary Arterial Pressure Among Sleep Apneics
T. PODSZUS and I. BECKER 241

Sleep Apnea Activity and General Morbidity in a Field Study
J. H. PETER, U. HESS, H. HIMMELMANN, U. KÖHLER, J. MAYER, T. PODSZUS, J. SIEGRIST, and E. SOHN 248

Breathing During Sleep in Normal Subjects
N. J. DOUGLAS 254

Sleep-Related Disordered Breathing, Daytime Hypertension, and Nocturnal Hypotension in Older Males
M. R. LITTNER, D. MCGINTY, and N. STERN 261

Part 6: Cardiorespiratory Disorders During Sleep and Hemodynamics

Nocturnal Hyopxemia and Pulmonary Arterial Blood Pressure
K. H. RÜHLE, and H. MATTHYS 271

Interaction of Sleep Apnea and Chronic Lung Disease
E. C. FLETCHER 279

The Role of Sleep-Related Breathing Disorders in Cardiorespiratory Disease: Hemodynamics
R. J. MARTIN 299

Part 7: Cardiovasular Risk and Sleep Apnea

Nocturnal Hemodynamics in Patients with Sleep Apnea
J. MAYER, H. GREB, B. HERRES, T. M. KLOSS, T. PENZEL, J. H. PETER, T. PODSZUS, and P. VON WICHERT 315

Plasma Levels of Catecholamines and Cardiovascular Parameters During Sleep in Patients with Sleep Apnea Syndrome
K. Ehlenz, U. Köhler, J. Mayer, J. H. Peter, P. von Wichert, and H. Kaffarnik 321

Echocardiographic Findings in Sleep Apnea
W. Motz, C. Bethge, M. Klepzig, H. Blanke, and B. E. Strauer 326

Bradyarrhythmias in Patients with Sleep Apnea
U. Köhler, W. Rasbach, and J. H. Peter 330

Part 8: Therapy

Treatment of Sleep Apnea by Prosthetic Mandibular Advancement
K. Meier-Ewert, and B. Brosig 341

Review of the Therapeutic Approaches to Sleep Apnea
D. Kurtz, and J. Krieger 346

Five Years' Experience with Home Nasal Continuous Positive Airway Pressure Therapy for the Obstructive Sleep Apnea Syndrome
F. Issa, R. Grunstein, J. Bruderer, L. Costas, V. McCauley, M. Berthon-Jones, and C. Sullivan 360

Problems in the Application of Nasal Continuous Positive Airway Pressure for the Treatment of Obstructive Sleep Apnea. Hypoxemia During Sleep on Nasal Continuous Positive Airway Pressure Treatment
J. Krieger, and D. Kurtz 366

Hemodynamics in Obstructive Sleep Apnea Syndrome Patients Treated by Continuous Positive Airway Pressure
O. Marrone, G. Ferrara, C. Macaluso, F. Milone, F. Cibella, V. Bellia, and G. Bonsignore 375

Reversibility of Severe Cardiac Arrhythmias in Sleep Apnea Under Nasal Continuous Positive Airway Pressure Therapy
H. Becker, M. Faust, U. Köhler, and J. H. Peter 380

Current Research in Sleep-Related Breathing Disorders: Conclusions for Internal Diagnostics and Therapy
J. H. Peter 388

Contributors

T. Åkerstedt
IPM & Stress Research, Karolinska Institute
Box 60205, S-10401 Stockholm, Sweden

P. Aubry
Service de Pneumologie, CHU d' Amiens - Université de Picardie, Hôpital Sud, Avenue Rene Laenec, Salouel 80480 Saleux, France

H. Becker
Medizinische Poliklinik - Zeitreihenlabor, University of Marburg, Baldingerstraße, D-3550 Marburg, FRG

I. Becker
Medizinische Poliklinik - Zeitreihenlabor, University of Marburg, Baldingerstraße, D-3550 Marburg, FRG

V. Bellia
Università Degli Studi di Palermo, Instituto di Medicina Generale e Pneumologia, University of Palermo, Via Trabucco 180, I-90146 Palermo, Italy

M. Berthon-Jones
Department of Medicine, University of Sydney, Sydney, NSW 2006, Australia

C. Bethge
Klinikum Marburg, Baldingerstraße, D-3550 Marburg, FRG

H. Blanke
Klinikum Marburg, Baldingerstraße, D-3550 Marburg, FRG

G. Bonsignore
Università Degli Studi di Palermo, Instituto di Medicine Generale e Pneumologia, University of Palermo, Via Trabucco 180, I-90146 Palermo, Italy

B. Brosig
Neurologische Klinik Hephata, D-3578 Schwalmstadt-Treysa, FRG

J. BRUDERER
Department of Medicine, University of Sydney, Sydney, NSW 2006, Australia

F. CIBELLA
Università Degli Studi di Palermo, Instituto di Medicina Generale e Pneumologia, University of Palermo, Via Trabucco 180, I-90146 Palermo, Italy

F. CIRIGNOTTA
Institute of Neurology, University of Bologna, Via U. Foscolo 7, I-40123 Bologna, Italy

L. COSTAS
Department of Medicine, University of Sydney, Sydney, NSW 2006, Australia

H.-G. DAUN
Medizinisches Zentrum für Nervenheilkunde, Neurologische Klinik und Poliklinik, University of Marburg, Rudolf-Bultmann-Str. 8, D-3550 Marburg, FRG

N. J. DOUGLAS
Department of Respiratory Medicine, University of Edinburgh, City Hospital, Greenbank Drive, Edinburgh EH10 5SB, UK

K. EHLENZ
Zentrum für Innere Medizin, Abteilung für Endokrinologie und Stoffwechsel, Baldingerstraße, D-3550 Marburg, FRG

B. EHRIG
Medizinische Poliklinik – Zeitreihenlabor, University of Marburg, Baldingerstraße, D-3550 Marburg, FRG

M. FAUST
Medizinische Poliklinik – Zeitreihenlabor, University of Marburg, Baldingerstraße, D-3550 Marburg, FRG

G. FERRARA
Università Degli Studi di Palermo, Instituto di Medicina Generale e Pneumologia, University of Palermo, Via Trabucco 180, I-90146 Palermo, Italy

E. C. FLETCHER
Department of Internal Medicine, Baylor College of Medicine, One Baylor Plaza, Texas Medical Center, Houston, Texas 77030, USA

E. FUCHS
Medizinische Poliklinik – Zeitreihenlabor, University of Marburg, Baldingerstraße, D-3550 Marburg, FRG

T. Gislason
Department of Lung Medicine, Akademiska Sjukhuset, Uppsala University, S-75185 Uppsala, Sweden

H. Greb
Medizinische Poliklinik - Zeitreihenlabor, University of Marburg, Baldingerstraße, D-3550 Marburg, FRG

R. Grunstein
Sleep Unit, Department of Thoracic Medicine, Royal Prince Alfred Hospital, Camperdown, NSW 2050, Australia

K. Heikkilä
Department of Public Health, University of Helsinki, Haartmaninkatu 3, SF-00290 Helsinki 29, Finland

B. Herres
Medizinische Poliklinik - Zeitreihenlabor, University of Marburg, Baldingerstraße, D-3550 Marburg, FRG

U. Hess
Medizinische Poliklinik - Zeitreihenlabor, University of Marburg, Baldingerstraße, D-3550 Marburg, FRG

G. Hildebrandt
Institut für Arbeitsphysiologie und Rehabilitationsforschung, University of Marburg, Robert-Koch-Str. 7 a, D-3550 Marburg, FRG

H. Himmelmann
Medizinische Poliklinik - Zeitreihenlabor, University of Marburg, Baldingerstraße, D-3550 Marburg, FRG

M. Hügens
Medizinische Poliklinik - Zeitreihenlabor, University of Marburg, Baldingerstraße, D-3550 Marburg, FRG

F. G. Issa
Department of Medicine, University of Sydney
Sydney, NSW 2006, Australia

H. Kaffarnik
Zentrum für Innere Medizin, Abteilung für Endokrinologie und Stoffwechsel, Baldingerstraße, D-3550 Marburg, FRG

J. Kaprio
Department of Public Health, University of Helsinki, Haartmaninkatu 3, SF-00290 Helsinki 29, Finland

M. KLEPZIG
Klinikum Marburg, Baldingerstraße, D-3550 Marburg, FRG

T. M. KLOSS
Medizinische Poliklinik - Zeitreihenlabor, University of Marburg, Baldingerstraße, D-3550 Marburg, FRG

U. KÖHLER
Medizinische Poliklinik - Zeitreihenlabor, University of Marburg, Baldingerstraße, D-3550 Marburg, FRG

W. P. KOELLA
Buchenstr. 1, CH-4104 Oberwil (BL), Switzerland

M. KOSKENVUO
Department of Public Health, University of Helsinki, Haartmaninkatu 3, SF-00290 Helsinki 29, Finland

J. KRIEGER
Service d'Explorations Fonctionelles du Système Nerveux, Centre Hospitalier Règional, Place de l'Hôpital, F-67091 Strasbourg Cédex, France

D. KURTZ
Service d'Explorations Fonctionelle du Système Nerveux, Hôpital Civil, F-67091 Strasbourg Cédex, France

P. LAVIE
Sleep Laboratory, Faculty of Medicine, Technion - Israel Institute of Technology, Gutwirth Building, Technion City, Haifa 32000, Israel

K.-O. LIEBMANN
The Griffin Hospital, Sleep Disorders Center, 130 Division Street, Derby, Connecticut 06418, USA

M. R. LITTNER
Sepulveda Veterans Administration Medical Center, 16111 Plummer Street, Sepulveda, California 91343, USA

E. LUGARESI
Institute of Neurology, University of Bologna, Via U. Foscolo 7, I-40123 Bologna, Italy

C. MACALUSO
Università Degli Studi di Palermo, Instituto di Medicina Generale e Pneumologia, University of Palermo, Via Trabucco 180, I-90146 Palermo, Italy

O. Marrone
Università Degli Studi di Palermo, Instituto di Medicina Generale e Pneumologia, University of Palermo, Via Trabucco 180, I-90146 Palermo, Italy

R. J. Martin
Pulmonary Physiology Unit, National Jewish Center for Immunology and Respiratory Medicine, 1400 Jackson Street, Denver, Colorado 80206, USA

H. Matthys
Robert-Koch-Klinik, Abteilung für Pneumologie, University of Freiburg, Hugstetter-Str. 55, D-7800 Freiburg, FRG

J. Mayer
Medizinische Poliklinik - Zeitreihenlabor, University of Marburg, Baldingerstraße, D-3550 Marburg, FRG

N. McCauley
Department of Medicine, University of Sydney, Sydney, NSW 2006, Australia

D. McGinty
Sepulveda Veterans Administration Medical Center, 16111 Plummer Street, Sepulveda, California 91343, USA

K. Meier-Ewert
Neurologische Klinik Hephata, D-3578 Schwalmstadt-Treysa, FRG

K. Meinzer
Zentrales Entwicklungs-Laboratorium für Elektronik, University of Marburg, Ernst-Giller-Str. 20, D-3550 Marburg, FRG

N. Meslier
Clinique de Pneumologie, CHU 49033 Angers Cedex, France

F. Milone
Università Degli Studi di Palermo, Instituto di Medicina Generale e Pneumologia, University of Palermo, Via Trabucco 180, I-90146 Palermo, Italy

P. Montagna
Institute of Neurology, University of Bologna, Via U. Foscolo 7, I-40123 Bologna, Italy

R. Moog
Institut für Arbeitsphysiologie und Rehabilitationsforschung, University of Marburg, Robert-Koch-Str. 7 a, D-3550 Marburg, FRG

W. Motz
Klinikum Marburg, Baldingerstraße, D-3550 Marburg, FRG

U. Müller
Zentrales Entwicklungs-Laboratorium für Elektronik, University of Marburg, Ernst-Giller-Str. 20, D-3550 Marburg, FRG

M. Partinen
Department of Neurology, University of Helsinki, Haartmaninkatu 3, SF-00290 Helsinki 29, Finland

R. Peled
Sleep Laboratory, Unit of Behavioral Biology, Faculty of Medicine, Technion - Israel Institute of Technology, Gutwirth Building, Haifa 32000, Israel

T. Penzel
Arbeitsgruppe Systemstrukturen und Thermodynamik, Institut für Theoretische Physik, University of Marburg, Renthof 7, D-3550 Marburg, FRG

J. H. Peter
Medizinische Poliklinik - Zeitreihenlabor, University of Marburg, Baldingerstraße, D-3550 Marburg, FRG

F. Pinciroli
Dipartimento di Elettronica, Politecnico di Milano, Piazza L. da Vinci 32, I-20133 Milano, Italy

T. Podszus
Medizinische Poliklinik - Zeitreihenlabor, University of Marburg, Baldingerstraße, D-3550 Marburg, FRG

J. L. Racineux
Clinique de Pneumologie, CHU 49033 Angers Cedex, France

W. Rasbach
Medizinische Poliklinik - Zeitreihenlabor, University of Marburg, Baldingerstraße, D-3550 Marburg, FRG

F. Raschke
Institut für Arbeitsphysiologie und Rehabilitationsforschung, University of Marburg, Robert-Koch-Str. 7 a, D-3550 Marburg, FRG

Z. Rida
Service de Pneumologie, CHU d'Amiens - Université de Picardie, Hôpital Sud, Avenue Rene Laennec, Salouel 80480 Saleux, France

D. Rose
Service de Pneumologie, CHU d'Amiens - Université de Picardie, Hôpital Sud, Avenue Rene Laennec, Salouel 80480 Saleux, France

R. Rossi
Dipartimento di Elettronica, Politecnico di Milano, Piazza L. da Vinci 32, I-20133 Milano, Italy

S. A. Rothenberg
New York University Medical Center, General Clinical Research Center, Sleep Research Laboratory, 550 1st Avenue, New York, NY 10016, USA

K. H. Rühle
Robert-Koch-Klinik, Abteilung für Pneumologie, University of Freiburg, Hugstetter-Str. 55, D-7800 Freiburg, FRG

S. Sarna
Department of Public Health, University of Helsinki, Haartmaninkatu 3, SF-00290 Helsinki 29, Finland

J. Siegrist
Institut für Medizinische Soziologie, Medical School, University of Marburg, Bunsenstr. 2, D-3550 Marburg, FRG

E. Sohn
Medizinische Poliklinik - Zeitreihenlabor, University of Marburg, Baldingerstraße, D-3550 Marburg, FRG

N. Stern
Sepulveda Veterans Administration Medical Center, 16111 Plummer Street, Sepulveda, California 91343, USA

B. E. Strauer
Klinikum Marburg, Zentrum für Innere Medizin, Schwerpunkt Kardiologie, Baldingerstraße, D-3550 Marburg, FRG

C. Sullivan
Department of Medicine, University of Sydney, Sydney, NSW 2006, Australia

T. Telakivi
Ullanlinna Sleep Disorders Clinic, SF-00290 Helsinki, Finland

M. J. Tobin
Division of Pulmonary Medicine, University of Texas, Health Science Center at Houston, 6431 Fannin, Suite 1.274, Houston, Texas 77030, USA

T. Veleine
Service de Pneumologie and Service de Neurophysiologie, CHU d'Amiens - Université de Picardie, Hôpital Sud, Avenue Rene Laennec, Salouel 80480 Saleux, France

L. Vergani
Dipartimento di Elettronica, Politecnico di Milano, Piazza L. da Vinci 32, I-20133 Milano, Italy

P. von Wichert
Zentrum für Innere Medizin, Medizinische Poliklinik, University of Marburg, Baldingerstraße, D-3550 Marburg, FRG

K. Weber
Medizinische Poliklinik - Zeitreihenlabor, University of Marburg, Baldingerstraße, D-3550 Marburg, FRG

M. Zahorka
Medizinische Poliklinik - Zeitreihenlabor, University of Marburg, Baldingerstraße, D-3550 Marburg, FRG

Part 1: Sleep and Disordered Sleep

Sleep - Introductory Notes

P. LAVIE

The Starting Point

The past few years have seen the rapid progress of a new subspeciality of medicine which can be rightly termed "sleep medicine." The emergence of this branch of medicine has been catalyzed by the awareness that certain physiological dysfunctions are state specific. Of these the most impressive example is the sleep apnea syndrome, the subject matter of the present book, in which breathing disorders are exclusively manifested during sleep.

This medical progress could not have been achieved without preparatory research on the nature of sleep itself and on its physiological characteristics. The concept of sleep as an active process worthy of physiological research has gained credence slowly. It may sound surprising, but almost until the mid-twentieth century sleep was considered to be a passive phenomenon caused by deafferentation of the cerebral cortex to incoming sensory stimulation. This view prevailed for almost two millennia, from the sleep theories of the classical period to the twentieth-century theories of Kleitman and Bremer (for a detailed review see [1]). The 1953 discovery of REM sleep (Rapid Eye Movement sleep) by Aserinsky and Kleitman [2] has overthrown these "passive" theories. This discovery has decisively changed scientific views on sleep, its causes, and its function.

The purpose of this brief introductory chapter is to provide the reader who is a novice in sleep research with some basic information about the sleep process and its regulating mechanisms and to familiarize him with "sleep" terminology.

The Infrastructure of Sleep

The structure of sleep follows a regular and deterministic chain of events, which can be monitored by a variety of physiological parameters. Three parameters are conventionally used to trace its progress: electroencephalogram (EEG), electrooculogram (EOG), and electromyogram (EMG) [3]. The division of sleep into different stages is based on simultaneous changes in all three parameters. While the wake state is characterized by a mixed-frequency, low-voltage EEG activity (beta activity of > 14 Hz), rapid eye movements, and a high tonic level of EMG activity, the transition from wake to sleep is signaled by a slowing down of the EEG toward the alpha (8–10 Hz) and theta bands (4–7 Hz), replacement of rapid

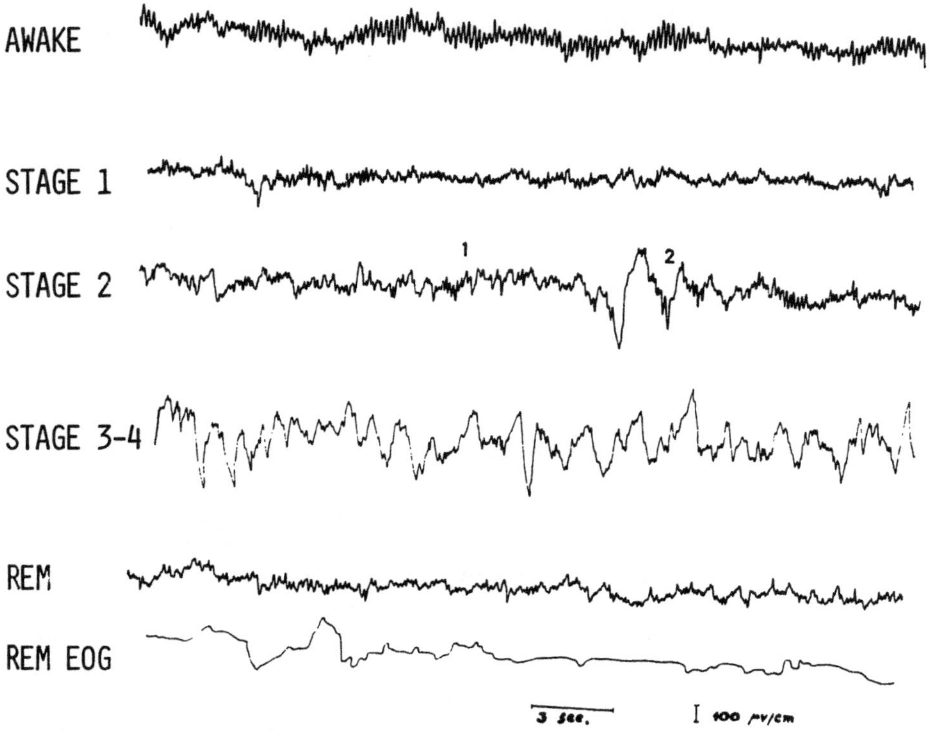

Fig. 1. EEG patterns during different sleep stages. *1,* Sleep spindles; *2,* K-complex

eye movements by slow rolling eye movements, and a gradual relaxation of muscular tonus relative to wakefulness (Fig. 1). This transition period, which may last from 2–10 min, is called stage 1 of sleep. Neurally, the slowing of EEG activity from low-voltage mixed frequency to synchronized theta activity represents the "switching on" of somnogenic structures, and the suppression of the influence of the brainstem reticular formation arousal system.

The end of the "transition period" and the appearance of "true" sleep coincide with the manifestation of two distinct EEG patterns superimposed on the continuing theta activity: the K-complex and the sleep spindle. The K-complex is a monophasic wave of approximately 150–200 μV lasting no more than 1–2 s. Although the K-complex is evoked endogenously, it can be elicited by external events such as environmental noises [4]. Therefore, it is considered to be a microarousal, particularly when it has a tail of alpha activity. The sleep spindle is a burst of approximately 12–14 Hz EEG activity at a rate of 2–5 per min whose function is still not completely understood. The appearance of K-complex and/or sleep spindle on a background of theta activity defines the occurrence of sleep stage 2. By that time the slow and rolling eye movements disappear, and muscle tonus is further depressed compared to stage 1. Although the awakening threshold in sleep stage 2 is higher than in stage 1, sleepers can still be easily aroused. The deepest stages of sleep are yet to come.

The physiological signs of deepening sleep are the gradual appearance of delta EEG activity (0.5–3 Hz). First, delta activity is sparse, appearing in clusters lasting no more than a few seconds. Gradually, delta activity consolidates until it dominates the entire record. Sleep stages 3 and 4, or slow-wave sleep (SWS), are characterized by almost continuous delta activity. Stages 3 and 4 are differentiated from each other only by the proportion of delta activity present in the record. In both, arousal thresholds are very high and autonomic activity very stable. In normal sleepers the progression from stage 1 to stage 4 takes about 15–20 min.

The process of gradual slowing of the EEG activity, and the increase in voltage are interrupted by the appearance of the fifth sleep stage, or REM sleep. Usually, the change from slow-wave sleep stage 4 to REM sleep is not a direct change. Stage 4 terminates in gross body movements, which are followed by gradual lightening of sleep, that is, a regression from stage 4 to stages 3 and 2. This finally leads the way to REM sleep.

The first REM period appears after approximately 90 min ± 11 min from sleep onset (Fig. 2). The time period from sleep onset to the appearance of the first REM period, which is termed "REM latency," has an important clinical value. The reason is that in certain sleep disorders as well as in affective disorders it may be dramatically modified (e.g., [5]). REM sleep is a unique combination of

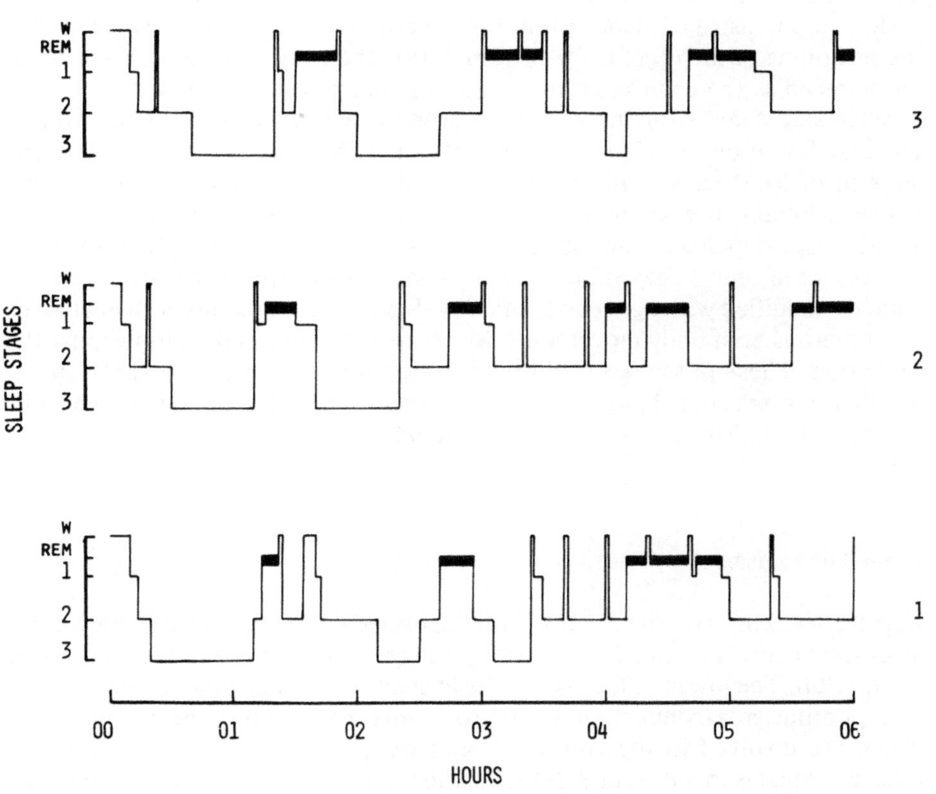

Fig. 2. Sleep hypnograms of a young adult who slept in the laboratory for 3 nights

physiological events, whose hallmarks are rapid eye movements, mixed-frequency, low-voltage EEG resembling stage 1, and muscular atonia. Besides these three prominent REM phenomena, there are a variety of additional REM-related phenomena such as a great instability of the autonomic regulating system [6] and a shift in the control mechanism of the respiratory system away from the metabolic controls and toward the voluntary respiratory system [7]. There is also a great change in core temperature regulation [8], an increase in brain oxygen consumption [9], an increase in the firing rate of cortical cells and increased transport along the brain visual pathways (see review [10]), and penile erections in males [11]. Subjects awakened from REM sleep usually report vivid and detailed dreams [12]. In view of this kaleidoscopic appearance, it is no wonder that REM sleep is also called "paradoxical sleep".

After completion of the first REM period, which lasts about 5–10 min, the sleep cycle restarts. Thus, the sleep process comprises of REM-NREM cycles with a period of approximately 1.5 h. Superimposed on this cyclic process are linear trends which modify the content of each cycle as the night progresses. The length of REM periods increases through the night, reaching an asymptote of 20–25 min in the fourth or fifth REM period, while reciprocally, the amount of "slow-wave sleep" or stage 3/4 decreases [13]. Thus, most of the sleep stage 3/4 appears in the first third of the sleep period, while most of the REM sleep appears in the last third of the sleep period. Besides the change in the content of the cycle, there is also a tendency toward shortening of the cycle from 90–100 min at the beginning of the night to 70–80 min during the early morning. This is not as pronounced as the changes in the sleep stages themselves, however.

Sleep stages and structure also show pronounced ontogenetic trends. During the first few months of life the amounts of REM sleep are largest [14]. The amount of REM sleep stabilizes at approximately 20%–25% of total sleep time between 10 and 20 years of age. In contrast to this stabilization, there is a progressive, age-dependent diminution of slow-wave sleep [15]. People in their 70s and 80s have only a few minutes of slow-wave sleep. Another feature of sleep which is modified with age is body motility. REM sleep in infants is characterized by numerous brief body movements, which are superimposed on tonic muscular inhibition. These phasic events are suppressed after the age of 10 years, an age which also marks the change toward an overall suppression of body movements in sleep (unpublished results from our laboratory).

Brain Mechanisms

Results of animal experimentation have identified several neural systems located at different levels of the CNS which participate in sleep–wake regulation (see review [16]). The lowest "sleep center" is located in the brainstem medullary area. The pontine area contains at least two regulating systems, the raphe nuclei, which are involved in the control of slow-wave sleep, and the locus ceruleus nucleus which is involved in REM regulation. Diencephalic and forebrain structures have also been shown to be involved in sleep induction and regulation.

Thus, it appears that during each phylogenetic stage of development a unique sleep stage evolves.

We recently reported on a unique case in which a localized brainstem lesion in the left pontine area, caused by shrapnel, was associated with a highly selective suppression of REM sleep [17]. This patient had a mean of less than 2% REM sleep in 15 whole-night, polyhypnographic recordings. Curiously enough, this patient did not show any of the typical signs of REM deprivation. This provides some confirmation of the animal experiments regarding the pontine control of REM sleep.

Temporal Aspects of Sleep and Waking

The sleep process obeys two periodic processes: the ultradian periodicity which characterizes the infrastructure of sleep described above, and the circadian periodicity which characterizes the alternation between sleep and waking. Both appear to be under the control of endogenous mechanisms: a brainstem ultradian oscillator and a diencephalic circadian oscillator. Under normal living conditions, the sleep-wake cycle is synchronized with the day-night cycle and with social life. Most people who are not shift-workers sleep during the dark hours and are active during the light hours. However, the oscillator governing sleep-wake behavior, which is thought to be located in the suprachiasmatic nucleus of the hypothalamus, continues to operate in isolation from all time cues. Its endogenous periodicity differs, sometimes widely, from 24 h, and may attain 28-30 h in length (for extensive review see [18]). In isolation, the placement and length of the sleep period is influenced by the periodicity of the sleep-cycle oscillator and its interaction with the circadian temperature oscillator. There have been several reports on persons living under normal conditions who display sleep-wake cycles as if they were in isolation, indicating the potential vulnerability of the coupling mechanism between the endogenous sleep-wake oscillator and the environmental synchronizing agents [19].

Summary

The process of falling asleep, which for centuries was thought to be passively induced by interference with brain activities, is in fact a complex and intricate process actively generated by specially evolved brain mechanisms. This requires delicate coordination between several brain areas subserving sensory perception, motor activity, and autonomic regulation. Some are inhibited throughout the entire sleep period, while others dramatically change their mode of operation in comparison to waking. In view of these changes, it is no wonder that the wake to sleep transition is not always smooth and uneventful. In some, the transition into sleep signals the appearance of a variety of disorders which, although sleepspecific, have a profound influence on the quality of life in general.

References

1. Moruzzi G (1964) The historical development of the deafferentation hypothesis of sleep. Proceedings of the American Philosophical Society 108:19–28
2. Aserinsky E, Kleitman N (1953) Regularly occurring periods of eye motility and concomitant phenomena during sleep. Science 118:273–274
3. Rechtschaffen A, Kales A (1968) (eds) A manual of standardized terminology, techniques and scoring system for sleep stages of human subjects (NIH publ. no. 204) US Government Printing Office, Washington D.C.
4. Roth M, Shaw J, Green J (1956) The form, voltage distribution and physiological significance of the K-complex. Electroencephalogr Clin Neurophysiol 6:385–402
5. Rechtschaffen A, Wolpert EA, Dement WC, Mitchell SA, Fisher C (1963) Nocturnal sleep of narcoleptics. Electroencephalogr Clin Neurophysiol 15:599–609
6. Snyder F, Hobson A, Morrison D, Goldfrank F (1964) Changes in respiration, heart rate, and systolic blood pressure in human sleep. J Appl Physiol 19:417–422
7. Phillipson E, Sullivan C (1978) Respiratory control mechanisms during non-REM and REM sleep. In: Guilleminault C, Dement WC (eds) Sleep apnea syndromes. Alan R. Liss, New York, pp 47–64
8. Parmeggiani PL, Rabini C (1967) Shivering and panting during sleep. Brain Res 6:789–791
9. Brebbia DR, Althuler KZ (1965) Oxygen consumption in rats and electroencephalic stage of sleep. Science 150:1621–1623
10. Steriade M, Hobson JA (1976) Neuronal activity during the sleep-waking cycle. Prog Neurobiol 6:155–376
11. Fisher C, Gross J, Zuch J (1965) Cycles of penile erection synchronous with dreaming (REM) sleep. Arch Gen Psychiatry 12:29–45
12. Dement WC, Kleitman N (1957) Cyclic variations in EEG during sleep and their relation to eye movements, body motility and dreaming. Electroencephalogr Clin Neurophysiol 9:673–690
13. Webb WB, Agnew HW (1971) Stage 4 sleep: influence of time course variables. Science 174:1354–1356
14. Roffwarg HP, Muzio JN, Dement WC (1966) Ontogenetic development of the human sleep-dream cycle. Science 152:604–619
15. Feinberg I, Heller N, Koresko RL (1967) EEG sleep patterns as a function of normal and pathological aging in man. J Psychiatr Res 5:107–144
16. Jouvet M (1967) Neurophysiology of the states of sleep. Physiol Rev 47:117–177
17. Lavie P, Pratt H, Sharf B, Peled R, Brown J (1984) Localized pontine lesion: nearly total absence of REM sleep. Neurology (NY) 34:118–120
18. Wever RA (1979) The circadian system of man. Results of experiments under temporal isolation. Springer-Verlag, Berlin
19. Wollman M, Lavie P (1986) A hypernychthemeral sleep-wake cycle: some hidden regularities. Sleep 9:324–334

Chronobiological Aspects of Sleep Disorders

G. HILDEBRANDT

The regular change between sleep and wakefulness or activity within the 24 h day is accompanied by variations in physiological functions so extensive that formerly it was believed to be the only reason for the day-night changes of bodily functions. Once modern chronobiology was able to prove that these daily rhythmic variations continue under constant conditions, even in a free-running sleep-wake cycle in isolation experiments, it became evident that the sleep-wake cycle is just one part or functional level of a complex circadian system, representing an endogenous rhythmicity which is synchronized by the action of the environment as zeitgeber.

On the other hand, sleep was formerly thought to be merely a consequence of prior wakefulness, leading daily to recuperation and restoration of physical capacity, as is true of other recovery processes.

Examining the time demands of the various recuperative (or hygiogenetic) processes, night sleep takes up a remarkably central position between the shorter periods of metabolic recuperation and processes of longer duration, such as compensation, healing, and adaptation, which lead to a higher level of adaptive capacity and health (Table 1).

Table 1. Time requirements of the various recuperative processes (hygiogenetic functions)

Hygiogenetic functions	Time demand
	year
Capacity adaptation	|
	month
Functional adaptation healing, reconvalescence	|
	week
Overcompensation	|
Night sleep	night
	|
Refill of energy stores metabolic recovery	hour
	|
Compensation of O_2-debts	minute
	|
	second
Membrane recovery	|

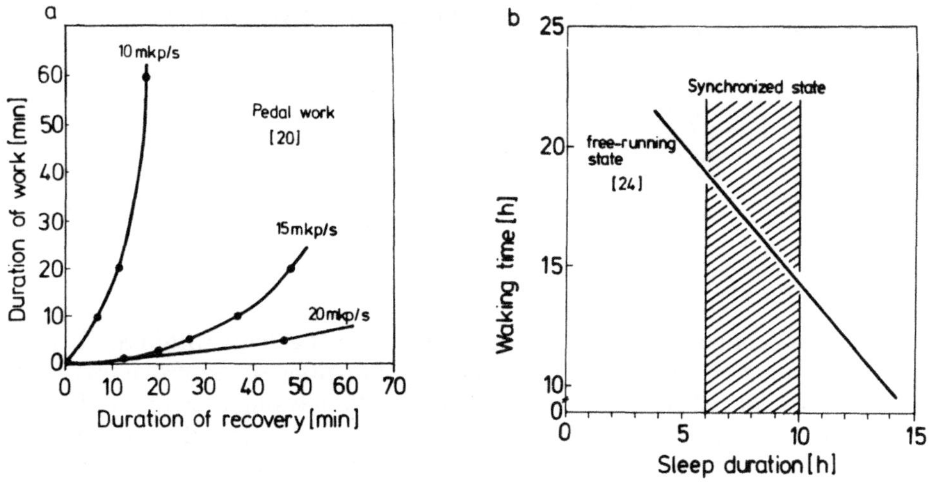

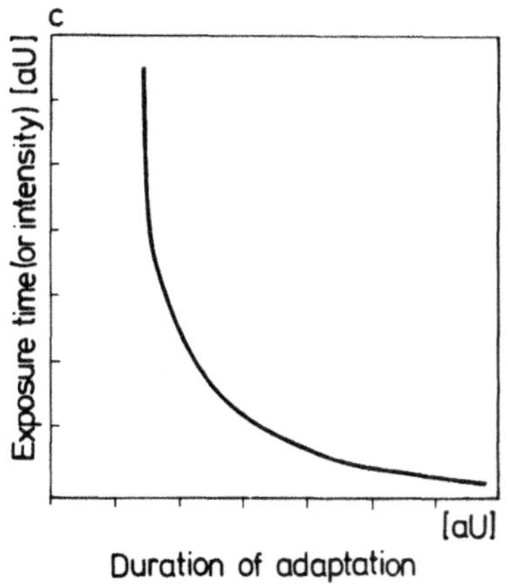

Fig. 1a–c. a Dependence of the duration of recovery on the duration of work under different work loads [20]; *mkp,* meter · kilopond. **b** Sleep duration as related to prior waking time in a synchronized state and in a free-running state of the circadian system [24]. **c** Principal scheme of the dependence of the duration of adaptation on the time of exposure to an adaptogenic stressor. *aU,* arbitrary units

Whereas in the briefer recovery processes the duration of recovery is positively related to prior load (Fig. 1) in the sense of an hour-glass mechanism, sleep duration is not related to the rate of strain or waking time of the previous day. This was shown by several studies including the results of Pöllmann [28] in our group. During isolation experiments in a free-running state of the sleep-wake cycle, even an inverse correlation between sleep duration and waking time became prominent, as seen in an increase of the $\alpha{:}\rho$ ratio [39]. This inverse relationship seems to prevail also in the range of the longer lasting adaptive processes, in which an increase of exposure time speeds up adaptive compensation, thus shortening adaptation time [3, 11].

On the other hand, as shown by the results of Pöllmann [28] (Fig. 2), it is the quality of sleep that depends on the strain of the day.

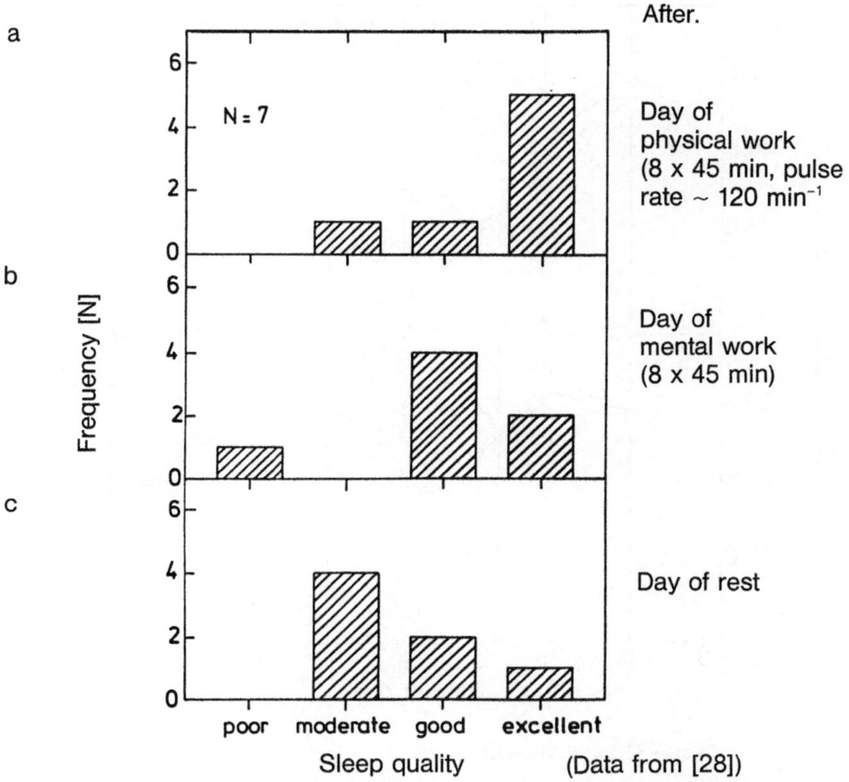

Fig. 2a–c. Frequency distribution of self-rated sleep quality following a day of physical work (**a**), of mental work (**b**), and of rest (**c**) in seven people [28]

From all of the above one can derive that under normal conditions night sleep firstly is not merely controlled by metabolic compensations and secondly does not simply represent a process of overcompensation or adaptation. As a substantial part of the circadian system, sleep and its disorders seem to be rather a chronobiological problem, and the issues here are those of biological rhythmicity.

There are at least three different chronobiological aspects to be considered:

1. Sleep Depends on the Circadian Rhythm

The circadian rhythm is synchronized to zeitgebers in the normal earthly environment. This assures that natural sleep time takes place at night, as is true for all diurnal organisms. (I will not consider circannual influences on sleep in this paper.)

Under synchronized conditions onset and end of night sleep are strongly related to the circadian phase of deep body temperature (Fig. 3). This also applies to people with different spontaneous phase positions (morning vs evening types)

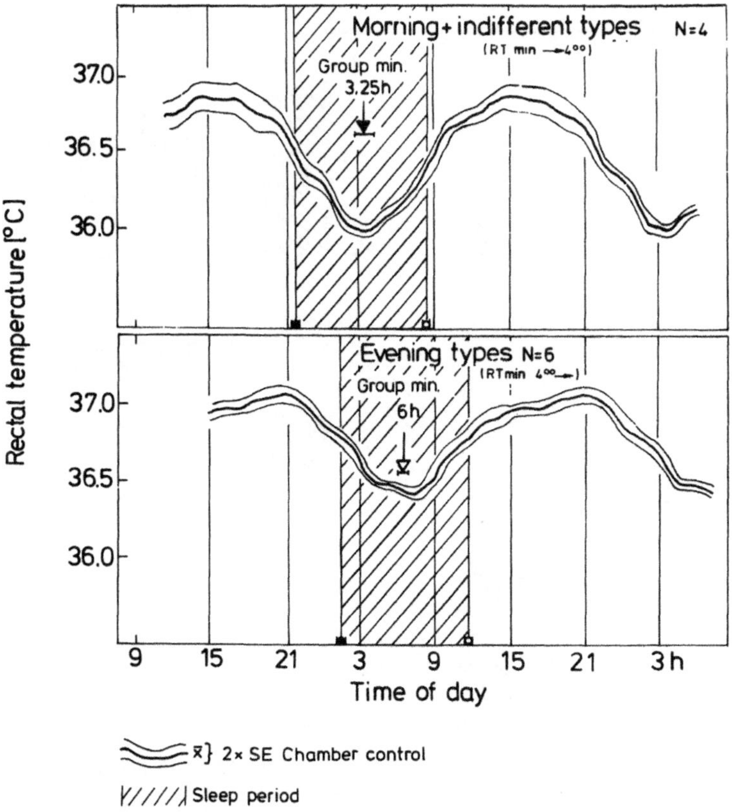

Fig. 3. Mean course of rectal temperature of morning- and indifferent-type *(above)* and of evening-types people *(below)* as compared to the average spontaneous main sleep period *(hatched areas)* under continuous resting conditions in a climate-controlled environment (data from Moog, unpublished)

and has been demonstrated under strictly controlled resting conditions in a climate-controlled sleep chamber.

However, this phase relationship can be disturbed in the state of internal desynchronization, such as may occur under free-running conditions in isolation experiments (Fig. 4). Here the sleep–wake cycle and the circadian rhythm of body temperature can each run freely and individually with different frequencies and therefore different rates of shift over the course of the day.

Menzel [25] was the first to show that sleep-disturbed patients undergo a frequency multiplication of the circadian system, exhibiting a 12-h cycle of several autonomous functions. In particular, the amplitude of the early afternoon dip increases ("postlunch dip" according to some) with increasing recovery deficit; thus the frequency of driving accidents caused by falling asleep shows an obvious 12-h cycle (Fig. 5). Furthermore, in engine drivers of the Deutsche Bundesbahn,

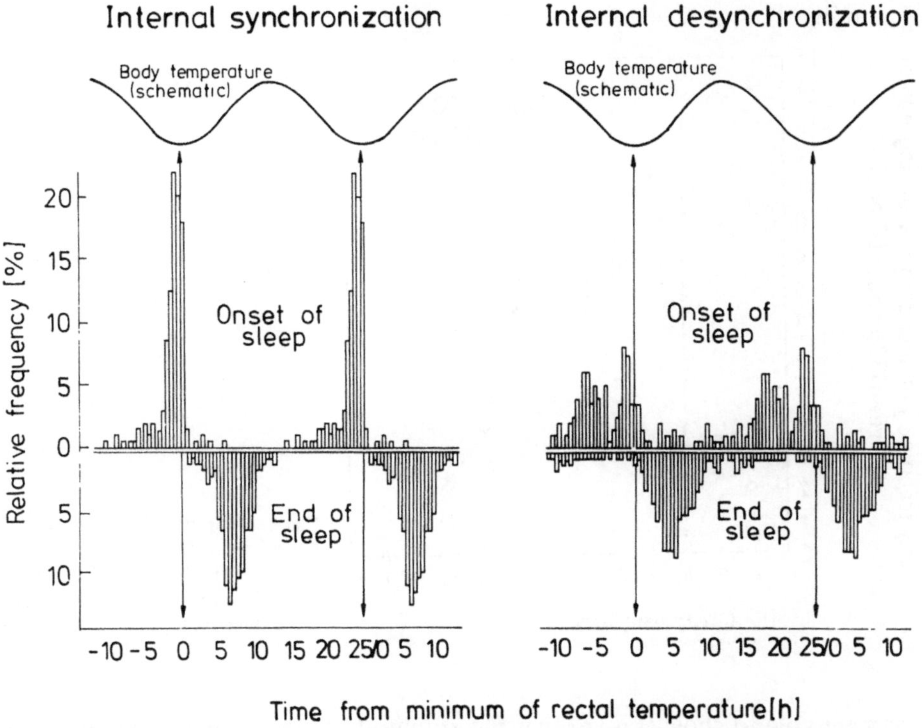

Fig. 4. Phase relationship between body temperature and onset and end of sleep in the state of internal circadian synchronization *(left)* vs internal desynchronization *(right)* [41]

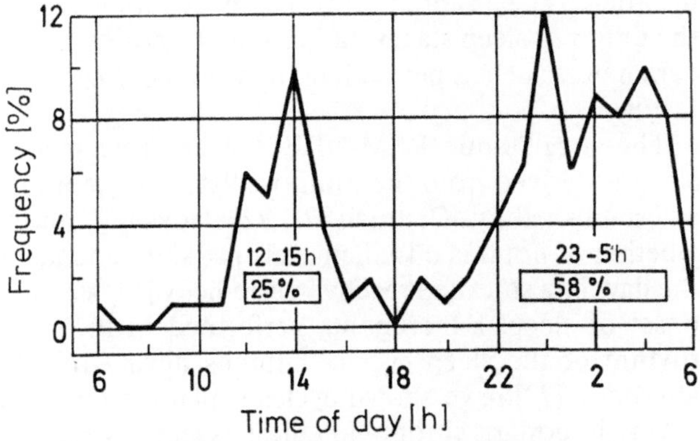

Fig. 5. Daily course of the frequency of car accidents caused by drivers falling asleep [30]

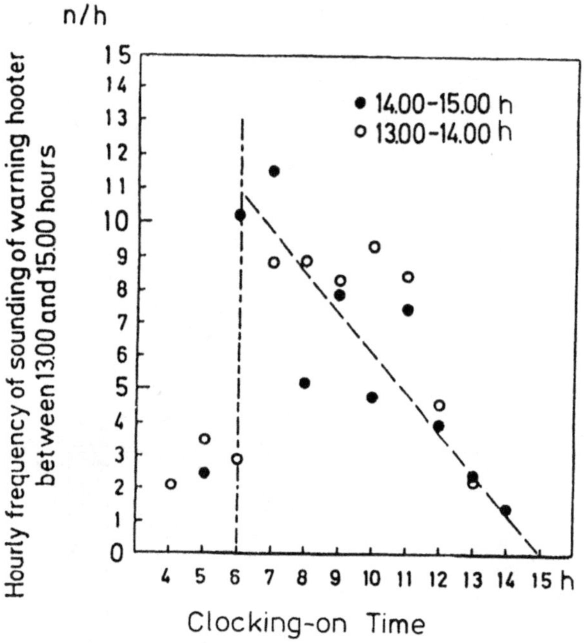

Fig. 6. Mean hourly frequency of sounding of the warning hooter between 13.00 and 15.00 h, as related to the time of day when shift started [19]

we were able to show (Fig. 6) that the amplitude of the early afternoon dip, as indicated by the frequency of handling errors, increases with tiredness, as a function of prior work duration.

Recent studies by Lavie [23] with sleep-deprived subjects have shown that the ultradian structure acts as a gate mechanism for falling asleep.

2. Sleep Itself is a Process which is Periodically Structured

I would like to stress the periodic structuring because assessment of normal and disordered sleep is primarily done by quantitative comparison of the segments of the different sleep stages, rather than by critical examination of chronobiological parameters such as period length of the sleep cycles, their amplitude, or damping factors.

The circa 90-min REM-NREM sleep cycle as a basic time structure of night sleep is derived from the multioscillatory system of the basic rest-activity cycle, as established by Kleitman [21, 22]. However, up to now it has not been clear whether or not this ultradian cycle is a spontaneous rhythm, running throughout the day, or a so-called reactive periodicity [10] which is triggered or evoked by the onset of sleep. Experiments performed in the morning have proven that the rhythm of the sleep cycle continues during the day, but observations in the afternoon [23] have shown cycles which are quite different.

One important chronobiological aspect has recently been confirmed by Broughton [2] who stated that the sleep cycle is part of a very complex system of

Table 2. Ultradian submultiples of the 24-h period

period length 24 h	Circadian period
12 h	Sleep deprivation
6 h 3 h	Frequent ultradian superimposition
90 min	REM-NREM-sleep cycle

frequency co-ordination of integer ratios of ultradian rhythms which are related to the 24-h period (Table 2) [14, 25]. The meaning of disorders of this time structure has not been considered up to now in sleep pathology. However, the fact that a basic rest–activity cycle can be maintained without sleep does point to the fact that the time structure of sleep is related only to one functional level taking part in its production.

3. Sleep Represents a Time-Ordering Process within the Organism

This process can be shown particularly in the time structure of the circulatory and respiratory systems. More than 30 years ago it was known that during night sleep the ratio of heart beat and respiration frequencies is adjusted to the normal integer ratio of 4:1. This applies irrespective of the direction of deviation during the day as well as of the individual level of the single frequencies [8] (Fig. 7). According to the results of Pöllmann [28], the frequency of the normal integer ratios (for 15-min averages) increases up to the end of night sleep, indicating that this enhancement of time order is a result of sleep rather than a precondition.

However, this nightly normalization of the integer frequency ratio of heart beat and respiration is only an isolated component of a complex time structure which is restored by sleep.

As shown by Raschke et al. [32], the frequency ratios between respiratory rhythm and blood pressure rhythm as well as those between the blood pressure rhythm and the 1-min rhythm of peripheral blood flow are likewise precisely adjusted to the whole-number ratio of 4:1 (Fig. 8).

The fact that the 1-min rhythm is also incorporated into this normalized time order during night sleep seems to be of interest with respect to the pathological disturbances of the time structure of the respiratory rhythm. As shown by example in Fig. 9, in a sleeping healthy subject the 1-min rhythm of skin blood flow goes along with rhythmic changes not only of the heart cycle but also of the respiratory rhythm, being incorporated into a cycle of higher order, which seems to be closely related to the time structure of pathological sleep apnea.

The time-ordering activity of sleep not only concerns the coordination of rhythm frequencies but also includes an intensification of phase coordination. Figure 10 showns the frequency distribution of 100 onsets of inspiration, each within the heart cycle from R peak to R peak of the ECG, before and during

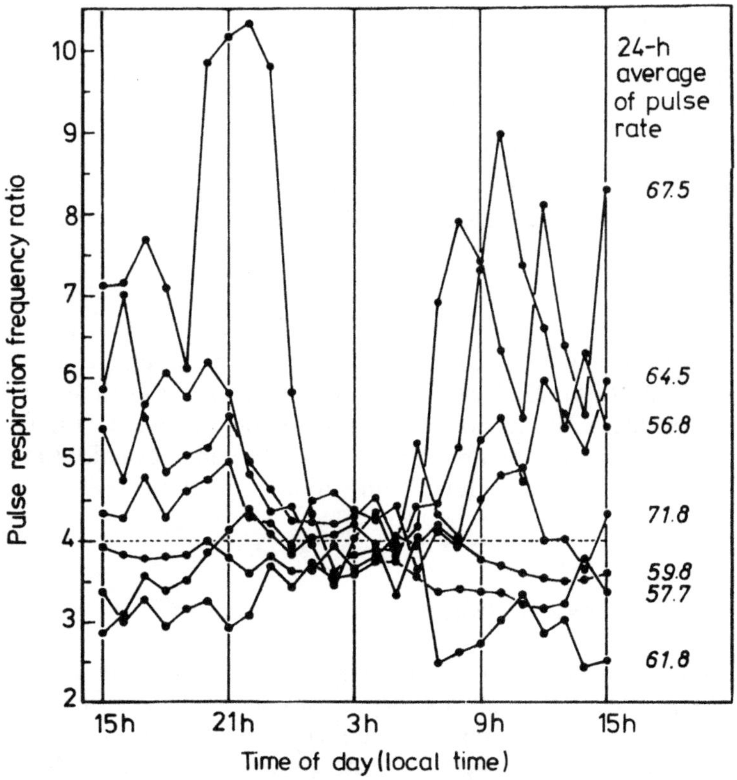

Fig. 7. Individual courses of the pulse–respiration frequency ratio at different levels of heart beat rate (24-h average). Hourly measurements of both were taken over at least 2 min. Healthy subjects in recumbency, eating identical meals at equal intervals [9]; *4,* normal value

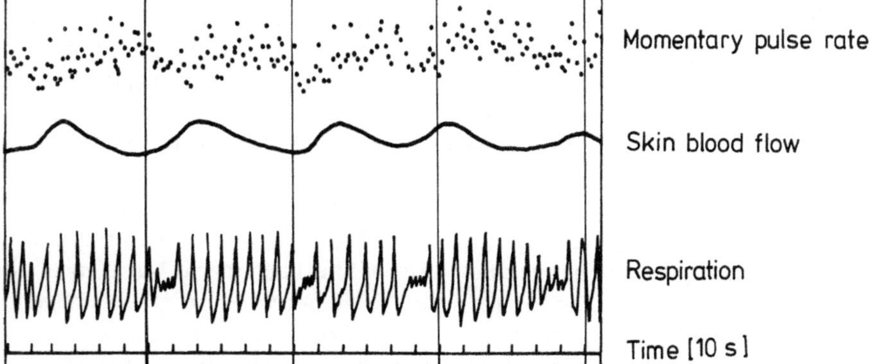

Fig. 9. Synchronous 1-min rhythmical variations of momentary pulse rate, skin blood flow (heat-clearance measurement), and respiration (air temperature in the nostrils) in a healthy resting subject [9]

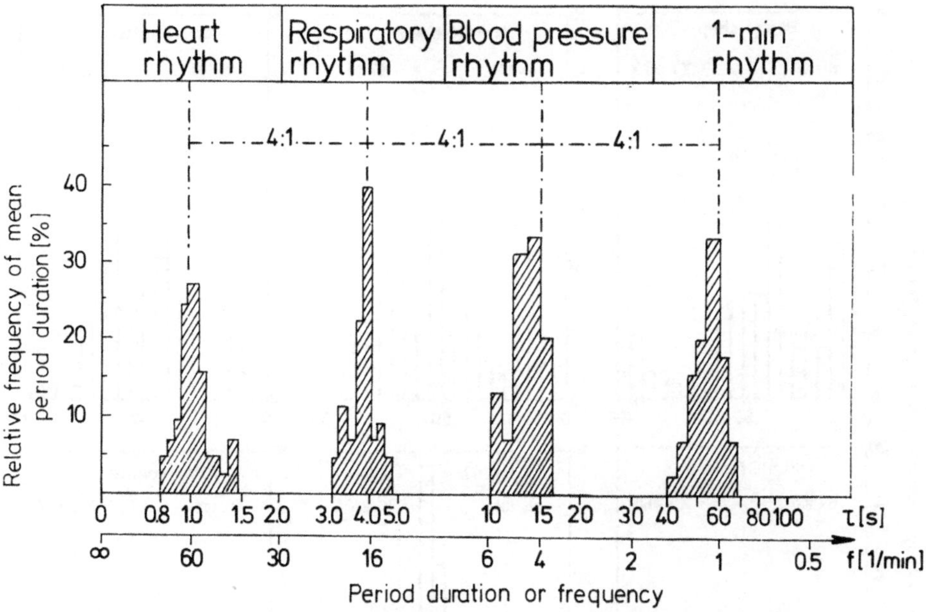

Fig. 8. Frequency histogram of the mean heart rate, respiration rate, blood pressure waves, and 1-min rhythms during night sleep of 18 healthy subjects, totalling 53 nights [31]

several hours of night sleep. After 4 h of sleep, inspiratory onsets become restricted to a certain phase of the heart cycle, whereas before sleep there are only small areas of phase preference.

Again, the intensification of phase coupling between heart beat and respiration is only one part of a general increase of phase coordination of the various rhythmic functions by which the organism improves its functional economy during sleep. As shown in Fig. 11, the coupling rates between certain other rhythmical functions also increase during the night.

This enhancement of the internal time order seems to be an important precondition for regeneration and sleep quality. In a preliminary study, Storch [37] from our group was able to observe that the spontaneous sleep duration was shorter the higher the nightly increase of the coupling rate between heart beat and inspiration.

Of course, sleep disorders concern all the different chronobiological aspects of sleep. Our knowledge so far is mainly restricted to the dependence of sleep on the state of the circadian system.

There are, on the one hand, sleep disorders which are caused by disturbances of the normal synchronization of the circadian system to time order in the environment. These can originate from an inability to sense the zeitgeber signals of the environment or respond to the zeitgeber stimulus. The first possibility applies primarily to the blind, who very frequently suffer from sleep disorders.

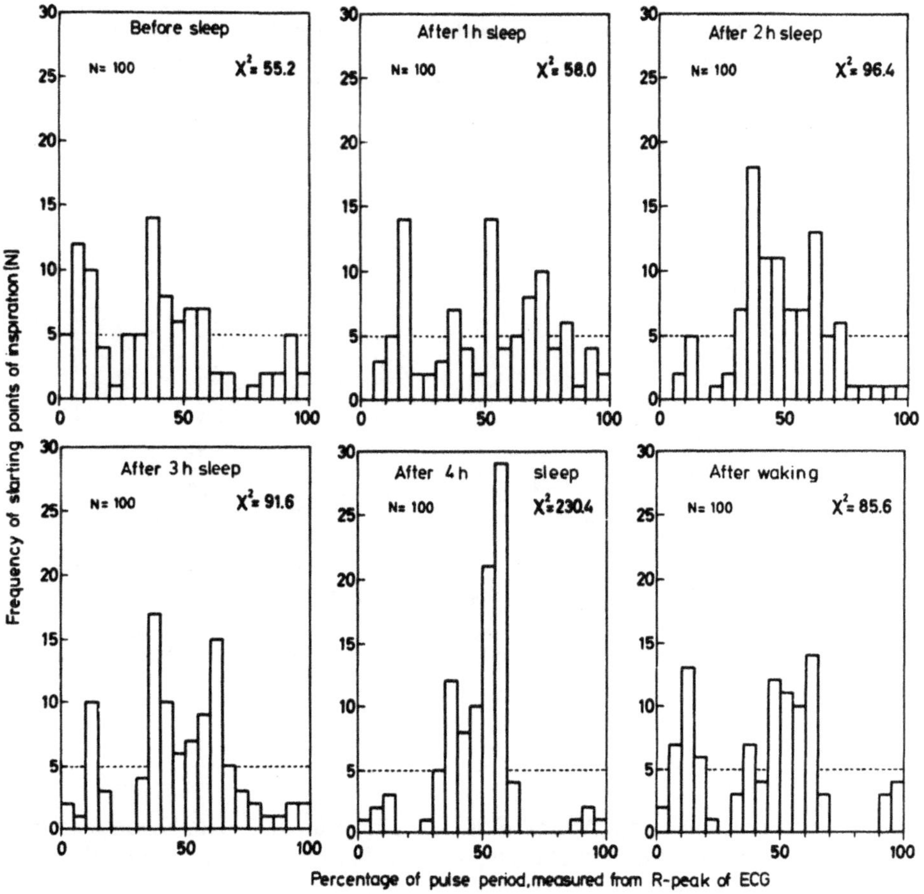

Fig. 10. Frequency distribution of 100 inspiratory onsets within the heart period. The latter is measured from R-peak to R-peak of the ECG and divided into 20 classes of 5%. Measurements before and during night sleep, as well as after waking, in a healthy subject. For evaluation of phase coupling, the χ^2 values are given (5 represents equal distribution) for which the $p = 0.05$ level of significance is attained at 30. 1 [37]

According to our own studies, performed by Moog et al. [27] under strict resting conditions in a climate-controlled chamber, blind subjects as compared to sighted (Fig. 12) exhibit much less strict phase preferences for the circadian maxima and minima of body temperature. Moreover, even if one synchronizes the individual daily courses of rectal temperature according to the minima, a reduction of the circadian amplitude becomes evident in the blind, the more so the more serious the sleep disorder (Fig. 13).

The ability to respond to a zeitgeber stimulus can be not only diminished or even completely lost in patients suffering from an inefficiency of the adrenocortical system, but may also vary physiologically with the circadian changes

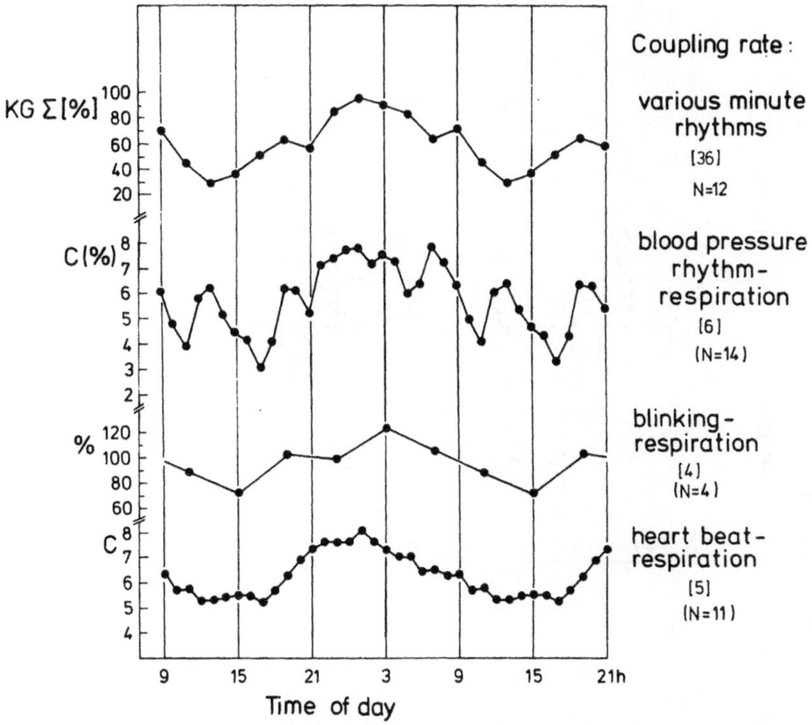

Fig. 11. Daily courses of coupling rates among various rhythmical functions [4–6, 36]

themselves. In a group of healthy subjects who rested in the dark for an 8-h period and then – at different times of day – were exposed to a defined light intensity (Fig. 14), the decrease of the eosinophil count caused by an increase of cortisol production as well as the nonspecific accompanying increase of heart rate were maximal at the normal (accustomed) time of morning activation; 12 h later in the evening, on the other hand, the same procedure elicited no response at all. Evidently, therefore, the very circadian variation of responsiveness to the zeitgeber stumulus assures that the organism itself contributes to the stabilization of the normal phase relationship by avoiding responses to ill-timed stimuli.

From all of this one can derive that a strict regulation of light and darkness must play an important role in the treatment of sleep disorders. In principle it is possible to strengthen the synchronization of the circadian system. This can be gathered from the temporal distributions of the daily maxima of various autonomous functions at the beginning and end of clinical treatment (Fig. 15).

Among those sleep disorders caused by rapid time shifts or by incoherencies of the synchronizing environment, the disturbances which are part of the "jet lag syndrome" are mostly taken for granted or as unavoidable; in any case they have not been sufficiently studied up to now. For example, we are not well informed

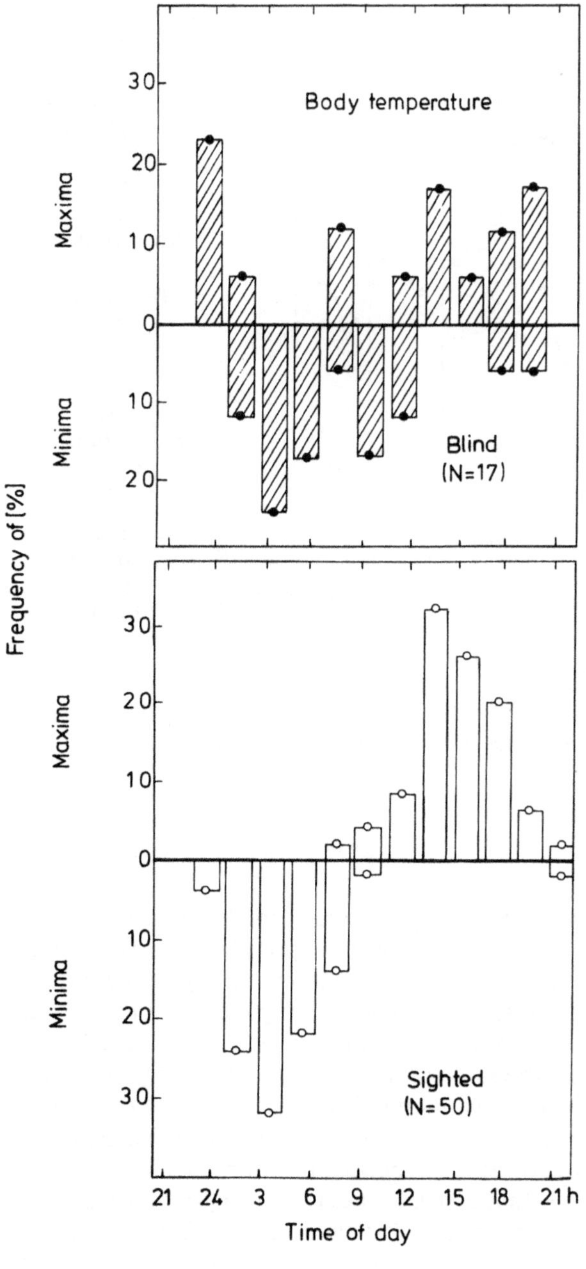

Fig. 12. Frequency distribution of daily maxima and minima of body temperature in blind *(above)* and sighted *(below)* subjects under constant resting conditions in a climate-controlled chamber (control days) [27]

about the detailed differences between east- und west-bound shifts, as well as about the interindividual differences between circadian phase types (morning and evening types).

More precise information is available on the sleep disorders caused by night and shift work, which result from contradictory incoherencies of the zeitgeber

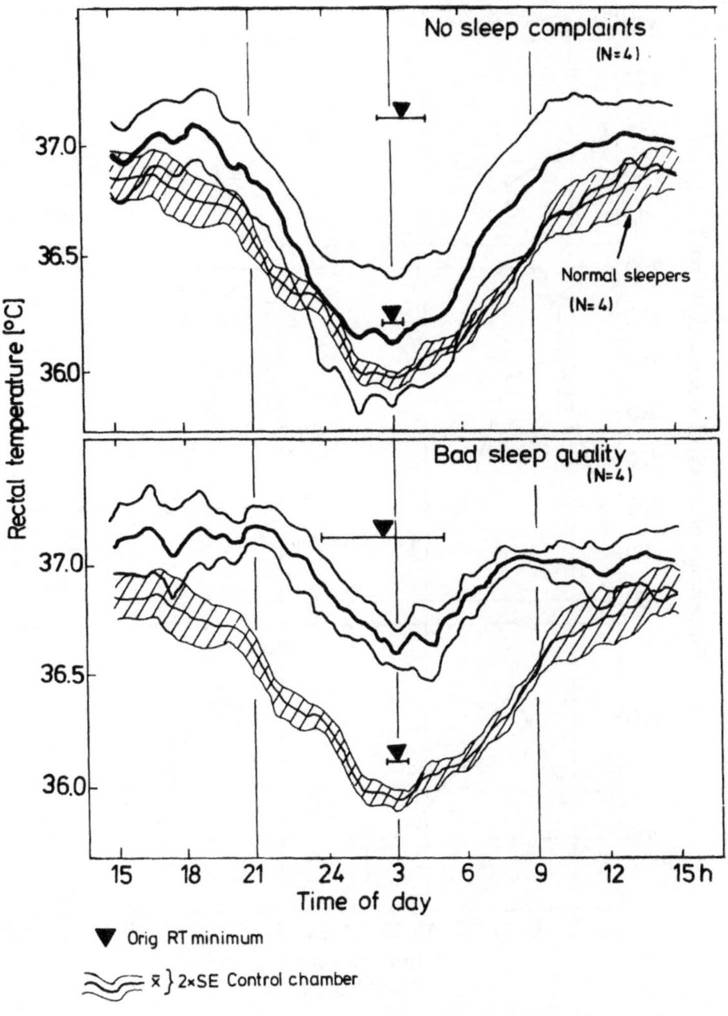

Fig. 13. Mean daily courses of rectal temperature in blind subjects who reported poor quality of sleep *(below)* and no sleep complaints *(above)* as compared to the corresponding ranges of sighted normal sleepers *(hatched area)* [27]; *arrowheads*, mean of minima ± SE.

regimen. Night work, at least initially, leads to an internal desynchronization between two circadian functions, the phase relationship of which represents an important precondition for recuperation and regeneration during night sleep.

As presented in Fig. 16, under normal conditions the nightly maximum of functional economy, as indicated by a maximum of the ergometrically measured physical working capacity, is carefully protected from exploitation by a synchronous circadian minimum of vigilance, as indicated by the longest reaction time. An arbitrary disruption of this phase relationship which provides the restoration of energy reserves must decisively worsen the quality of sleep and lead to recovery deficits.

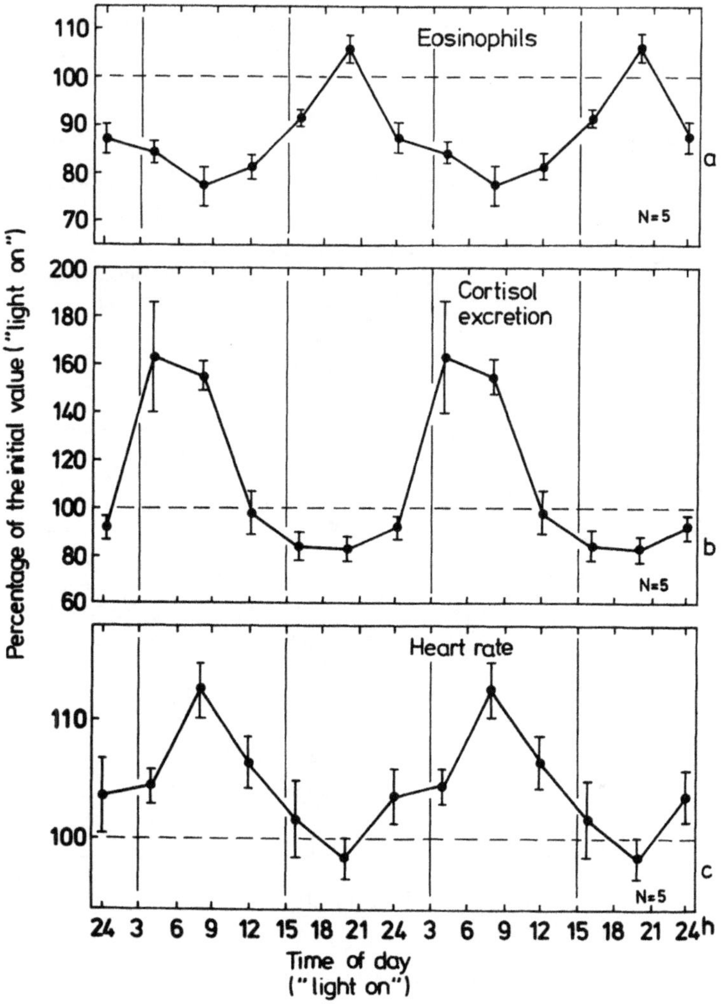

Fig. 14a–c. a Average daily course of change in the number of eosinophils after 2 h of exposure to light, following an 8-h period of darkness, in five healthy subjects. **b** Average daily course of cortisol excretion (urine) during the first 2 h of light exposure. **c** Average daily course of heart rate deviation during the 1st h of exposure to light. The *ordinates* are scaled in percentage of the initial values at light-on. The *brackets* indicate the range of standard errors. For clarity the curves are plotted twice [18]

In accordance with this, field studies, as performed by Rutenfranz et al. [35], have shown that the frequency of sleep disorders is much higher among night workers than day workers (Fig. 17). A concomitant, significant reduction of sleep duration, however, is not only caused by chronobiological reasons but also aggravated by social factors, disturbances by noise, etc. [17]. From the theoretical point of view, one should expect that the frequency of sleep disorders in night workers is reduced when phase adaptation of the circadian system proceeds.

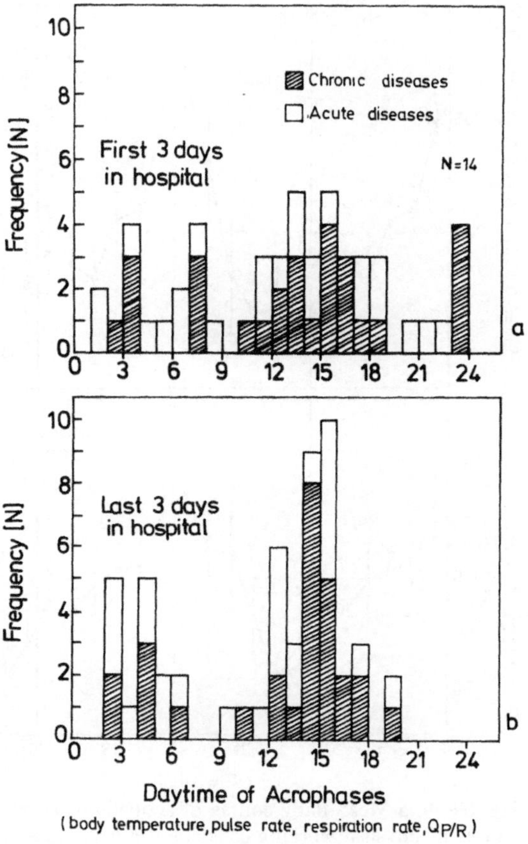

Fig. 15a, b. Distribution of circadian acrophase of body temperature, pulse rate, respiration rate, and pulse–respiration frequency ratio ($Q_{P/R}$) in patients suffering from acute *(clear)* or chronic *(hatched)* diseases, during the first 3 days (**a**) and the last 3 days (**b**) of hospitalization [34]

However, according to our experience, as gained under strict resting conditions in a climate-controlled environment (for a review of the literature see [15]), only evening-type people are able to achieve a satisfactory phase adaptation to night work (Fig. 18). This can be seen from the shift of the spontaneous sleep period as well as from the minima of body temperature on the control days. It will be discussed in more detail by Moog (this volume). In morning-type people, on the other hand, no phase adaptation and consequently no tolerance to night work is observed. In this case an increasing recovery deficit leads to frequency multiplication of the circadian system and to the typical subjective complaints of nontolerant night workers who are continuously forced to sleep during a circadian phase which does not favor recovery processes.

It is important to note that the chronobiological disorder in the nonadapting night worker is not restricted to the circadian system but seemingly includes the whole time structure of the organism. This becomes evident from the fact (Fig. 19a) that (as shown by Pöllmann [29]) the normalization of the integer frequency ratio of heart rate and respiratory rate is progressively disturbed after inversion of the life schedule to night work and is restored after returning to

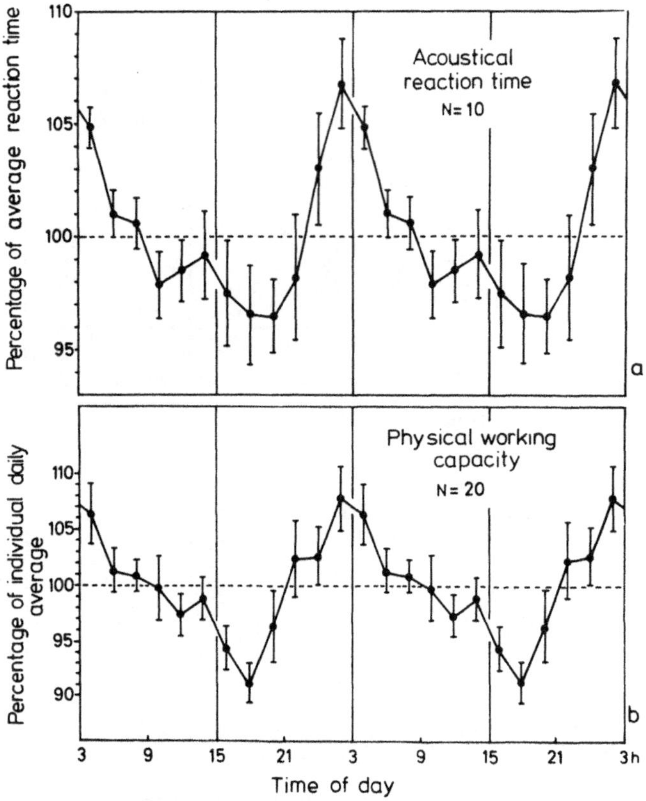

Fig. 16a, b. a Mean daily course of acoustic reaction time in 10 healthy subjects. **b** Mean daily course of physical working capacity at a heart rate of 170 beats/min (PWC 170) [12, 38]

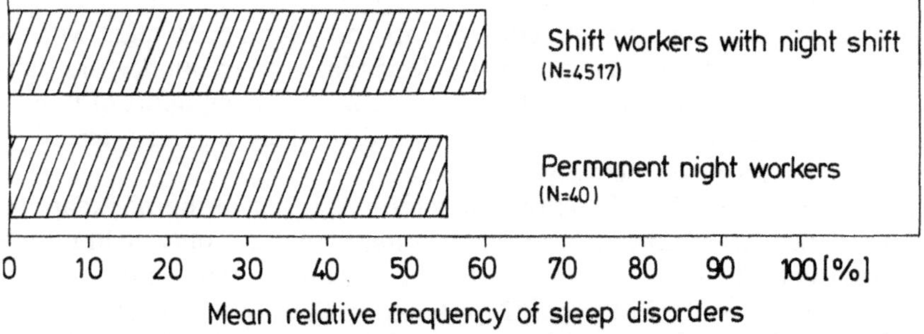

Fig. 17. Mean relative frequency of sleep disorders among workers in different shift systems as compared to day workers [35]

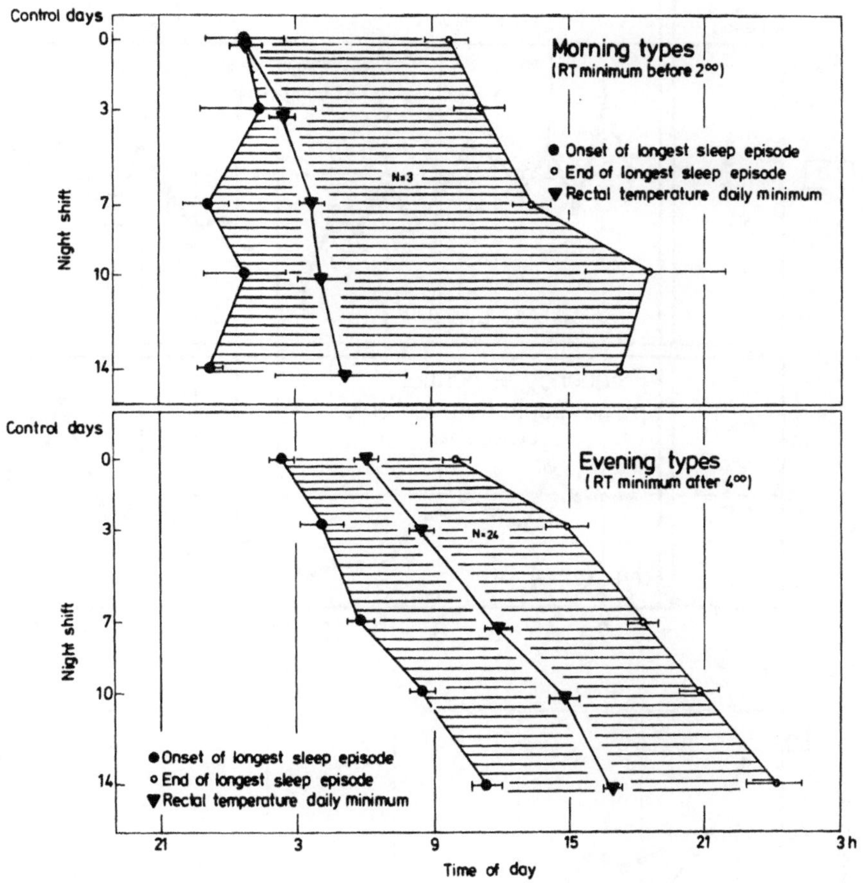

Fig. 18. Mean onset and end of the longest sleep periods and of the daily rectal temperature minimum on control days during a night-shift period in groups of different individual circadian phase positions. *Brackets indicate standard errors [17, 26]*

normal routines. In Fig. 19b, the average of the ratio within the last 2 hours of sleep deviates from the norm 4:1 during the night-work period; a return to the norm takes approximately 6 days.

Finally, if we consider all the different aspects of the chronobiological preconditions of sleep we must conclude that the treatment of sleep disorders cannot deal only with sleep itself, but rather must include the entire time structure of the organism. We have already shown that diurnal behavior can influence sleep quality, which in principle has recently been confirmed by the animal studies of Guilleminault [7]. It is, therefore, not surprising that spa cure treatment, for instance during which the entire regimen of the day is regulated and controlled, can considerably reduce the frequency of sleep disorders. This is shown in Fig. 20 in the results of three different authors. On the other hand, this mode of

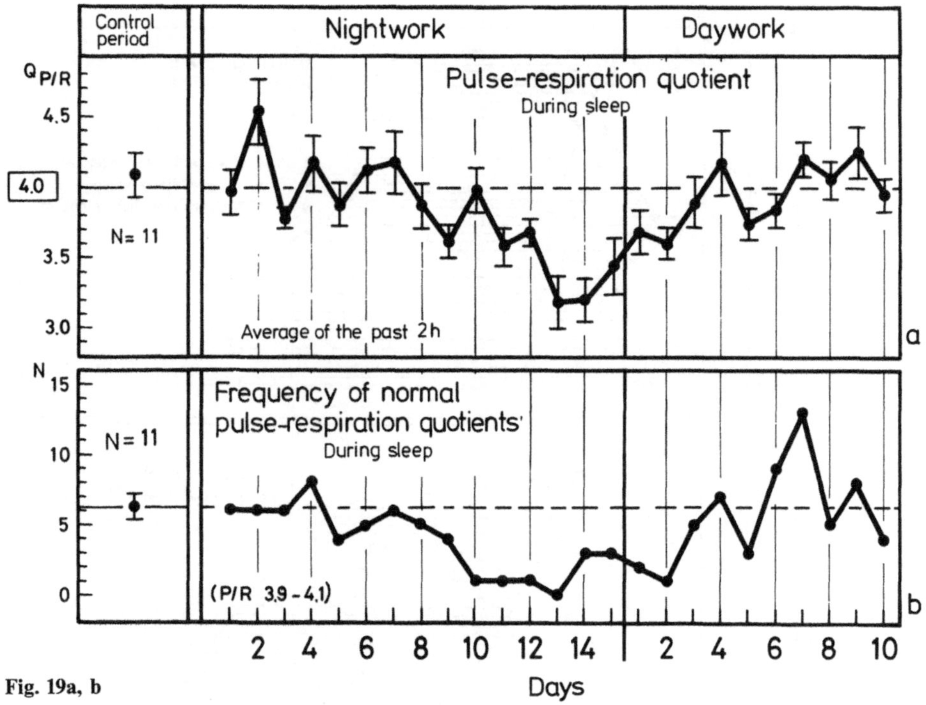

Fig. 19a, b

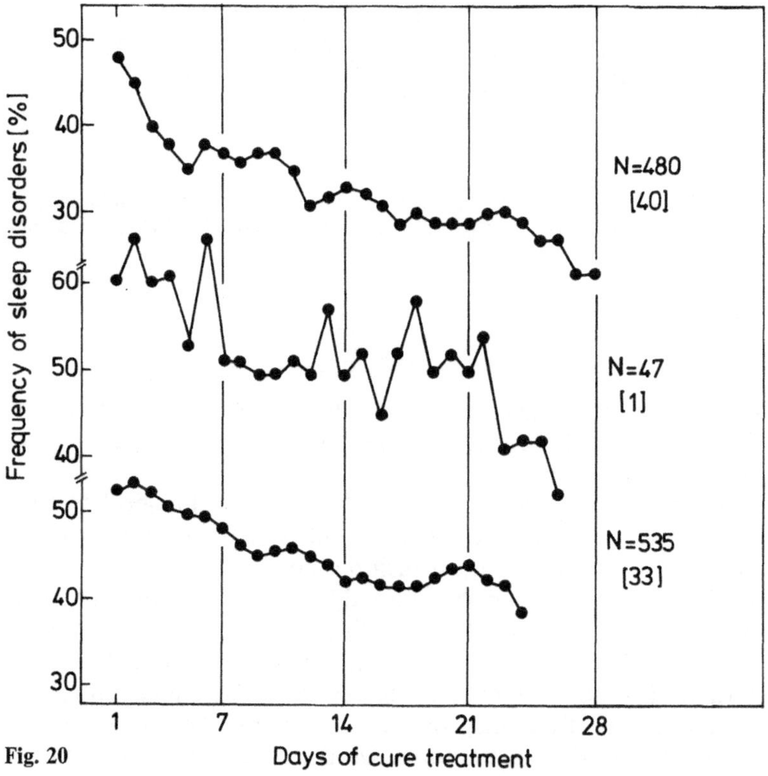

Fig. 20

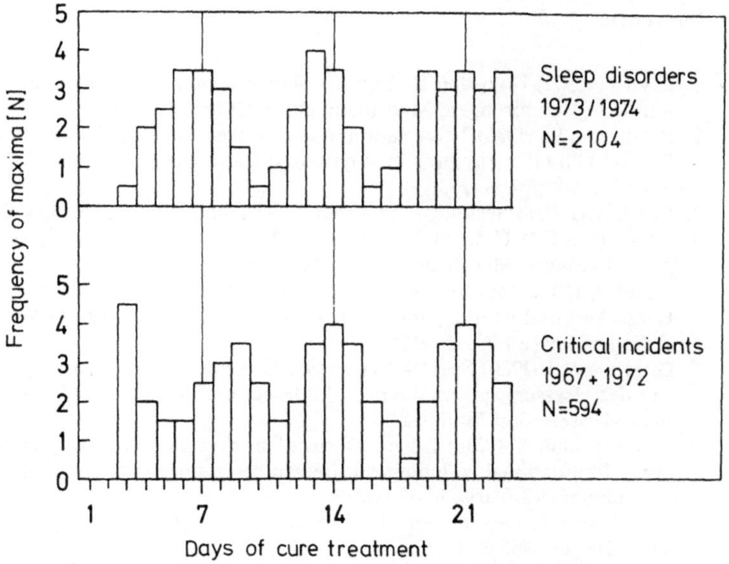

Fig. 21. Maximal frequencies of sleep disorders and of critical incidents in groups of patients undergoing 4-week cure treatments [13, 33]

treatment leads to periodic variations in the autonomous system which are structured by characteristic circaseptan periodicity (Fig. 21). Roughly every 7th day, a critical ergotropic phase occurs in this system, leading to frequency multiplication in the circadian system and, as a consequence, to maximal occurrence of sleep disorders as well as other critical incidents; thus there is a complex influence of the autonomous system on sleep or its preconditions.

All in all, sleep in its different parameters is strongly dependent on various components of the complex time structure of the organism; this must be taken into consideration for a better understanding of sleep disorders and when planning their mode of treatment.

Fig. 19a, b. a Mean pulse-respiration frequency ratio (average of 15-min totals from the last 2 h of sleep) during a 15-day period of night work and subsequent return to day work [29]. **b** Frequency of normal pulse-respiration frequency ratio. $Q_{P/R}$, pulse-respiration ratio; *4*, normal value

Fig. 20. Relative frequency of sleep disorders in three different groups of patients during a 4-week cure treatment, as found by different authors [40, 1, 33] from top to bottom, respectively

References

1. Baier H (1971) Über den Einfluß der aktivierenden Kurbehandlung auf funktionelle Herz- und Kreislaufstörungen. Med Inaug-Dissertation Marburg
2. Broughton RJ (1985) Three central issues concerning ultradian rhythms. In: Schulz H, Lavie P (eds) Ultradian rhythms in physiology and behavior. Springer, Berlin Heidelberg New York Tokyo, pp 217–233
3. Brück K (1969) Physiologische Aspekte der Anpassung. Arch Phys Ther 21:217–224
4. Engel H (1973) Untersuchungen über die Koordination des Lidschlages mit Herz- und Atemrhythmus. Med Inaug-Dissertation, Marburg
5. Engel P, Hildebrandt G, Voigt ED (1969) Der Tagesgang der Phasenkoppelung zwischen Herzschlag und Atmung und seine Beeinflussung durch dosierte Arbeitsbelastung. Internat Z Angew Physiol 27:339–355
6. Goldmann B (1980) Spektralanalytische Untersuchungen zum Tagesgang der Schwankungen des Herzschlages im Atem-, Blutdruck- und Minutenrhythmus beim Menschen. Med Inaug-Dissertation Marburg
7. Guilleminault C (1986) Effects of circadian rhythm and activity on the sleep-wakefulness cycle. International colloquium ultradian respiratory and metabolic rhythms of mean and low frequencies, Paris, 10–12 April
8. Hildebrandt G (1953) Über die rhythmische Funktionsordnung von Puls und Atmung. Z Klin Med 150:445–454
9. Hildebrandt G (1961) Rhythmus und Regulation. Med Welt 1961:73–81
10. Hildebrandt G (1962) Reaktive Perioden und Spontanrhythmik. Reports VII. Conference of the International Society for Biological Rhythm, Siena 1960. Panminerva Medica, Torino, pp 75–82
11. Hildebrandt G (1967) The time factor in adaptation. In: Tromp SW, Weihe WH (eds) Biometeorology 2, proceedings of the III. international biometeorology congress, Pau 1963. Pergamon, Oxford, pp 258–275
12. Hildebrandt G (1976) Chronobiologische Grundlagen der Leistungsfähigkeit und Chronohygiene. In: Hildebrandt G (ed) Biologische Rhythmen und Arbeit. Springer, Vienna New York, pp 1–19
13. Hildebrandt G (1978) Kurkrisen und reaktiver Kurprozeß. Z Phys Med 7:145–159
14. Hildebrandt G (1979) Rhythmical functional order and man's emancipation from the time factor. In: Schaefer KE, Hildebrandt G, Macbeth N (eds) Basis of an individual physiology. Futura, New York, pp 15–43
15. Hildebrandt G (1980) Survey of current concepts relative to rhythms and shift work. In: Scheving LE, Halberg F (eds) Chronobiology: principles and applications to shifts and schedules. NATO-advanced study institutes, series D, no 3. Sijthoff and Noordhoff, Alphen aan den Rijn, pp. 261–292
16. Hildebrandt G (1985) Therapeutische Physiologie, Grundlagen der Kurortbehandlung. In. Amelung W, Hildebrandt G (eds) Balneologie und medizinische Klimatologie, vol 1. Springer, Berlin Heidelberg New York Tokyo
17. Hildebrandt G (1986) Individual differences in susceptibility to night- and shift work (introductory remarks). In: Haider M, Koller M, Cervinka R (eds) Night- an shiftwork, longterm effects and their prevention. Lang, Frankfurt, pp 109–122
18. Hildebrandt G, Lowes EM (1972) Tagesrhythmische Schwankungen der vegetativen Lichtreaktion beim Menschen. J Interdiscipl Cycle Res 3:289–301
19. Hildebrandt G, Rohmert W, Rutenfranz J (1974) 12&24 h rhythms in error frequency of locomotive drivers and the influence of tiredness on it. Int J Chronobiol 2:175–180
20. Karrasch K, Müller EA (1951) Das Verhalten der Pulsfrequenz in der Erholungsperiode nach körperlicher Arbeit. Arbeitsphysiologie 14:369–382
21. Kleitman N (1963) Sleep and wakefulness. University of Chicago Press, Chicago
22. Kleitman N (1983) Basic rest-activity cycle – 22 years later. Sleep 4:311–317
23. Lavie P (1985) Ultradian rhythms: gates of sleep and wakefulness. Exp Brain Res [Suppl] 12:148–164
24. Lucas R (1973) Untersuchungen über den Nachtschlaf des Menschen bei circadian frei laufendem Schlaf-Wachzyklus. Med Inaug-Dissertation, Marburg

25. Menzel W (1955) Therapie unter dem Gesichtspunkt biologischer Rhythmen. In: Lampert H, Heupke W, Kühnau J, Schliephake E (eds) Ergebnisse der physikalisch-diätetischen Therapie, vol 5. Steinkopff, Dresden, pp 1–38
26. Moog R (1983) Sleep patterns in morning- and evening types during night shift. 4th international congress of sleep research. APSS, Bologna
27. Moog R, Endlich H, Hildebrandt G, Martens H (1985) Circadian rhythms in blind persons. J Interdiscipl Cycle Res 16:295
28. Pöllmann L (1972) Der Einfluß der Tagesbelastung auf die Frequenzkoordination von Herzschlag und Atmung sowie auf Blutdruck und Spontanbewegungen im Nachtschlaf gesunder Versuchspersonen. Med Inaug-Dissertation, Marburg
29. Pöllmann L (1975) Continuous measurements of heart and respiratory rate during a long-term experiment with inverted activity cycle. In: Colquhoun P, Folkard S, Knauth P, Rutenfranz J (eds) Experimental studies of night- and shift-work. Westdeutscher, Opladen, pp 244–253
30. Prokop O, Prokop L (1955) Ermüdung und Einschlafen am Steuer. Dtsch Z Gerichtl Med 44:343
31. Raschke F (1982) Analysis of the frequency and phase relationships of circulatory and respiratory rhythms during adaptive processes. In: Hildebrandt G, Hensel H (eds) biological adaptation. Thieme, Stuttgart, pp 52–63
32. Raschke F, Bockelbrink W, Hildebrandt G (1977) Spectral analysis of momentary heart rate for examination of recovery during night sleep. In: Koella WP, Levin P (eds) Sleep. Karger, Basel, pp 298–301
33. Riedel E (1977) Kurzwischenfälle und subjektiver Befindensverlauf von Herz- und Kreislaufkranken bei konventioneller Badekur und vorwiegend trainierender Kurbehandlung. Med Inaug-Dissertation, Marburg
34. Rippert R (1983) Untersuchungen über die Veränderungen tagesrhythmischer Funktionsparameter während der stationären Behandlung von akut und chronisch Kranken. Med Inaug-Dissertation, Marburg
35. Rutenfranz J, Knauth P, Angersbach A (1979) Shift work research issues. Paper presented at a symposium sponsored by the National Institute for Occupational Safety and Health and Office of Naval Research: Variations in work-sleep schedules: effects on health and performance. San Diego, September
36. Sinz R (1978) Zeitstrukturen und organismische Regulation. Akademie, Berlin
37. Storch J (1967) Methodische Grundlagen zur Bestimmung der Puls-Atem-Koppelung beim Menschen und ihr Verhalten im Nachtschlaf. Med Inaug-Dissertation, Marburg
38. Voigt ED, Engel P, Klein H (1968) Über den Tagesgang der körperlichen Leistungsfähigkeit. Int Z Angew Physiol 25:1–12
39. Wever RA (1979) The circadian system of man. Results of experiments under temporal isolation. Springer, Berlin Heidelberg New York
40. Zipp C (1981) Kureffekt und Kurerfolg bei Patienten mit und ohne Psychotherapie. Med Inaug-Dissertation, Marburg
41. Zulley J, Wever R, Aschoff J (1981) The dependence of onset and duration of sleep on circadian rhythm of rectal temperature. Pflugers Arch 391:314–318

Critical Assessment Issues in Disordered Sleep and Wakefulness

K.-O. LIEBMANN

The purpose of this paper is to introduce internists and other medical practitioners to critical issues in the assessment of disturbed sleep and wakefulness. The emphasis will be on listening, clinical observation, a careful history, and attention to epidemiology as necessary elements of diagnosis so that the polysomnogram and other laboratory findings are put into their proper context. Physicians need to be mindful that biological and psychosocial factors play a role in causing and sustaining disordered sleep. This awareness will heighten their ability to recognize, treat, and properly refer patients with these afflictions.

The diagnosis of sleep disorders begins, like any other diagnosis in medicine, with the presenting complaint. Patients present with two typical major complaints, namely, insufficient sleep or insomnia and excessive sleep or somnolence.

Those same complaints are used in the Diagnostic Classification of Sleep and Arousal Disorders [1] to form the basis for two of the four major nosological categories:

1. Disorders of initiating and maintaining sleep (DIMS) or insomnias and
2. Disorders of excessive somnolence (DOES) or hypersomnias. The two remaining categories are:
3. Disorders of the sleep-wake schedule (including "jet lag" and work shift schedule changes)
4. Dysfunctions associated with sleep, sleep stages, or partial arousals (parasomnias). They include sleep walking, pavor nocturnus, enuresis, dream anxiety attack (nightmares), and other functional disturbances during sleep. These phenomena do not usually affect the quality and architecture of sleep. They may, however, be quite dramatic and disruptive.

This diagnostic classification was developed by the Association of Sleep Disorders Centers and published in 1979 in the journal *Sleep* [1]. It provides thorough descriptions of the syndromes subsumed under each category. While subject to modification and clarification, it is a basic reference both for the newcomer and the advanced clinician.

Prevalence

Reports on the prevalence of sleep disorders vary somewhat depending on the nature of the survey but present a relatively consistent picture. In 1979, a study on the use of sleeping pills, sponsored by the National Academy of Sciences and summarizing previous surveys, notes that about one-third of the adult population of the United States of America "would report some sleep disturbance in any given year." However, "only 15 to 20 percent of those reporting any sleep problem, or six percent of the adult population, would bring it to the attention of a physician, who would prescribe a sleeping pill for about half of them" [2]. Since the emergence of specialized centers or laboratories for the study of sleep-wake disorders, an unknown yet growing portion of these patients are being studied using both the new classification and the polysomnogram. In 1982, Coleman [3] reported a survey covering a 2-year period (1978–1980) based on almost 5000 patient records from Sleep Disorders Centers in the United States of America using the new nosology. Typically, patients referred to these centers have had persistent rather than transient sleep pathology. A second report [4], based on a 1-year period (1981–1982) and involving 18 centers in the United States of America and over 3000 new cases, noted a remarkably consistent frequency for the four main categories. Excluding nocturnal penile tumescence studies which constitute about one-sixth of the total, the remaining sample consists of nearly 6500 cases. Of these, almost one-half are DOES, one-third are DIMS, one-fifth to one-sixth are parasomnias, and only a few percent fall under schedule disturbances. Incidence and prevalence figures may vary with different surveys and between clinics and laboratories which specialize in one or another aspect of these disorders. The following discussion will focus on the more commonly seen DIMS and DOES without disputing the considerable and probably growing importance of the other categories.

The Presenting Complaint

The type of complaint gives a first diagnostic clue. The insomniac may have difficulty falling asleep, wake up frequently, wake up too early in the morning, and complain of insufficient sleep or total sleeplessness. He may feel tired, fatigued, irritable, and exhausted during the day. The somnolent patient may report falling asleep at inappropriate times during the day (e.g., while driving) or feeling excessively sleepy and groggy. Often, he can be strangely unconcerned about his predicament. The complaints of either sleepiness or fatigue during the day describe two distinctly different experiences, namely, the uncontrollable tendency to fall asleep as opposed to the inability to sleep or rest when desired. Also, typically, the insomniac complains of his predicament much more than the somnolent patient.

The History

Having defined the type of presenting complaint or dysfunction, the clinician proceeds to obtain the history: onset, duration, frequency of occurrence, intensity or disrupting effect, and precipitating or associated factors. Onset, duration, and usually precipitating factors differentiate the transient from the persistent sleep disorders.

Transient disruptions of sleep or, less commonly, increased sleepiness, by definition lasting not longer than 3 weeks beyond the events that caused them, may be due to acute emotional arousal caused by anxiety, grief, guilt, joy, excitement, fearful or hopeful anticipation, and strong conflicting feelings. These sleep disturbances are universal, the precipitating stress can usually be discovered, and further laboratory workup is rarely requested or required. Transient arousals which may be massive or barely perceived also occur due to withdrawal from sedatives including alcohol (even small amounts), with the use of stimulants (caffeine, amphetamines, cocaine), and with pain and other strong sensory stimuli (light, heat, cold). Acute psychosis is typically accompanied by loss of sleep. Again, the history provides the clue.

Any acute sleep disturbance can become chronic if the precipitating stresses cannot be removed or for other reasons as yet poorly understood. Usually, physicians encounter chronic or *persistent* rather than transient sleep disorders. They last from months to decades, often with insidious onset, fluctuating intensity, remissions, and exacerbations, with or without clear precipitants. Their adverse effect on the patient's mental and physical functioning may be subtle or profound, resulting in mild but continuous dysfunction or severe impairment.

The following sections will briefly describe common and often grave disturbances of sleep and wakefulness which occur with psychiatric illness and psychological dysfunction and may first come to the attention of internists and general medical practitioners.

Disorders of Initiating and Maintaining Sleep

Slightly over one-third of DIMS are associated with psychiatric illness, another 15% with psychophysiological insomnia, and about 12% with drug and alcohol dependency. In total, in almost two-thirds of insomnia cases psychological or as yet largely unknown biological factors play a significant role. The only other DIMS found in more than 10% of people in this category is nocturnal myoclonus [3].

Among DIMS related to *psychiatric* conditions, 50% in Coleman's study [3] were due to major affective disorders, 45% to personality disorders including neuroses, and 5% to psychosis.

The diagnosis of affective or mood disorder, predominantly unipolar (recurrent) depression and bipolar (manic depressive) illness, is based mainly on history and observation. However, in the differential diagnosis between primary (endogenous) affective disorder and depression secondary to medical illness, the sleep EEG can assist the clinician. Typically, sleep in unipolar depression is characterized by shortened REM latency (less than 40 min), a shift of REM sleep to the first half of the REM period, marked increase in phasic REM activity and mixing of stage NREM with REM sleep [5]. Manic depressive illness is accompanied by similar changes in sleep architecture. During the manic phase the patient is insomniac while during the depressed phase he is hypersomniac. The extended wakefulness phase is characterized by euphoria, irritability, and other signs of excessive mental and physical energy in contrast to the profound anergia of the depressed phase [8].

Difficulty in falling asleep and staying asleep also characterizes neuroses and personality disorders, usually those with anxiety at their core. Attention to signs and symptoms associated with these disorders may reveal somatization, hypochondriasis, obsessive thinking, compulsive behavior, and histrionic, paranoid, schizoid, and avoidant traits. The personal histories of these patients may be marked by social isolation, superficial or unstable social relationships, or chaotic lives. Highly prevalent among conditions accompanied by trouble falling or staying asleep are generalized anxiety disorders [6], which are also marked by persistent anxiety, apprehension, and signs of excessive vigilance, autonomic hyperactivity, and motor tension [7]. Recurrent dream anxiety attacks and disturbed sleep are found in posttraumatic stress disorders which develop as an acute or delayed response to massive psychological trauma [8].

The second most common insomnia, constituting about 15% of DIMS, is persistent psychophysiological insomnia, defined as "a sleep onset and intermediary sleep maintenance insomnia that develops as a result of the mutually reinforcing factors of chronic, somatized tension - anxiety and negative conditioning to sleep" [1, p. 24]. The sleep of these patients can be characterized by increased sleep latency, decrease in slow-wave sleep, and atypical α-activity. Organic or major psychological abnormalities may be strikingly absent [9]. Typically, patients report poor, fitful, light sleep, chronic fatigue, ache, and multiple somatic complaints.

Another large group of insomnias is associated with the intermittent or prolonged use of prescribed or otherwise available and abused drugs and substances, including ethanol. Their often disruptive and long-lasting impact upon the architecture of sleep and upon daytime wakefulness will be discussed elsewhere in this book (see chapter by Koella). Beyond obtaining the history of their use from the patient and recognizing their effect upon sleep, the clinician needs also to be aware of factors such as tolerance, habituation, dependence, short- and long-term withdrawal syndromes, and the emergence of underlying and hitherto camouflaged medical and psychological disorders.

Disorders of Excessive Somnolence

Among DOES referred to sleep laboratories in the United States of America, almost one-half belong to the group of sleep apneas. Since sleep apnea syndromes and accompanying daytime sleepiness are being described by other authors in this book (see chapters by Douglas, Lavie, Lugaresi, Peter), they will not be elaborated upon here. Another one-quarter to one-fifth of the same sample were diagnosed as narcolepsy and almost one-tenth as "idiopathic CNS hypersomnia" [3]. Both disorders are marked by recurrent daytime sleepiness. The sleep attacks of the narcoleptic, accompanied by abnormal manifestations of REM sleep during waking hours, typically consist of short but refreshing naps with dreams. Idiopathic CNS hypersomnia lacks manifestations of REM and naps are generally lengthy, nonrefreshing, and without dreams [1]. Excessive need for sleep and daytime sleepiness associated with mood disorders, though seen uncommonly in most sleep laboratories, deserve clinical attention since unrecognized and untreated depression can lead to suicide. Beyond the depressed phase of manic depressive illness already described under DIMS, there is evidence that for instance young depressed patients sleep significantly more than age-matched controls [10]. Besides depressed mood and hypersomnia, there may be changes in appetite and bowel functions, unexplainable aches and pains, loss of interest, and the typical inability to experience joy and pleasure in any activity (anhedonia).

Conclusion

Sleep disorders are highly prevalent in the general population and warrant thorough medical evaluation. Insomnia frequently can be traced to psychological and psychiatric disorders, whereas hypersomnia is more often associated with organic and neurological dysfunction. The diagnosis of disordered sleep and wakefulness is one stage in a continuing process, not a final result. Making the diagnosis begins with the complaint. It does not end in the sleep laboratory or with the polysomnogram. Recording all-night sleep together with other physiological variables may offer striking findings which seem to explain the complaint fully. At other times, test results may be entirely "normal" or offer only partial, conflicting, cryptic, and as yet undecipherable responses to the seemingly simple question of why patients complain of being sleepless, tired, or sleepy.

In summary, then, the diagnosis cannot be one-dimensional or unifactorial. Understanding the patient's problem requires the diagnostician to consider biological, psychological, and social factors and also to remember that our knowledge of any of these factors and their interplay is incomplete. Consultation with specialists in related fields will increase this knowledge. Making a diagnosis, therefore, demands continuing attention to the many facets of a sleep complaint from the first interview to the final disposition.

References

1. Association of Sleep Disorders Centers (1979) Diagnostic classification of sleep and arousal disorders, 1st ed. Sleep 2
2. Institute of Medicine (1979) Sleeping pills, insomnia, and medical practice. National Academy of Sciences, Washington DC, p 48
3. Coleman RM et al (1982) Sleep-wake disorders based on a polysomnographic diagnosis - a national cooperative study. JAMA 247 (7):997-1003
4. Coleman RM (1983) Diagnosis treatment and follow-up of about 8,000 sleep/wake disorder patients. In: Guilleminault C, Lugaresi E (eds) Sleep/wake disorders: natural history, epidemiology, and long-term evolution. Raven, New York
5. Kupfer DJ, Foster FG (1978) EEG sleep and depression. IN: William R, Karacan I (eds) Sleep disorders diagnosis and treatment. Wiley, New York, pp 163-204
6. Weissmann MM, Merikangas KR (1986) The epidemiology of anxiety and panic disorders: an update. J Clin Psychiatry 47 (6) [Suppl]: 11-17
7. Lesser IM, Rubin RT (1983) Diagnostic considerations in panic disorders. J Clin Psychiatry 47 (6) [Suppl]:6

8. Diagnostic and statistical manual of mental disorders, 3rd edn (1980) American Psychiatric Association, Washington DC, pp 236–238
9. Hauri P, Fisher J (1986) Persistent psychophysiologic (learned) insomnia. Sleep 9 (1):38–53
10. Hawkins DR, Taub JM, Van de Castle RL (1985) Extended sleep (hypersomnia) in young depressed patients. Am J Psychiatry 142:905–910

Suggested Reading

Roffwarg H, Erman M (1985) Evaluation and diagnosis of the sleep disorders: implications for psychiatry and other clinical specialties. In: Hales RE, Frances AJ (eds) Psychiatry update: American Psychiatric association annual review, vol 4. American Psychiatric, Washington DC, pp 294–328

Hauri P (1982) Current concepts. The sleep disorders, 2nd edn. Upjohn, Kalamazoo

The Interaction of Drugs with Sleep

W. P. KOELLA

Introduction

Many drugs produce, in addition to their primary therapeutic action or their pleasure-generating effects, a more or less pronounced influence on sleep; this side effect may manifest itself in the first place by alterations of the quantity of sleep. On the one hand a drug may hinder the onset, disrupt the continuity, and/or (rather rarely) cause early termination of sleep and thus reduce total sleep time, i.e., insomnia, and concomitant reduction of sleep's "detiring" effect. On the other hand, some agents may produce supersomnia; they prolong sleep time and, in addition, induce somnolence during the intersleep periods of waking.

In turn, one finds, particularly if using adequate diagnostic probes, that the "sleep effects" of drugs are rather qualitative in nature in that the structure of sleep is deranged. The drugs affect the "preprogrammed" relation between, and the temporal order of, the various sleep stages. In other words, drugs may cause dyssomnia. In the majority of cases of drug-induced sleep disturbances, one encounters a combined effect; the structure and the duration of sleep deviate from the pattern observed under nondrugged conditions.

We shall present and discuss in this chapter such drug-induced sleep effects as observed in both humans and animals. Rather than being exhaustive and review all the drugs that have been found to affect sleep to any extent, we prefer to be selective and describe the effects induced by only a few classes of agents. This approach offers a better chance of discerning some basic principles inherent in such effects. Furthermore, by selecting classes of agents about which we have at least some notion concerning their principle locus and mechanism(s) of action, we may arrive at some conclusions about the ways and means in which such compounds are liable to affect sleep in addition to their (desired) therapeutic or pleasure-inducing action. These aspects will be dealt with in the third section.

In the next section we shall describe first the sleep effects of the following six classes of drugs:

1. Hypnotics and anxiolytics
2. β-Adrenoceptor antagonists (β-blockers)
3. Antidepressant drugs
4. Stimulants (amphetamine-type agents)
5. antipsychotics, neuroleptics
6. Psychodelics, narcotics, alcohol.

Phenomenology of Sleep Effects

Hypnotics and Anxiolytics

It is of course a truism if one states that hypnotics and most of the anxiolytics enhance sleep. They usually shorten sleep latency; they reduce "fragmentation" and delay termination of sleep. Yet these, at first glance, beneficial effects must usually be "bought" at the cost of several drawbacks. Virtually all hypnotics (and the anxiolytics used as hypnotic agents) presently available lose, to a smaller or greater degree and slowly or more quickly, their efficacy with repeated administration regimes. A typical consequence of this habituation is usually a pronounced insomnia rebound appearing with the withdrawal of the drug. Just as importantly, they rarely, if at all, are capable of correcting abnormal structural trends, such as signs of (a priori) disturbed sleep (before administration of a drug). In fact, hypnotics often are liable to produce their own dyssomnia, in that they depress (or enhance to abnormally high levels) to a smaller or larger degree one or several stages of sleep. In particular, REM and stages NREM-3 and -4 are often found to succumb to the perturbing influence of these agents. Evidently the majority, if not all, of the presently available hypnotics exert an influence on sleep not only in a beneficial, but also to some extent in an adverse manner. A few examples from the pertinent literature should suffice to illustrate this point.

A study of Kales and coworkers [31] showed the effect of pentobarbital (100 mg/die) on sleep of sleep-disturbed subjects. These authors observed a moderate depressing effect on REM sleep, mainly in the later stages of treatment, with a slight rebound after withdrawal. Stage NREM-4 - a priori reduced in these insomniacs - was almost totally eliminated (Table 1).

With modern benzodiazepines such dyssomnic side effects, in addition to their sleep-promoting influence, are also the rule, although in general to a lesser extent. Nicholson and coworkers [49] have observed that in normal sleepers diazepam (total dose 10 mg) reduced REM sleep by 15%. Oxazepam (0.77 and 2.3 mg/kg) was found to bring down REM sleep from its control level of 24.7% (of

Table 1. Effect of pentobarbital (100 mg) (%) on the sleep stages of four insomniac subjects in a 47-night study [31]

	Base-line		Drug nights			Withdrawal			
	2–4	5–7	16	17–18	30	31–32	33–35	45	46–47
REM sleep	22.5	21.6	21.7	20.3	17.9	23.4	24.6	19.3	22.7
Stage NREM 1	6.4	4.4	5.1	4.5	4.6	5.5	6.5	5.1	7.1
2	63.4	69.0	66.1	67.5	68.6	61.3	57.3	64.3	60.4
3	6.3	5.0	7.0	6.9	6.0	6.7	8.3	6.9	6.8
4	1.6	0.0	0.1	0.7	2.9	3.0	3.2	4.4	3.0
REM latency (min)	112.7	86.0	98.6	88.0	81.1	89.0	69.4	124.8	76.4

Table 2. Effect of flurazepam (30 mg) (%) on sleep stages of four insomniac subjects in a 47-night study [31]

	Base-line	No. of drug nights				Withdrawal			
	2–4	5–7	16	17–18	30	31–32	33–35	45	46–47
REM sleep	26.2	22.9	20.4	19.4	19.3	22.2	25.5	24.3	26.3
Stage NREM 1	4.3	1.8	2.7	1.7	1.6	2.0	2.9	4.5	3.6
2	53.2	66.1	70.1	71.7	71.5	70.3	65.6	60.1	57.2
3	9.8	4.1	6.1	6.8	6.7	4.7	5.5	6.2	6.3
4	6.6	5.0	0.7	0.4	0.9	0.8	0.5	4.9	6.7
REM latency (min)	69.8	107.3	76.9	114.6	125.3	101.1	81.5	92.9	62.7

total sleep) to 18.8% and 15.1%, respectively, and to reduce stage NREM-4 from its original 48 to 32 and 27 min, respectively [18]. The somnogenic and dyssomnogenic effects of flurazepam (30 mg) in insomniac patients during a long-term study are illustrated in Table 2. This dosage reduced total waking time, although with some habituation in the 5th week of the study. There also was a slight reduction of REM sleep, but with no withdrawal rebound, and a marked suppression of stage NREM-4 [31]. Nitrazepam in doses of 10 and 20 mg reduced REM sleep by 50% and 65%, respectively, during the first 6 h of the drug night and doubled REM latency; it did not have much effect on stages NREM-3 and -4 [23]. In another study of normal subjects 10 mg of nitrazepam were found to have little influence on REM sleep (23.7% to 22.9%) but a pronounced effect on stage NREM-3 and -4 (18.6% to 12.0%) [20]. Flunitrazepam, in doses of 2 and 6 mg, has been shown to have a marked, dose-dependent influence on REM sleep in normal subjects. These dosages reduced REM sleep from 23% (control) to 13.2% and 5.8%, respectively, with little rebound after withdrawal. The percentage of the combined stages NREM-3 and -4 decreased from the control level of 20.7% to 17.6% and 10.1%, respectively [20]. In insomniacs 1 mg of this compound was ineffective as a sleep promotor; still, it curtailed stage NREM-4 by 90%. The (hypnogenically) effective dose of 2 mg reduced REM sleep by 70% and suppressed completely stage NREM-4 [10]. Midazolam, a short-acting benzodiazepine, was shown in doses of 5, 10, and 20 mg to reduce sleep latency in insomniacs in a dose-dependent fashion and to enhance sleep efficiency (% sleep in relation to recording time). It also increased the percentage of stage NREM-2, but reduced REM sleep slightly and left stages NREM-3 and -4 virtually unchanged [26].

Of interest also in the present context is a study of Gaillard and Phelippeau [19], who investigated the effect of flunitrazepam on dream content in normal sleepers. This benzodiazepine, besides its action on stages NREM-3 and -4 and REM sleep, had a rather pronounced influence in the sense that it made dreams more "unpleasant," enhanced "verbal and physical aggressivity," and increased "sexuality."

β-Adrenergic Receptor Antagonists

In general, β-blocking agents are said to have anxiolytic if not sedating effects besides their therapeutic action, particularly in diseases of the circulatory system [21, 37, 47]. There are also numerous reports stating that β-blockers produce disturbances of sleep, such as difficulty in staying asleep, restlessness during the night, early waking, and unpleasant, often frightening dreams [8]. Newer studies clearly indicate that a number of selected β-blockers produces a disturbed sleep pattern, as shown in electrographic investigations, in humans and animals. Betts and Alford [9] studied sleep with the use of EEG, EOG, and EMG in 10 women (20–27 years old) under the influence of atenolol (50 and 100 mg), propranolol (80 and 120 mg), metoprolol (50 and 100 mg), pindolol (10 and 50 mg), and placebo. After two baseline nights, the subjects were kept for 2 nights on the low dose, for 4 nights on the high dose, and for 2 nights on placebo (withdrawal). A questionnaire concerning subjective appreciation of the quality of sleep was completed every morning. Of the four active drugs, propranolol, metoprolol, and pindolol - all lipophilic - increased the subjective recollection of awakenings and of dreaming, while no such effect was noted after the hydrophilic atenolol. On the basis of the electrical recordings, it was noted that pindolol, and to a considerably lesser extent metoprolol and propranolol, enhanced waking time (Table 3). Under high-dose conditions, pindolol and, again to lesser extent propranolol and atenolol, reduced REM sleep, whereas metoprolol had hardly any effect (Table 3). Pindolol led to a considerable REM rebound during the first withdrawal night.

Hilakivi and co-workers [27] have shown that in cats propranolol curtailed paradoxical sleep and that propranolol and pindolol reduced deep slow-wave sleep and enhanced drowsy waking time. The latter effect is probably the result of a combination of the sedating effect of the β-blocker and the "replacing pressure" from the deeper to the lighter stages of sleep. Adrian and collaborators [2] also found that β-blockers inhibited the appearance of paradoxical sleep (in cats).

Table 3. The influence of β-adrenoceptor antagonists on sleep [9]

	Baseline	Low dose	High dose	Withdrawal
Effects on waking scores (group means, minutes; $n = 10$)				
Placebo	3.00 ± 0.82	3.90 ± 1.80	4.20 ± 2.20	5.72 ± 4.40
Atenolol	4.14 ± 0.90	4.50 ± 2.90	4.40 ± 2.60	3.30 ± 1.38
Propranolol	4.40 ± 1.94	6.25 ± 6.39	9.60 ± 8.20	4.47 ± 2.80
Metoprolol	3.78 ± 1.30	5.39 ± 8.00	6.10 ± 4.26	5.80 ± 6.40
Pindolol	4.50 ± 0.58	18.50 ± 25.4*	12.70 ± 14.80*	3.60 ± 1.30
Effects on REM sleep (means of percentages; high dose only)				
Placebo	20.16 ± 4.38		20.50 ± 3.89	20.25 ± 4.70
Atenolol	20.16 ± 4.38		17.30 ± 6.80**	17.20 ± 4.40
Propranolol	20.16 ± 4.38		16.50 ± 3.00**	19.60 ± 4.60
Metoprolol	20.16 ± 4.38		20.00 ± 6.10	20.10 ± 5.90
Pindolol	20.16 ± 4.38		13.30 ± 8.97***	27.70 ± 5.20

* $p < 0.01$; ** $p < 0.05$; *** $p < 0.001$ (compared with baseline)

Antidepressant Drugs

The effects of antidepressant drugs on sleep are of particular interest as depressed patients – the most frequent users of this class of agents – often, if not commonly, suffer from insomnia combined with marked dyssomnia. Depressed patients tend to have a prolonged sleep latency; during the night, they spend longer time in the waking and drowsy state; their total sleep time as well as their slow-wave sleep percentage are reduced; their (first) REM latency (in normals around 80–90 min) is extremely shortened; and their first REM-period is prolonged, while their total REM percentage may be enhanced or somewhat reduced. Normally, the most obvious effect of antidepressant drugs is a reduction of REM sleep, whereas little of this effect is seen in depressed patients.

Zung [67] studied the effect of desipramine on the sleep of seven healthy volunteers. He found that this drug (25 mg tid) decreased REM and markedly enhanced NREM-4 percentage (Table 4). It also increased the number while shortening the duration of the REM-periods. It reduced the number of stage shifts per hour from a control mean of 5.4 to about 4.6 (mean of 4 drug nights). In depressed patients Zung [68] noted that desipramine (4 × 25 mg/day) increased percentage time of stage NREM-4, decreased the number of stage shifts, and prolonged the sleep cycles from a (pretreatment) mean of about 30 min to 1–2 h (Table 4). The substantial drop in the SDS-index showed that the patients also improved clinically under the treatment. However, the drug hardly affected the total REM-quota in these patients.

Ritvo and co-workers [58] investigated the effect on sleep of imipramine in seven enuretic (but otherwise normal) boys. The drug, given before bedtime in a single dose of 25 mg (50 mg in one especially heavy youngster), reduced REM sleep from the original 24.8% to 12.3%; it enhanced time spent in stage NREM-2 (from 46.6% to 60.4%); it prolonged REM latency by almost 100%; but it did not

Table 4. The effect of 3 × 25 mg/day of desipramine on the percentage of the various sleep stages in the adult normal volunteer [67] and of 4 × 25 mg/day of desipramine on the percentage of the sleep stages in the depressed patients [68]. (The original stage designation has been retained; yet A, B, C, D, E can be replaced without much error by awake, NREM-1, 2, 3 and 4, respectively)

	stage percentage of total sleep time					
	A	B	C	D	E	REM
Normal volunteers						
1 - 4 control	0.5	12.3	26.8	15.8	21.5	23.1
5 drug	0.5	11.4	39.4	14.7	21.0	13.0
6 drug	1.0	13.4	30.5	18.2	26.1	10.8
7 drug	0.7	14.7	29.8	14.2	26.0	14.6
8 drug	0.9	14.8	27.1	14.4	27.2	15.6
Depressed patients						
before treatment	6.4	32.7	18.7	10.7	15.2	16.3
week 1	1.2	22.6	23.1	18.2	20.4	14.5
week 4	0.2	23.1	20.0	14.6	24.0	18.1

affect stage NREM-4. Hartmann and Cravens [24] investigated the effect of amitriptyline on the sleep pattern of normal young men. The experimental series was extended to 25 days, followed by an "off-drug period" of 25 days. This agent (in a dose of 50 mg/day) again clearly increased total sleep time and slow-wave sleep time, reduced waking time, and markedly depressed REM time (d-sleep in Hartmann's nomenclature), both in regard to absolute time measures as well as their percentages. Most of these effects were more pronounced in the first days than in the later days of the experimental period. Also, all these parameters tended to show a rebound (in the opposite direction of the drug effect) after cessation of treatment. Dürrigl [15] studied the effect of maprotiline on sleep of depressed patients. In the course of the 3 placebo-, 5 drug-, 2 recovery-, and 5 additional drug-days regimen, it was noted that this tetracyclic compound decreased waking time, enhanced somewhat stage NREM-2, reduced stage NREM-4 (and slightly stage NREM-3), and enhanced the (initially low) REM sleep. Pakesch and Saletu [52] investigated the effect on sleep of diclofensine, a new antidepressant structurally related to nomifensine, but with an additional dopamine-reuptake action. The work was carried out in 12 healthy volunteers. Although chemically different from the "classical" tricyclic agents, diclofensine (one dose of 60 mg) was also found to prolong REM-latency and to reduce REM-percentage, while slightly enhancing stage NREM-2.

The monoamine oxidase inhibitor phenelzine (in a daily dose of 60–90 mg), but not nialamide, all but abolished the signs of REM sleep in two male volunteers. Withdrawal of phenelzine was followed by a pronounced REM rebound. Also, this drug reduced restlessness during sleep throughout the treatment period, while on withdrawal it caused pronounced insomnia [3].

Brebbia and co-workers [11] investigated in healthy volunteers the effect of lithium on sleep, using 3 placebo- and 8 drug-days as the whole experimental series. In this study no effect of the compound on sleep was observed. Chernik and Mendels [12] studied five depressed patients who showed reduced δ-activity in their EEG and a rather increased REM percentage before treatment. Under lithium (1200–1800 mg/day) REM sleep was reduced, REM latency was prolonged, and δ-sleep (stage NREM-3 and -4) was increased. Of interest is also the observation in this study that these sleep effects began within 24 h after the start of treatment. In Kupfer and co-workers' study [36] lithium (300–2400 mg/day) was shown to decrease REM sleep, mostly by shortening REM episodes, to prolong REM latency, and to enhance stages NREM-3 and -4 (δ-sleep).

Whatever had been found concerning the effect of antidepressants on the sleep pattern of (normal) humans has been – more or less – confirmed in (normal) experimental animals. Obal and co-workers [50] studied the effects of amitriptyline on the sleep of rats. The drug was given for 5 days in doses of 2×1, 5, or 15 mg/kg per day. Amitriptyline was found to increase, in a dose-dependent fashion, NREM sleep and to decrease REM sleep and waking time. After withdrawal there was a tendency towards a rebound of these variables. Riou-Merle and Depoortere [55] investigated the effect of imipramine (10 mg/kg per day) for 14 days on the sleep pattern of rats (Sprague-Dawley strain). This agent dramatically reduced the total duration of paradoxical sleep and the frequency of paradoxical sleep episodes; it enhanced REM-latency, and reduced the dominant

ϑ-frequency of the EEG. Wallach and co-workers [64] noted that in the cat such tricyclic drugs as amitriptyline (10–15 mg/kg), desmethylimipramine (10 mg/kg), and imipramine (10–15 mg/kg) suppressed paradoxical sleep from the normal quota of about 13% (per 24-h day) to 0%. They also reduced waking (by roughly one-half) and enhanced slow-wave sleep from 50% to 75%–82% (of the whole day). Scherschlicht and co-workers [61] studied, in the cat, the effect on sleep of a whole series of antidepressants. The drugs used were tertiary (amitriptyline, clomipramine, imipramine, cyanopramine) and secondary (desipramine, nortriptyline) tricyclics, tertiary (citalopram, iprindole) and secondary (maprotiline) nontricyclics, as well as bicyclics (binodaline, diclofensine, nomifensine, zimelidine), tetracyclics (mianserin), MAO-inhibitors (pargyline, moclobemide), chemically atypical antidepressants (femoxetine, fluvoxamine, paroxetine, viloxazine), and morphine, d-amphetamine, and phenobarbitone. In lower doses all of these drugs selectively reduced paradoxical sleep on the day of administration; in higher doses they, in addition to their REM-depressing effect, also tended to augment NREM sleep (Fig. 1). Concerning their paradoxial sleep suppressing effect, the tertiary amines, such as clomipramine, proved to be more potent than secondary amines, e.g., desipramine or nortriptyline. The paradoxical sleep suppressing effect in cats of a variety of MAO-inhibitors has been demonstrated also by Jouvet and collaborators [30]. In the macaque monkey Reite and co-workers [54] noted that iproniazid significantly reduced the amount, and prolonged the latency, of paradoxical sleep. The other MAO-inhibitor tested, namely tranylcypromine, prolonged the latency, but had no effect on the total amount of paradoxical sleep.

Stimulants

Stimulants, as is well known, inhibit falling asleep; they suppress to various degrees REM sleep and reduce or, in some rare instances, even increase the amount of slow-wave sleep.

Rechtschaffen and Maron [53] studied the effect of d-amphetamine on sleep in eight healthy volunteers. Two doses, 10 and 15 mg, were used, and both prolonged REM latency, decreased the total amount of REM sleep, increased - though not to any significant degree - the number of awakenings, prolonged sleep latency, and increased the number of (intrasleep) body movements. In Feinberg and co-workers' study [16] dextroamphetamine (10 and 20 mg, in two each of four healthy subjects respectively) was found to prolong during the 2 drug nights both sleep-latency and REM latency, decreased the total amount of sleep, and reduced REM sleep. After withdrawal, the total sleep time, REM sleep and rapid eye-movements increased to levels above control. According to Oswald

Fig. 1. Effect of 20 antidepressant drugs, with potential or clinically proven effectiveness, on sleep–wake cycle of cats, in comparison to morphine, D-amphetamine, and phenobarbitone. The bars represent percentage of predrug controls (= 100%). They give means of at least 3 animals for every drug. Doses in mg/kg body weight, given i.p. This figure was kindly supplied by the authors of [61]

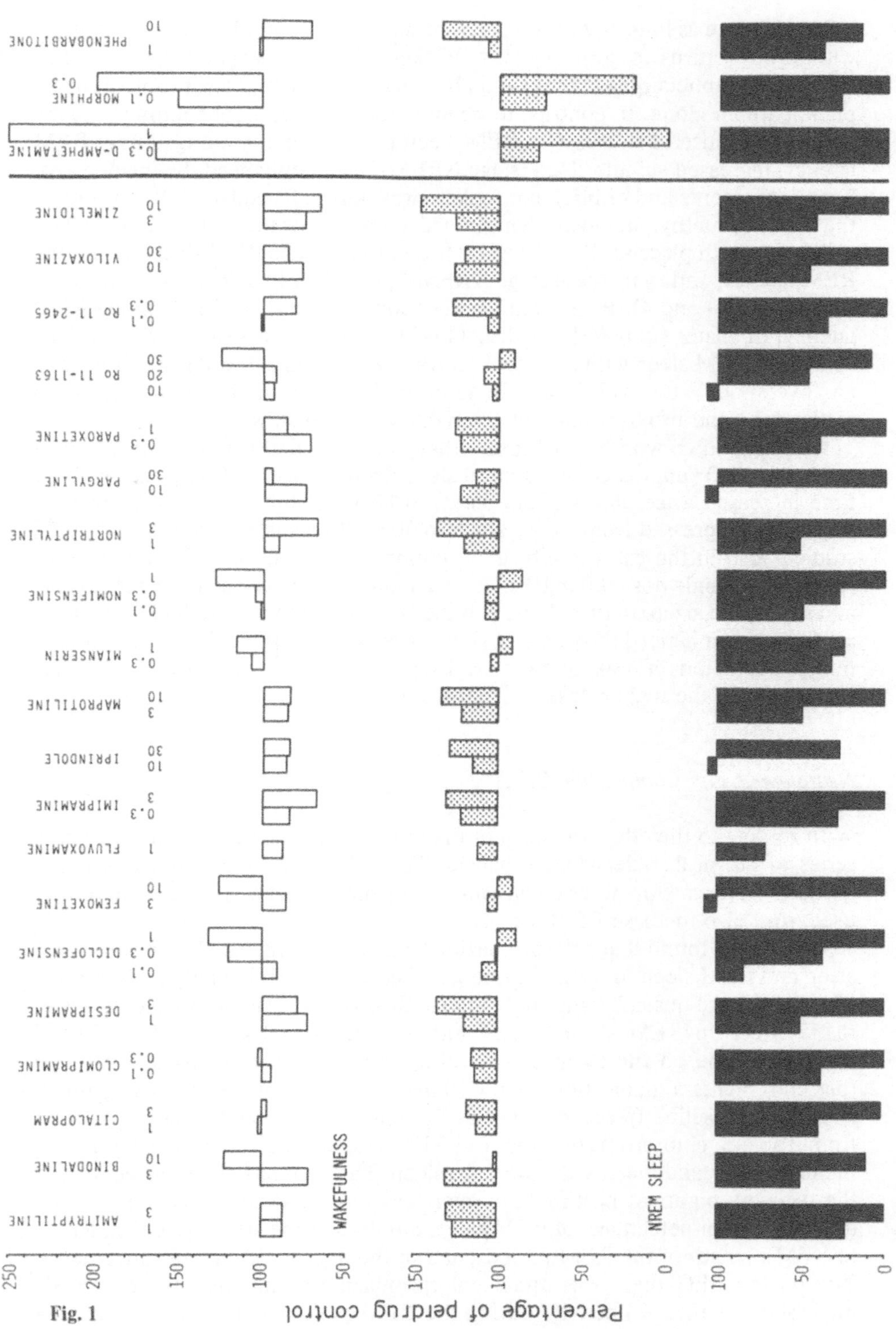
PHENOBARBITONE 1 10
0.1 MORPHINE 0.3
0.3 D-AMPHETAMINE 1
ZIMELIDINE 3 10
VILOXAZINE 10 30
Ro 11-2465 0.1 0.3
Ro 11-1163 10 20 30
PAROXETINE 0.3 1
PARGYLINE 10 30
NORTRIPTYLINE 1 3
NOMIFENSINE 0.1 0.3 1
MIANSERIN 0.3 1
MAPROTILINE 3 10
IPRINDOLE 10 30
IMIPRAMINE 0.3 3
FLUVOXAMINE 1
FEMOXETINE 3 10
DICLOFENSINE 0.1 0.3 1
DESIPRAMINE 1 3
CLOMIPRAMINE 0.1 0.3
CITALOPRAM 1 3
BINODALINE 3 10
AMITRIPTILINE 1 3
WAKEFULNESS
NREM SLEEP
REM SLEEP
250 200 150 100 50
150 100 50 0
100 50 0
Percentage of perdrug control

Fig. 1

[51] it may take as long as 2 months before the REM rebound after amphetamine withdrawal returns to control levels. Baekeland [5] investigated the combined effect of d-amphetamine (15 mg) and phenobarbital (100 mg) against placebo and phenobarbital alone. In contrast to phenobarbital alone, amphetamine plus the barbiturate caused a decrease in REM sleep percentage, a prolongation of REM latency, increased spindle sleep (stage NREM-2), and enhanced the incidence of body movements and of brief and longer awakenings. Baekeland [4] also studied the effect of methylphenidate (5 mg) on sleep in six healthy subjects in a balanced design with placebo. This drug was found to decrease REM sleep, to prolong REM latency, and to increase stage NREM-2; it had, in this dose, no effect on δ-sleep (stages 3 and 4). Fenfluramine was found by Lewis [40] to prolong REM latency. In a later study [41] this drug (40–80 mg, daily, for several days) initially decreased REM sleep with a gradual return towards control while "on drug" and an "overshoot" after withdrawal. In addition, fenfluramine increased intrasleep restlessness and bruxism but had a variable effect on slow-wave sleep.

Wallach and co-workers [64] found that in the cat methamphetamine (single dose, 4 mg/kg) suppressed paradoxical sleep (from 1.5% to 0.5%) and at the same time increased wakefulness (from 36.5% to 88.5% of the 24-h day). Slow-wave sleep was suppressed from 52.0% down to 11.0%. Johnson and collaborators [29] studied, also in the cat, the effects of amphetamine and of fenfluramine. Amphetamine (single dose, 1.0 mg/kg, i.p.) significantly suppressed both paradoxical and slow-wave sleep. In turn, fenfluramine (2.5 and 7.5 mg/kg) reduced paradoxical sleep but enhanced the quota of slow-wave and total sleep time with a concomitant reduction of waking time. A REM rebound was observed only after withdrawal of the higher doses of the two drugs.

Neuroleptics and Comparable Drugs

With respect to the effect on sleep of major tranquilizers, there again is a whole series of classical, older-vintage papers. They all agree in that these drugs in humans enhance slow-wave sleep and, in dependence of dose and type of drug used, may also increase REM sleep.

Toyoda [63] found that chlorpromazine (12.5–50 mg) enhanced both slow-wave sleep and REM sleep. In turn, Feinberg and co-workers [17] noted that in schizophrenics a large dose (200 mg) only increased slow-wave sleep and had no systematic effect on REM sleep. Lester and co-workers [38] studied the effect of chlorpromazine on the sleep of 12 healthy medical students, using 3 baseline (placebo) nights, 1 medication night (150 mg of CPZ), 1 post-drug recovery night, and 1 final baseline (placebo) night as the entire experimental series. As seen from Table 5, chlorpromazine reduced REM latency and the number of movement arousals, and increased slow-wave sleep. These effects were carried over to the recovery night. At no time, however, was there a systematic change in the total amount or percentage of REM sleep, duration of the sleep cycle (i.e., REM-to-REM), length of the REM periods, and in the density of the eye movements. Yet, on the EEG there was under chlorpromazine treatment a trend towards increased fast (i.e., β-) activity during the REM periods and reduced σ-spindle

Table 5. The effect of chlorpromazine on various sleep variables in healthy young male adults [38]

	Baseline		CPZ		Recovery	
Stage or variable	$\overline{X}$	s	$\overline{X}$	s	$\overline{X}$	s
W (%)	5.0	2.4	4.5	3.4	6.3	5.2
NREM-1 (%)	2.7	1.7	2.2	1.6	2.8	1.7
NREM-2 (%)	54.3	4.0	51.6	6.1	49.9	5.4
NREM-3+4 (%)	18.4	3.8	21.6	5.8	22.8	4.4
REM (%)	24.6	2.9	24.3	2.9	24.5	3.3
Sleep latency (min)	4.6	1.8	5.0	3.4	8.1	2.9
REM latency (min)	90.7	22.0	75.1	16.8	78.3	24.8
Average duration of Rem episode (min)	28.3	4.3	26.6	3.2	26.6	4.8
Sleep cycle (min)	102.7	15.7	100.4	10.3	100.6	15.5
No movement arousals	50.0	8.5	33.8	10.6	40.6	21.3

activity. Hartmann and Cravens [25] investigated its effect on the sleep of young adult male volunteers (21–35 years old). In a dose of 50 mg daily given over a period of 28 days, chlorpromazine clearly reduced wakefulness and enhanced total sleep time with a carryover into the first 2 days of the postmedication placebo period. However, marked changes as to percentage of either slow-wave sleep or REM sleep were not found. Risberg and co-workers [57] investigated in a first experiment the effects of a single dose of promethazine (50, 100, or 200 mg) on the sleep of ten healthy volunteers. In the second experiment a dose of the same drug (100 mg) was given for 9 (drug)nights after 3–6 baseline nights, and followed by several recovery nights. In the "one-shot" experiment, promethazine was found to suppress, in a dose-dependent fashion, REM sleep (from 20.7% to 16.3%, 13.5%, and 11.4% using 50, 100, and 200 mg, respectively). There also was a slight increase in stage NREM-2 and – with the highest dose only – of stages NREM-3 and 4, and a prolongation of the REM latency. In the second experiment, the 100-mg dose initially suppressed REM sleep to levels comparable to those seen in the first experiment. With the continuation of drug administration, the REM-suppressing effect was gradually attenuated and reached zero level (i.e., control level) by the 7th night of application. This phase of adaptation was followed, upon withdrawal, by a pronounced REM rebound. Risberg and co-workers [56] also studied the effect of dixyrazine, another phenothiazine derivative, on sleep in ten normal volunteers. Three doses (12.5, 25, and 50 mg) were used. Again, this drug in the higher two doses suppressed REM sleep in the first night of application, while during the following nights the effect gradually diminished. Yet there was no rebound upon withdrawal.

Hartmann and Cravens [24] studied the effect on sleep of reserpine during a long-term administration regime. They noted that under a dose of 0.5 mg daily, total REM sleep time and the number of REM periods (per night) clearly increased. These effects were prominent from day 3 through the 2nd week of application. At the same time REM latency and the length of the sleep cycle (REM-to-REM) were shortened. During the first 3 days of application, reserpine slightly enhanced total sleep time and shortened the sleep latency. Total slow-wave sleep time was also slightly reduced for the first few days. All these changes were paralleled by an increased feeling of fatigue and a decrease in vigor during the daytime.

Concerning the effects on sleep of neuroleptics in animals, the following three reports are of special interest. Wallach and co-workers [64] noted that in cats chlorpromazine (15 mg/kg) virtually completely suppressed paradoxical sleep (from control levels of 13.5% down to 1.3%) on the 1st day, with a slow return towards control levels in the course of the 6-day continued treatment. In turn, slow-wave sleep was increased to close to 200% and 160% on days 1 and 2 respectively. Perphenazine (4 mg/kg), investigated in the same study, minimally suppressed paradoxical sleep, while slow-wave sleep increased by about 50% on day 1. Reite et al. [54] studied the effect on sleep of reserpine in the macaque monkey. They showed that this rauwolfia alkaloid enhanced paradoxical sleep in a highly significant manner (from control levels of 13.7% to 20.7%). It also increased the number of paradoxical sleep periods and shortened paradoxical sleep latency from a mean of 65 to 22 min. These effects were noted during the 1st day and continued throughout the 7-day period of drug administration. Total sleep time and total awake time were not markedly influenced by reserpine. These results are somewhat in conflict with the findings of Jouvet's group [13, 44]; the latter showed that reserpine in the cat suppressed slow-wave sleep and the tonic signs (muscular atonia and activity pattern in the cortical EEG) of paradoxical sleep while enhancing the rate of the so-called ponto-geniculo-occipital spikes (PGOs). More recently though, Stern and Morgane [62] have shown that in the same species the effect of reserpine seems to depend on the route of administration. Peripheral (e.g., intraperitoneal) application leads rather to depression of paradoxical sleep, while central (i.e., intraventricular) injection of reserpine is followed by a clear increase in paradoxical sleep. As yet, we have no good explanation for this discrepancy.

Psychodelics, Narcotics, Alcohol

These three classes of drugs have rather varied effects on sleep; general statements thus cannot be made.

Marijuana seems to produce a kind of stage NREM-4 deprivation, with little influence on REM-sleep. Barratt and co-workers [7] investigated in eight young male human subjects (21–26 years) its effect on sleep. All subjects were experienced marijuana users. After 3 baseline nights with no drug intake, the experimental subjects smoked for 10 nights a marijuana "joint" (containing 0.2 mg/kg bodyweight Δ 9-tetrahydrocannabinol) before bedtime, while the control subjects smoked "placebo-joints". The experiment concluded with 3 postdrug nights. All subjects were instructed not to smoke marijuana or ingest any other drug outside the laboratory. The sleep patterns were monitored using ordinary electrographic probes. Slow-wave sleep increased somewhat during the first 4 experimental days and then progressively decreased to reach levels significantly below baseline-night levels; it remained low during the 3-day postdrug period

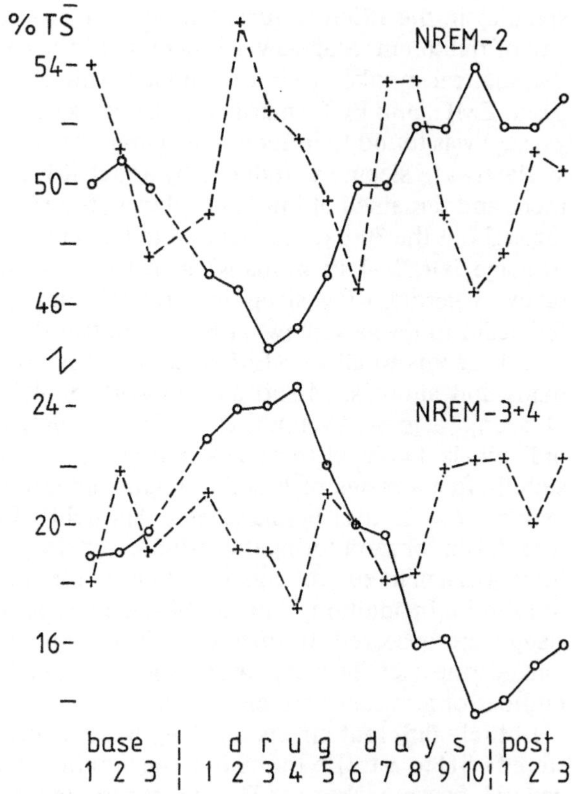

Fig. 2. The effect of marijuana on the sleep of young healthy adults. The experimental design included 3 baseline *(base)* days, 10 drug days and 3 postdrug days *(Post)*. Note initial increase, then drop, of stages NREM-3+4 (slow-wave sleep) and inverse behavior, virtually compensating for gain or loss of stages NREM-3+4, of stage NREM-2-sleep. All values in relation to total sleep (% means). O------O, experimental data; +------+, control data. This figure was drawn using the tabular data of [7]

(Fig. 2). Stage NREM-2 in general changed in a fashion opposite to stages NREM-3 and -4. However, no significant effects of marijuana on REM-sleep were noted. Total sleep time was somewhat reduced in the 1st drug night in both the experimental and the control subjects. Barrat and Adams [6] studied the effect of oral marijuana (distillates with 2.74 mg/kg Δ 9-tetrahydrocannabinol) on the sleep of cats ($n = 6$) prepared for EEG-, EMG-, and EOG-recordings. The drug was given daily for a period of 180 days with 5 predrug and 40 postdrug days. Two additional animals received only 0.342 mg/kg and one was given placebo. Electrographic recordings (for 11 h each day) were made during all baseline days, on days 1, 5, 10, 15, 20, 40, 80, 120, 160, and 180 of the experimental period, and on days 1, 5, 10, 15, 20, and 40 of the postdrug period. In the course of the 6-months drug period, slow-wave sleep gradually declined to about 60 to 50% of its baseline value. This level was reached at about day 20. A similar pattern emerged for spindles in the EEG. In turn, "drowsy" light sleep was enhanced from the first day of treatment. Stage-awake increased to levels about 50% above baseline. In the squirrel monkey ($n = 6$) supplied with electrodes for the recording of the EEG, EMG, and EOG, marijuana (1.2 mg/kg Δ 9-tetrahydrocannabinol, given by gavage) was found to influence also mainly stage NREM-4. What was referred to as slow-wave sleep was reduced by about 10% during the first few days of treatment and remained at low levels during the rest of the experimental period and throughout the 30-day recovery period. Conversely, "drowsy" sleep (comparable to stage NREM-1 in humans) increased and stayed elevated throughout the recovery period. REM sleep first dropped slightly, increased (by day 8), and then fell again to levels somewhat below control [1].

LSD seems to affect REM sleep, but obviously in a different manner in humans and animals. Muzio and co-workers [48] studied the effect on sleep of D-lysergic acid diethylamide (LSD-25, or simply LSD) in 12 psychiatrically sound individuals. Doses of from 0.08 to 0.73 μg/kg (6–40 μg, total dose) were administered after a series of baseline nights, alternating with placebo, either before bedtime or 1 h after falling asleep. All-night EEG, EMG, and EOG recordings were taken for monitoring the structure of sleep. On 21 of 36 occasions with LSD there was a marked prolongation of either the first or the second REM period, up to 141 min. In addition, short REM sleep episodes interrupting periods of NREM sleep were observed. In turn, the REM sleep periods following a markedly prolonged one usually were rather short. Under LSD body movements and the number of arousals were enhanced.

Entirely different effects on sleep were reported by Hobson [28] who administered LSD to cats. He found that the duration of the paradoxical sleep periods in general became shorter. During continuing paradoxical sleep periods there occurred many arousals. Furthermore paradoxical sleep was in general "poorly differentiated" from slow-wave sleep; many spindles and slow-wave activity disturbed the ordinary paradoxical sleep pattern of the EEG. In turn, slow-wave sleep episodes often showed a considerable admixture of low voltage fast activity unaccompanied though by changes in EMG-activity. In one cat, however, a low dose of LSD (2 μg/kg) produced an increase of paradoxical sleep percentage. Furthermore, susceptibility to arousal by incidental external stimuli was clearly increased and awakenings also occurred spontaneously during periods of slow-wave sleep, usually when these seemed to be evolving towards paradoxical sleep. According to Loew and co-workers [43], LSD in rats delayed the occurrence of sleep in general and of paradoxical sleep in particular. There were during paradoxical sleep episodes more brisk body movements in comparison with control animals.

Narcotics seem to suppress both slow-wave sleep and REM sleep. Kay and co-workers [33] investigated the effect of morphine in three doses (7.5, 15, and 30 mg) on the sleep of eight male nondependent opiate addicts; the drug was tested against placebo in a randomized crossover design. Morphine produced, in a dose-dependent fashion, an enhancement of the waking state with an associated increase in muscle tone. The drug decreased total REM time, mainly by prolonging REM latency and shortening individual REM episodes. Furthermore it reduced stages NREM-3 and 4 (δ-sleep) and increased stage NREM-1 ("drowsiness"). In addition, morphine tended to modify the EEG-pattern in that it reduced the amplitude of the δ-waves and of the σ-spindles; effects which made in the authors' view, staging, somewhat unreliable. Lewis and co-workers [42] investigated the effect of heroin (7.5 mg) on sleep in four male volunteers during 4 successive nights. They found a drastic reduction of the REM sleep percentage from about 22% to less than 10% of total sleep (mean of four individuals) following the first application, with a tendency towards control level during nights 2 and 3. Upon withdrawal there was a moderate to marked rebound, in particular during the first 3 h of the recovery nights. In addition there was, during the drug nights, an increase in stage NREM-1, and there were more shifts towards NREM-1 and awakening. Stages NREM-2 and 3+4 were not significantly affected by heroin, but stage NREM-2 was clearly increased during the first 3 h of the recovery nights.

In the cat, morphine increased waking time and reduced NREM sleep, REM sleep, and the REM/NREM ratio [60]. The effects obtained by two different doses of morphine are shown in Table 6 which was composed using Scherschlicht and co-workers' data [60].

Finally, a few notes on the effects of alcohol on sleep and the typical sleep patterns in alcoholics are in order. Obviously, alcohol affects REM sleep and, in a kind of compensatory fashion, also stage NREM-2. Kay and co-workers [32] and Williams and Salamy [65] have reviewed these matters. We cite here only a few examples. Yules and collaborators [66] investigated in three healthy subjects the effect on sleep of 1 g/kg bodyweight of ethyl alcohol (given just before bedtime) in the course of a 4 baseline, 5 alcohol, and 4 recovery-nights experiment. The REM sleep percentage dropped during the first drug night, increased to reach levels well above control by the 5th experimental night, and then returned towards control in the course of the recovery nights 3 to 4. This pattern was evident regardless of whether or not one considered the REM sleep percentage for the whole night, or separately for the first (the one with highest alcohol levels) and second halves of the night. Stage NREM-2 followed an inverse time course, while stages NREM-3 and -4 remained rather constant. REM latency varied rather inconsistently during the 5 drug nights. Rundell and co-workers [59] investigated in ten healthy volunteers the effect of a single dose (0.9 g/kg) of 95% alcohol on sleep. This dose significantly reduced REM sleep during the first part of the night, but not over the whole night. Sleep latency as well as duration of the first REM period were shortened. During recovery, sleep latency was prolonged and REM latency shortened. In a second study, the same group investigated the

Table 6. The effect of morphine (0.1 and 0.3 mg/kg, i.p.) on sleep of cats. Control values = 100%. This table was compiled using data from [60]

	0.1 mg/kg	0.3 mg/kg
waking	↑ 147%	↑↑ 198%
NREM sleep	↓ 73%	↓↓ 20%
REM sleep	↓ 32%	↓↓ 0%
REM/NREM ratio	↓ 50%	↓↓ 0%

effect on sleep of the same dose of alcohol but given for a total of 3 nights. The results were virtually the same.

Lester and co-workers [39] compared the sleep of alcoholics who went without a drink for at least 3 weeks, with that of age-matched normal controls. Alcoholics, in comparison with controls, had more frequent arousals, more of a light-drowsy stage, more stage shifts, and more frequent REM disruptions. REM sleep percentage was increased, due to increased rates of REM sleep episodes, but not prolonged mean REM periods. In particular younger alcoholics had less stage NREM-3 and -4, as compared with older alcoholics and controls.

On the Loci and Mechanisms of Action

Basic Aspects

The very diversity of the sleep effects described in the preceding section makes it rather probable that the influence of drugs on sleep is exerted via a variety of different loci and mechanisms of action. Furthermore, it is not unlikely that at least the mechanisms of (sleep)action are related to, if not identical with, those responsible for the therapeutic (and in a few cases, reward-producing) effects of these drugs. That is to say, the agents under consideration can (or must) be assumed to affect, via similar mechanisms, both, the "systems" that are pathologically deranged and those that control the organization and eventual realization of the various behavioral manifestations of sleep. This overlap in pharmacologically induced effects is obviously the consequence of poor system-related selectivity of the drugs. However, this lack of selectivity brings the advantage that one can apply the knowledge about the mechanisms of the therapeutic (or rewarding) action of a given drug towards the elucidation of the mechanism(s) of action responsible for side effects, with special reference to sleep effects.

In first approximation, it can be postulated that any effect on sleep is due to a central action of a given drug. Most (if not all) of the centrally acting agents (or agents with at least a powerful central component of action) exert their influence via interaction with one or more of the many and manifold "wet" neurotransmission mechanisms (making up the bulk of the central nervous signal carriers). Thus, one can postulate further that the sleep effects are the manifestation of those drugs' interference with one or several of these neurohumoral transmission mechanisms. More specifically, it can be assumed that drugs that affect sleep act directly (or, rarely, indirectly) on those parts of the central nervous system that comprise on the one hand the neuronal, reflex-type machinery which organizes and regulates sleep and, on the other, the neuronal effector networks which put into effect the particular profiles of activity in the various extroversive and internal behavioral systems, referred to as the behavioral semeiology of sleep.

In a recently published review article we have developed, on the basis of a rather vast variety of experimental and clinical data and relying heavily on the general rules of bio-organization, an integrated model, comprising this sleep-organizing and -regulating apparatus (SORA) and effector networks [35]. This model was based in principle on our novel General Theory of Vigilance [34]. A multitude of mainly wet neurotransmitter and purely neurohumoral network elements were assigned their presumed functional role within the whole of this sleep-organizing and -regulating machinery. A simplified version of this model is depicted in Fig. 3. This model appears to be well-suited to serve as a functional foundation for at least a tentative - in some cases rather safe - interpretation concerning the loci and mechanisms of action through which the various drugs produce their sleep effects. For the sake of simplicity and clarity we shall discuss these putative loci and mechanisms of action separately for the various stages of sleep.

The making of Changes in REM-Sleep

REM-sleep is characterized, in terms of functional behavioral conditions, by

a) a high level of responsiveness, i.e., vigilance, in the higher and lower function systems handling the majority of internal behaviors;
b) a rather low level of vigilance in most of the mainly extroversive motor systems (except, of course, the oculomotor apparatus and the respiratory muscles); and
c) a kind of noncontrol, or low vigilance in the greater part of the vegetative-autonomic system.

This REM-specific profile of vigilances is the manifestation of a similar profile of reactivities in the respective neuronal effector networks that subserve the making of these extroversive and internal behaviors. A low-voltage, fast, irregular cortical EEG pattern is the manifestation of high reactivity in the cortex which contains most of the effector networks in charge of the higher and lower functions. Rapid eye movements, muscular atonia, areflexia, and, e.g., in the cat, PGOs (ponto-geniculo-occipital spikes) and a pronomed theta pattern in the hippocampies are additional signs of the REM sleep state.

This profile of vigilances and reactivities is induced and maintained by a set of controlling instruments, consisting in the main of monoaminergic pathways. There is ample evidence that a high level of (ascending) cholinergic and a moderately high level of noradrenergic (β-mediated) activity, emerging from the center (see Fig. 3) are the important conditions for the maintenance of high reactivity in the cortical and limbic networks. This vigilance-enhancing output is supported by - certainly in the highly reactive areas - a low serotonergic and (probably) a low dopaminergic output. Furthermore, it can be assumed that this particular set of output activities is produced and controlled by the activity in the REM, or PS-subprogram, a pertinent component of the center (Fig. 3; for further details, see [14, 35]). With this multitude of controlling instruments, any change in the level of REM sleep as induced by drugs is liable to result from several different loci and mechanisms of action of the various sleep-active agents.

A reduction or inhibition of REM-sleep (attenuation of the REM signs, prolongation of REM latency, shortening of the REM periods) can be effected by,

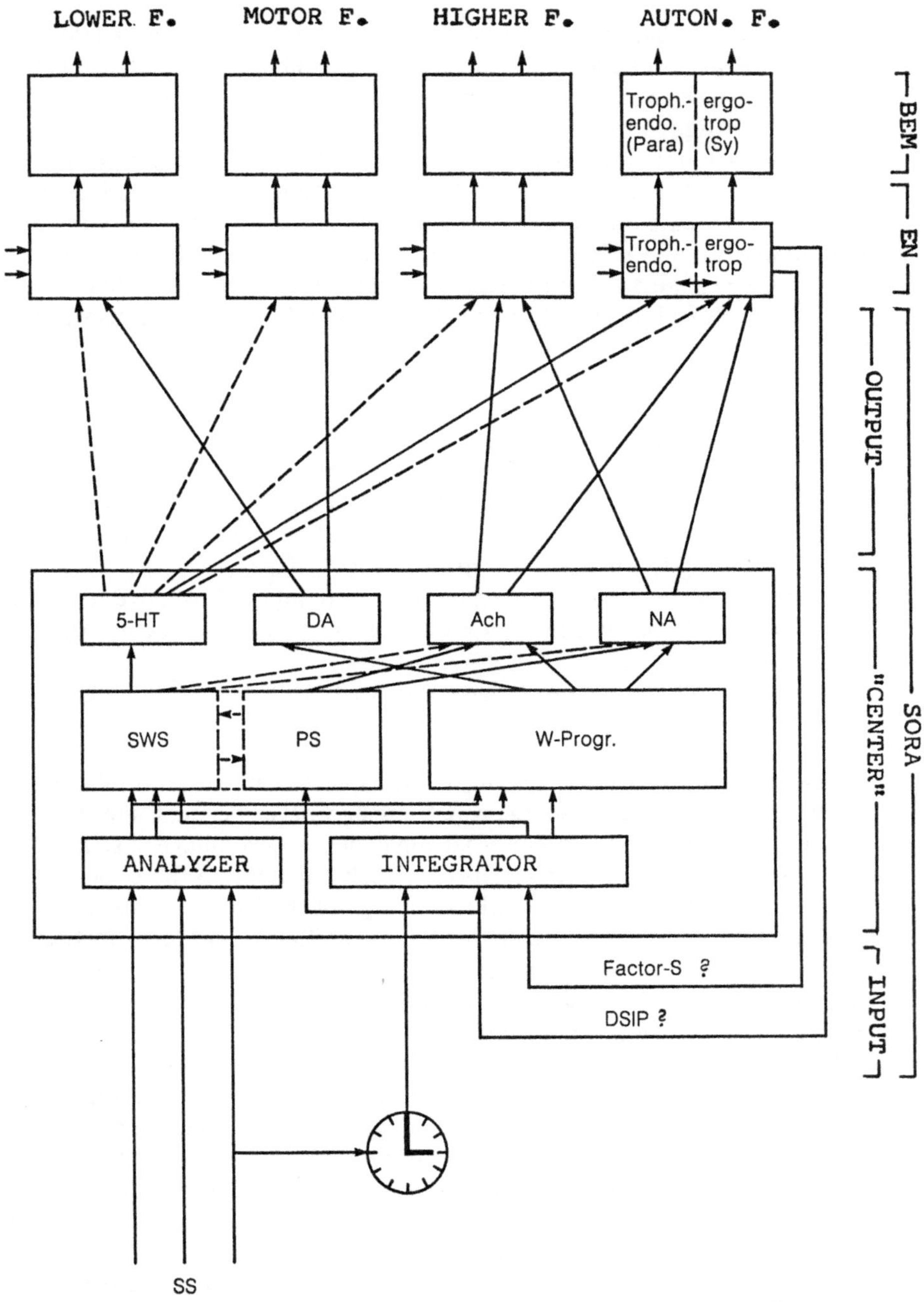

Fig. 3. Model of the sleep-organizing and -regulating apparatus *(SORA),* the effector networks *(EN),* and the behavioral executive mechanisms *(BEM)* – simplified version of the model proposed by Koella [35]. Note the reflex-type structure of SORA, with an input, a central coordinating (the *"center"*), and an output component. ENs subserve the making of particular behavioral patterns, here represented globally by higher, lower, motor, and autonomic functions. The autonomic sphere is subdivided into the areas subserving ergotropic (preponderance of peripheral sympathoadrenergic tone) and trophotropic-endophylactic "strategies" (prepon-

e.g., elevation of the ascending noradrenergic activity to the highest levels. This is accomplished, for example, through inhibition of noradrenaline reuptake by antidepressants, through facilitation of noradrenaline release by amphetamine and related drugs, and probably (and if so, indirectly) by opiates. However, inhibition of REM sleep may also be the consequence of a marked reduction of (β-)adrenergic transmission. This typically is the case for the REM-curtailing effect of (mainly lipophilic) β-blockers. Furthermore, the manifestations of REM sleep can be inhibited, or better, deactivated through suppression of cholinergic activity; it is more than likely that the notorious (but not always recognized) anticholinergic properties of most of the antidepressants are an important factor here.

An increase in dopaminergic output is also liable to inhibit REM sleep, at least as concerns its motor manifestations (muscular atonia, areflexia). The facilitation of dopamine release obviously is the (or one of the) mechanism(s) by which stimulants, such as amphetamine, can curtail REM sleep, or at least its muscular signs. Excessive serotonergic transmission activity, as accomplished, e.g., through the inhibition of 5-hydroxytryptamine reuptake by a variety of antidepressants, is a further mechanism that should lead to a reduction of REM sleep.

Finally, excessive and untimely reduction in activity in the PS-subprogram is also an important factor involved in the curtailing of REM sleep. There can be little doubt that this network includes as pertinent inhibitory elements a large number of (short-axoned) GABA-ergic neurons. GABA-ergic transmission and thus inhibition of postsynaptic neurons is markedly facilitated by all benzodiazepines [22, 45]. The characteristic, often marked, often lesser, suppression of REM sleep, as produced by such drugs as diazepam, flurazepam, and flunitrazepam, could well be the result of such GABA-induced excessive inhibition within the REM-organizing network.

An enhancement of REM sleep is seen occasionally with LSD (in humans) and neuroleptics. The inhibition of serotonergic activity by LSD (both via suppression of activity of serotonergic neurons and block of 5-hydroxytryptamine

---

derance of peripheral parasympathocholinergic tone). Note at least three types of regulating and timing inputs to the center: a feedback from the effector networks (represented, possibly, by such humoral sleep factors as *factor-S* or *DSIP*); a "clock" input, supplying information about (circadian) time; and collaterals from sensory afferent pathways *(SS)*. The center contains a wake-(W-) program and a sleep-(S-)program, the latter being subdivided into a *SWS*- (or NREM-) and a *PS*-(or REM-)subprogram (with mutually inhibiting interconnection). The center also contains an "analyzer" handling proper response to incoming sensory stimuli. It further contains the "roots" of the (mainly) monoaminergic output lines. These outputs - here only four of a putatively much larger number are shown - control reactivity in the ENs in order to establish a proper vigilance in the respective behavioral systems. Noradrenergic and cholinergic outputs appear to control (in a positive fashion) reactivity in the "higher function" systems. Dopaminergic pathways are likely to control (again in a positive fashion) the reactivity (and thus, vigilance) in the *"lower"* and *"motor"* functional systems. In turn, serotonergic *(5-HT)* pathways appear to exert a reactivity (and vigilance)-suppressing influence on mainly the higher, lower, and possibly also the motor function systems. They also seem to support reactivity in the trophotropic-endophylactic part of the *autonomic* functions. *DA,* dopamine; *Ach,* acetylcholine; *NA,* noradrenaline; 5-HT, serotomin.

receptors) could properly explain, by a process of disinhibition the emergence of enhanced REM activity. Neuroleptics may facilitate REM sleep through their (rather weak) blocking action of (mainly α-)adrenergic receptors.

The REM rebound, as observed after withdrawal of many REM inhibivting drugs, is probably due to up- or downwards overshoot of a multitude of systems which, during drug application, have become adapted (sub- or supersensitivity of receptors). After withdrawal of a drug, the systems, based on this "new state," are bound to react excessively in response to physiological signals to produce a higher propensity of REM sleep.

The Making of Changes in NREM sleep

Slow-wave sleep is characterized, in terms of functional/behavioral conditions, by
a) a markedly reduced level of vigilance in the systems of higher (and lower), functions;
b) a rather high level of vigilance in practically all motor systems, as evidenced by high muscular tone, high reflex excitability, and proneness towards somnambulistic activity; and
c) a shift of high vigilance from the ergotropic to the trophotropic-endo-phylactic aspects of the vegetative-autonomic system.

Again, as with REM sleep, this slow-wave sleep specific profile of vigilances is the manifestation of a similar profile of reactivities in the effector networks that subserve the organization and realization of the various extroversive and internal behaviors. A high-voltage, slow electrocorticogram signifies low reactivity in the (cortical) networks that subserve higher function behaviors. Motor quiescence is the manifestation of the absence of motor stimuli rather than, as indicated, of reduced motor vigilance. It can be postulated that this profile of reactivities and vigilances is induced and maintained by rather high levels of (ascending) 5-hydroxytryptamine activity. This is supported, in a permissive manner, by reduced noradrenergic and cholinergic activity. Again, this output profile is the result of the organizing activity in the SWS-subprogram in the center (see Fig. 3).

A reduction in slow-wave sleep can be assumed to be due to a variety of different mechanisms of action of the respective drugs. An enhancement of noradrenergic synaptic activity, as produced via inhibition of reuptake by most antidepressants, is bound to inhibit slow-wave sleep effectively. So is the enhancement of (dopamine and) noradrenaline release as effected by stimulants, such as amphetamine. A mechanism of action via activation of opiate receptors could be envisioned to explain the slow-wave sleep inhibiting effect of morphine. The slow-wave sleep (and the general sleep-) inhibiting effect of the β-adrenoceptor antagonists has now a plausible explanation after it was shown that most (lipophilic) β-blockers antagonize not only β-adrenergic but also serotonergic receptors [46]. The intimate cause of the reduction of slow-wave sleep in these cases clearly is due to a block of serotonergic transmission activity.

Concerning the often pronounced slow-wave sleep curtailing effects of benzodiazepines, we have to turn back again to the mechanism discussed in connection with the REM-suppressing action of these compounds. It seems to be the facilitated GABAergic activity – this time in the SWS-Subprogram – that reduces and deranges signal flow within, and output from, this subprogram network and thus curtails the emergence of the signs of slow-wave sleep. As to the stage NREM-4-suppressing effect of marijuana, we have no ready explanation. Neither do we have a plausible hypothesis for the action of alcohol on slow-wave sleep. Here, interaction with enzymes and thus interference with the metabolism of the various "wet" neurotransmitters may turn out to be the pertinent factor.

General Principles

As outlined in the foregoing two sections, there is a multitude of loci and mechanisms of action that (tentatively) may be held responsible for the actions of the various drugs on REM and/or NREM sleep. Even with a given single drug, there are often several mechanisms available which are capable of explaining this agent's (often parallel, often opposite) effects on the various stages of sleep. It seems indeed that a particular effect (e.g., a curtailing of REM sleep) of a given drug quite probably is the resultant sum of a multitude of influences on the sleep systems, it is probably the finely balanced impact of all actions that is responsible for a given effect, regardless of whether this is a change of REM or NREM sleep, and whether the effect is up or down. It comes as no surprise then to learn that the sleep effects of different drugs do vary to no small extent. Just whatever factor or action turns out to be the preponderant one (thus determining quality, quantity, and direction of the sleep effect) depends to a great extent on the type of drug, the dosage used, and the route of application, in addition to such factors as the level of adaptation (after previous applications of the same drug), the particular experimental setting, and the momentary level of responsiveness in the various systems.

Concluding Remarks

All of the drugs covered here affect sleep to a lesser or greater degree; yet they do this in directionally and qualitatively different manners. REM sleep appears to be the main target of such agents. Many drugs tend to suppress this stage of sleep which often leads to a REM rebound after withdrawal. However, a few drugs have been found to enhance REM sleep directly (i.e., not via rebound). Quite a few drugs have been found to enhance or suppress slow-wave sleep. These effects may occur either in isolation or together with the effects on REM sleep. Often, stage NREM-2 is found to increase when a given drug reduces REM and/or slow-wave sleep, as if the main role of stage NREM-2 were to "compensate" for the loss of either one or both of the latter stages.

It is quite obvious indeed that in many cases these side effects are not desired, even utterly disturbing. They are liable to reduce the actual value of a given drug or at least limit the choice of dosage and time of application.

Still, there are a few cases where these sleep effects are rather of desired nature in that they may add to the spectrum of therapeutic actions or perhaps open avenues towards novel uses. Concerning the former possibility, one tends to think of, e.g., the notorious REM depressing effect of antidepressants (at least in subjects in whom the REM quota is not a priori reduced). This REM curtailing action may in fact be an important factor supporting (or possibly even constituting) the antidepressant action of these compounds. It has been shown that REM deprivation can generate a marked, although short-lived antidepressant effect. Concerning new uses of drugs with sleep effects, we may mention the case of the neuroleptics which, with their slow-wave (and REM-) sleep enhancing effect, became quite useful hypnotics, particularly in older people. There is also the case of stimulants that can be applied quite successfully for the (symptomatic) treatment of some cases of narcolepsy.

It seems then that proper study of possible or established sleep effects of virtually all drugs is well-indicated. The results would add to our set of information about a given drug's side effects and thus provide a foundation for the establishment of countermeasures when necessary. The findings of sleep studies should produce the basis for making good use of such side actions. Finally, studies on sleep with a variety of drugs may furnish some novel information about the particular loci and mechanisms of action involved in sleep effects which could then be applied again to explain the mechanisms responsible for their primary therapeutic action. It is for this latter reason that we have made an effort to discuss - albeit in a rather simplified fashion - the putative loci and mechanisms of action that are (possibly) involved in generating sleep effects.

References

1. Adams PM, Barratt ES (1975) Effect of chronic marijuana administration on stages of primate sleep-wakefulness. Biol Psychiatry 10:315–322
2. Adrien J, Lanfumey L, Dugovic C (1985) Effects of beta-adrenergic antagonists and agonists on sleep. In: Wauquier A, Gaillard J-M, Monti JM, Radulovacki M (eds) Raven, New York, pp 93–106
3. Akindele MO, Evans JI, Oswald I (1970) Mono-amine oxidase inhibitors, sleep and mood. Electroencephalogr Clin Neurophysiol 29:47–56
4. Baekeland F (1966) The effect of methylphenidate on the sleep cycle in man. Psychopharmacologie 10:179–183
5. Baekeland F (1967) Pentobarbital and dextroamphetamine sulfate: effects on the sleep cycle in man. Psychopharmacologia 11:388–396
6. Barratt ES, Adams PM (1973) Chronic marijuana usage and sleep-wakefulness cycles in cats. Biol Psychiatry 6:207–214
7. Barratt ES, Beaver W, White R (1974) The effects of marijuana on human sleep patterns. Biol Psychiatry 8:47–54
8. Betts TA (1981) Adrenoceptor drugs and sleep. In: Wheatley D (ed) Psychopharmacology of sleep. Raven, New York, pp 199–212
9. Betts TA, Alford C (1985) β-blockers and sleep: a controlled trial. Eur J Clin Pharmacol 28 [Suppl]:65–68
10. Bixler EO, Kales A,. Soldatos CR, Kales JD (1977) Flunitrazepam, an investigational hypnotic drug: sleep laboratory evaluation. J Clin Pharmacol 17:569–578
11. Brebbia DR, Altschuler KZ, Kline NS (1969) Lithium and the electroencephalogram during sleep. Dis Nerv Syst 30:541–546

12. Chernik DA, Mendels J (1974) Longitudinal study of the effects of lithium carbonate on the sleep of hospitalized depressed patients. Biol Psychiatry 9:117–123
13. Delorme F, Jeannerod M, Jouvet M (1965) Effets remarquables de la réserpine sur l'activité EEG phasique ponto-géniculo-occipitale. CR Soc Biol (Paris) 159:900–903
14. Depoortere H (1985) Adrenergic agonists and antagonists and sleep-wakefulness stages. In: Wauquier A, Gaillard J-M, Monti JM, Radulovacki M (eds) Sleep, neurotransmitters and neuromodulators. Raven, New York, pp 79–92
15. Dürrigl V (1973) Some problems of the therapy of sleep disturbances in depressed patients. In: Koella WP, Levin P (eds) Sleep; proceedings of the 1st European congress of sleep research. Karger, Basel, pp 132–139
16. Feinberg I, Hibi S, Braun M, Cavness C, Westerman G, Small A (1974) Sleep amphetamine effects in MBDS and normal subjects. Arch Gen Psychiatry 31:723–731
17. Feinberg I, Wender PH, Keresko RL, Gottlieb F, Piehuta JA (1969) Differential effects of chlorpromazine and phenobarbital on EEG sleep patterns. J Psychiatr Res 7:101–109
18. Gaillard J-M, Aubert C (1975) Specificity of benzodiazepine action on human sleep confirmed. Another contribution of automatic analysis of polygraph recordings. Biol Psychiatry 10:185–197
19. Gaillard J-M, Phelippeau M (1976) Benzodiazepine-induced modifications of dream content: the effect of flunitrazepam. Neuropsychobiology 2:37–44
20. Gaillard J-M, Schulz P, Tissot R (1973) Effects of three benzodiazepines (nitrazepam, flunitrazepam, and bromazepam) on sleep of normal subjects, studied with an automatic sleep scoring system. Pharmacopsychiatry 6:207–217
21. Gosling RH (1977) Oxprenolol in der Behandlung von Angstzuständen - ein Bericht über klinische Erfahrungen in Großbritannien. In: Kielholz P (ed) Betablocker und Zentralnervensystem. Huber, Bern, pp 127–133
22. Haefely W, Polc P, Schaffner R, Keller HH, Pieri L, Möhler H (1978) Facilitation of GABA-ergic transmission by drugs. In: GABA-neurotransmitters, Alfred Nenzon symposium. Munksgaard, Copenhagen, pp 357–375
23. Haider I, Oswald I (1971) Effects of amylobarbitone and nitrazepam on the electrodermogram and other features of sleep. Br J Psychiatry 118:519–522
24. Hartmann E, Cravens J (1973) The effects of long term administration of psychotropic drugs on human sleep: II. The effects of reserpine. Psychopharmacologia 33:169–184
25. Hartmann E, Cravens J (1973) The effects of long term administration of psychotrophic drugs on human sleep: IV. The effects of chlorpromazine. Psychopharmacologia 33:203–218
26. Hauri P, Roth T, Sateia M, Zorick F (1983) Sleep laboratory and performance evaluation of midazolam in insomniacs. Br J Clin Pharmacol 16 [Suppl 1]:109S–114S
27. Hilakivi I, Mäkelä J, Leppävuori A, Putkonen PTS (1978) Effects of two adrenergic β-receptor blockers on sleep cycle of the cat. Med Biol 56:138
28. Hobson JR (1964) The effect of LSD on the sleep cycle of the cat. Electroencephalogr Clin Neurophysiol 17:52–56
29. Johnson DN, Funderburk WH, Ward JW (1971) Effects of fenfluramine on sleep-wakefulness in cats. Psychopharmacologia 20:1–9
30. Jouvet M, Vimont P, Delorme F (1965) Suppression élective du sommeil paradoxal chez le chat par les inhibiteurs de la monoamine oxydase. CR Soc Biol (Paris) 159:1595–1599
31. Kales A, Kales JD, Bixler ED, Scharf MB (1975) Effectiveness of hypnotic drugs with prolonged use: flurazepam and pentobarbital. Clin Pharmacol Ther 18:356–363
32. Kay DC, Blackburn AB, Buckingham JA, Karacan I (1976) Human pharmacology of sleep. In: Williams RL, Karacan I (eds) Pharmacology of sleep. Wiley, New York, pp 83–210
33. Kay DC, Eisenstein RB, Jasinski DR (1969) Morphine effects on human REM state, waking state, and NREM sleep. Psychopharmacologia 14:404–416
34. Koella WP (1982) A modern neurobiological concept of vigilance. Experientia 38:1426–1437
35. Koella WP (1984) The organization and regulation of sleep. A review of the experimental evidence and a novel integrated model of the organizing and regulating apparatus. Experientia 40:309–338
36. Kupfer DJ, Reynolds CF, Weiss BL, Foster FG (1974) Lithium carbonate and sleep in affective disorders: further considerations. Arch Gen Psychiatry 30:79–84

37. Lader M (1974) The peripheral and central role of the catecholamines in the mechanisms of anxiety. Int Pharmcopsychiatry 9:125–137
38. Lester BK, Coulter JD, Cowden LC, Williams HL (1971) Chlorpromazine and human sleep. Psychopharmacologia 20:280–287
39. Lester BK, Rundell OH, Gowden LG, Williams HL (1973) Chronic alcoholism, alcohol, and sleep. Adv Exp Med Biol 35:261–279
40. Lewis SA (1970) Comparative effects of some amphetamine derivatives on human sleep. In: Costa E, Garattini S (eds) Amphetamines and related compounds. Raven, New York, pp 873–888
41. Lewis SA, Oswald I, Dunleavy DLF (1971) Chronic fenfluramine administration: some cerebral effects. Br Med J 3:67–70
42. Lewis SA, Oswald I, Evans JI, Akindele MO, Tompsett SL (1970) Heroin and human sleep. Electroencephalogr Clin Neurophysiol 28:374–381
43. Loew DM, Depoortere H, Vigouret JM (1970) Wirkungen von D-Lysergsäure-diäthylamid (LSD-25) und 2-Brom-D-Lysergsäure-diäthylamid (BOL-148) auf das Schlafverhalten der Ratte. Naunyn Schmiedebergs Arch Pharmacol 266:394
44. Matsumoto J, Jouvet M (1964) Effets de réserpine, dopa et 5HTP sur les deux états de sommeil. CR Soc Biol (Paris) 158:2137–2140
45. Mendelson WB (1985) GABA-benzodiazepine receptor-chloride ionophore complex: implications for the pharmacology of sleep. In: Wauqier A, Gaillard J-M, Monti JM, Radulovacki M (eds) Sleep, neurotransmitters, neuromodulators. Raven, New York, pp 229–236
46. Middlemiss DN, Blakeborough L, Leather SR (1977) Direct evidence for an interaction of beta-adrenergic blockers with the 5-HT receptor. Nature 267:289–290
47. Middlemiss DN, Buxton DA, Greenwood DT (1981) Beta-adrenoceptor antagonists in psychiatry and neurology. Pharmacol Ther 12:419–437
48. Muzio JN, Roffwarg HP, Kaufman E (1966) Alterations in the nocturnal sleep cycle resulting from LSD. Electroencephalogr Clin Neurophysiol 21:313–324
49. Nicholson AN, Stone BM, Clarke CH (1976) Effect of diazepam and fosazepam (a soluble derivative of diazepam) on sleep in man. Br J Clin Pharmacol 3:533–541
50. Obál F Jr, Benedek G, Lelkes Z, Obál F (1985) Effects of acute and chronic treatment with amitriptyline on the sleep-wake activity of rats. Neuropharmacology 24:223–229
51. Oswald I (1980) Sleep studies in clinical pharmacology. Br J Clin Pharmacol 10:317–3236
52. Pakesch G, Saletu B (1986) Die Wirkung von Diclofensin auf den Schlaf und die verschiedenen Wachaktivitäten normaler Probanden: Somnopolygraphische und psychometrische Studien. In: Schmid-Burgk W, Koella WP (eds) Neue Aspekte der Therapie mit Antidepressiva. Fischer, Stuttgart, pp 163–179
53. Rechtschaffen A, Maron L (1964) The effect of amphetamine on the sleep cycle. Electroencephalogr Clin Neurophysiol 16:438–445
54. Reite M, Pegram GV, Stephens LM, Bixler EC, Lewis OL (1969) The effect of reserpine and monoamine oxidase inhibitors on paradoxical sleep in the monkey. Psychopharmacologia 14:12–17
55. Riou-Merle F, Depoortere H (1985) The action of chronic imipramine treatment on the sleep-wakefulness cycle and on the quality of paradoxical sleep in rats. In: Koella WP, Rüther E, Schulz H (eds) Sleep 1984; proceedings of the 7th European congress of sleep research. Fischer, Stuttgart, pp 301–303
56. Risberg A-M, Risberg J, Elmqvist D, Ingvar DH (1975) Effects of dixyrazine and methaqualone on sleep pattern in normal man. Eur J Clin Pharmacol 8:227–231
57. Risberg A-M, Risberg J, Ingvar DH (1975) Effects of promethazine on nocturnal sleep in normal man. Psychopharmacologia 43:279–284
58. Ritvo ER, Ornitz EM, LaFranchi S, Walter RD (1967) Effects of imipramine on the sleep-dream cycle: an EEG study in boys. Electroencephalogr Clin Neurophysiol 22:465–468
59. Rundell OH, Lester BK Griffith WJ, Williams HL (1972) Alcohol and sleep in young adults. Psychopharmacologia 26:201–218
60. Scherschlicht R, Marias J, Schneeberger J, Steiner M (1981) Model insomnia in animals. In: Koella WP (ed) Sleep 1980; proceedings of the European congress of sleep research. Karger, Basel, pp 147–155

61. Scherschlicht R, Polc P, Schneeberger J, Steiner M, Haefely W (1982) Selective suppression of rapid eye movement sleep (REMS) in cats by typical and atypical antidepressants. In: Costa E, Racagni G (eds) Typical and atypical antidepressants: molecular mechanisms. Raven, New York, pp 264–359
62. Stern WC, Morgane PJ (1973) The effects of reserpine on sleep and brain biogenic amine levels in the cat. Psychopharmacologia 28:275–286
63. Toyoda J (1964) The effects of chlorpromazine and imipramine on human nocturnal sleep electroencephalogram. Folia Psychiatry Neurol Jpn 18:198–221
64. Wallach MB, Winters WD, Mandell AJ, Spooner CE (1969) Effects of antidepressant drugs on wakefulness and sleep in the cat. Electroencephalogr Clin Neurophysiol 27:574–580
65. Williams HL, Salamy A (1972) Alcohol and sleep. In: Kissin B, Begleiter H (eds) The biology of alcoholism. Physiology and behavior. Plenum, New York, pp 435–483
66. Yules RB, Freedman DX, Chandler KA (1966) The effect of ethyl alcohol on man's electroencephalographic sleep cycle. Electroencephalogr Clin Neurophysiol 20:109–111
67. Zung WWK (1968) Effect of antidepressant drugs on sleeping and dreaming: II. On the adult male. Excerpta Med Intern Congress Series 150:1824–1826
68. Zung WWK (1969) Effect of antidepressant drugs on sleeping and dreaming: III. On the depressent patient. Biol Psychiatry 1:283–287

Part 2: Measurement

Measurement of Sleep Fragmentation

S. A. Rothenberg

Introduction and Background

It has been widely observed that a period of good sleep leaves a person refreshed, frequently energetic, enthusiastic, and in good spirits; on the other hand, poor sleep is associated with daytime sleepiness, lethargy, and frequently mild to moderate forms of ill-temper. However, the specific set of variables that determines the quality of sleep remains elusive. It is the premise of this chapter that the fragmentation (or continuity) of sleep is one of the variables contributing to the quality of a period of sleep and thus a measurement technique for this parameter would be useful for analyzing sleep studies and testing hypotheses. Sleep fragmentation may be thought of as the pessimist's view of sleep continuity insofar as decreasing sleep fragmentation is equivalent to increasing sleep continuity, and vice versa. As one sometimes views the world with a pessimist's eye and sometimes with an optimist's eye, both terms will be used interchangeably in this chapter.

There are several relatively standard variables, reported in most sleep studies, that characterize well the average structure of a sleep period:

A. **Period of study**
- ☐ Total time in bed
- ☐ Total recording time
- ☐ Total sleep period

B. **Quantity and quality**
- ☐ Total sleep time (TST)
- ☐ Sleep efficiency

C. **Architecture**
- ☐ Sleep stages in min
- ☐ Sleep stage percentage of TST
- ☐ Latency to sleep onset
- ☐ Latency to stage REM

D. **Continuity or fragmentation**
- ☐ Total awake time
- ☐ Awake time after sleep onset
- ☐ Number of awakenings
- ☐ Number of stage changes

Group A variables are used to describe the period of observation in a sleep study and are also used as the baseline in the calculation of some derived variables, for example sleep efficiency. Group B contains variables used to describe the overall quantity and quality of a period of sleep. Group C gives more specific information about the stages of sleep in terms of total amount or percentage of total sleep time (TST) and some information about the position of that sleep within the observation period. Although these variables provide accurate summaries of many sleep events, most measures emphasize the amount of sleep rather than its continuity. Sleep continuity or fragmentation is defined by the fluctuation in sleep stage resulting from regular NREM/REM cycling and all other factors. The group D variables begin to describe the continuity of sleep. The last variable in group D, the number of stage changes, is a good measure of the overall level of sleep fragmentation. However, none of the variables listed describes how time is distributed within one stage of sleep. That is, one cannot tell whether 60 min of any stage of sleep occurred as one uninterrupted 60-min period or as 60 1-min periods. A thorough analysis of sleep fragmentation should contain both the number of times each stage of sleep occurred and the duration of each occurrence.

The question of how sleep stages are distributed within a sleep period has lately received greater attention, in part because of the increased awareness of the prevalence of sleep disorders in which disruptions of the sleep cycle are common. Recent studies involving the obstructive sleep apnea syndrome (OSAS) and periodic movements during sleep, both of which disrupt the sleep cycle, have focused attention on the role of sleep fragmentation [1, 2, 3]. In addition, studies in which sleep was fragmented experimentally suggest that daytime behavior and sleep physiology may be affected by fragmentation of the sleep process [4, 5]. Nowhere is the fragmentation of sleep more dramatic than in OSAS, where it has been shown that frequent and sometimes prolonged cessations of breathing are ended by arousal responses that interrupt sleep. There may be several hundred such disruptions each night, shortening the longest uninterrupted period of sleep to several minutes or to as little as 10–20 s in extreme cases [6, 7].

For the past several years an extremely effective treatment, nasal continuous positive airway pressure (nCPAP), has been used to eliminate apneas in OSAS [8, 9]. When nCPAP was used to eliminate apneas, and traditional methods of analysis were applied to the sleep records of OSAS patients before and during treatment, significant increases in the total number of minutes spent in stages NREM-3 and 4 and REM sleep were observed [10–13]. Similar findings have been reported for patients with OSAS who were studied pre- and posttracheostomy [14]. However some studies found no significant differences in TST and in the number of minutes of stage NREM-2 [10, 11].

When making the comparison of fragmented to continuous sleep it was difficult to reconcile the qualitative differences in sleep before and during nCPAP treatment, with the absence of statistically significant differences in TST and total amount of stage NREM-2. Primarily, sleep occurred in longer, more continuous episodes that were not being reflected well in the measures of total minutes of each stage or sleep. This is especially interesting because differences from normal sleep structure in untreated OSAS have been related to hypersomnolence during waking, which is frequently the first symptom presented by patients with OSAS [7]. With the exception of variables related to body movement and the total number of stage changes, apnea studies have tended not to focus on the differences in sleep fragmentation between treatment conditions [12, 13, 15]. Interest in characterizing the highly periodic disruption or fragmentation of sleep that occurs with the cessation of breathing in OSAS and the equally dramatic changes during treatment with nCPAP led to the development of an analysis in our sleep research laboratory for the measurement of sleep fragmentation. This analysis was called the frequency analysis of consecutive epochs (FACE) [10, 11].

Methods

Physiological Monitoring

Subjects were screened during an afternoon nap study for symptoms of OSAS and for ability to tolerate the nCPAP mask. Seven subjects (six male and one female; mean age 42 years, range 21–67 years) who had moderate to severe, predominantly obstructive apneas (apnea index greater than 35 per h), in whom nCPAP reduced the occurrence of apnea, and who tolerated the nCPAP mask, were selected for this study.The apnea index was defined as the number of apneas per h of study.

Each subject was studied on 2 consecutive nights, the first night in the chronic untreated state and the second with nCPAP treatment for the first time. Sleep variables monitored were EEG, EOG, chin EMG, and ECG. Arterial oxygen saturation (SaO_2) was recorded using an ear oximeter (Biox II, Ohmeda, Boulder, Colorado). Thoracic and abdominal movements were measured by inductance plethysmography (Respitrace, Ambulatory Monitoring, Ardsley, New York). Oral and nasal airflow were monitored using thermistors in the pretreatment study. While receiving nCPAP, fluctuations in mask pressure and flow were used as indices of nasal airflow; a thermistor confirmed the absence of oral airflow. CPAP was delivered via a nasal mask [9]. With the exceptions noted above and the presence of the nCPAP mask on the second night, physiological monitoring was the same on each night. Subjects were placed in light- and sound- attenuated sleep rooms at 11 p.m. and were awakened at 7 a.m. the following morning unless the study was ended earlier because of spontaneous awakening.

Sleep Stage Scoring

NREM and REM sleep stages, movement time, and awake periods were manually assigned to 20-s epochs of the sleep record based on the activity from the EEG, EOG, and EMG electrodes in accordance with international conventions [16]. Any epoch containing muscle activity that obscured or distorted less than 50% of the page was staged conventionally and counted as a body movement.

Any epoch containing muscle activity that neither obscured nor distorted the EEG waveform was staged conventionally and counted as a twitch. Sleep stage scores were entered directly into a computer terminal using a program that structured the data in a format convenient for subsequent analysis. Differences in conventional data were analyzed by paired t-tests.

Frequency Analysis of Consecutive Epochs

The unit of analysis in this method is consecutive epochs. Starting with the first epoch in the comparison period, the number of epochs with the same stage score is counted until the stage score changes. In Fig. 1 B for example, the first three epochs are scored as stage NREM-1, and as there is a stage change at epoch 4, they are counted as one occurrence of three consecutive epochs of stage NREM-1 sleep. Similarly epochs 4 and 5 are counted as one occurrence of two consecutive epochs of stage NREM-2 sleep, and epochs 6 and 7 are counted as one occurrence of two consecutive epochs of stage REM sleep. This process repeats at every stage change until the end of the record or the end of some fixed comparison period, if more than one record is being analyzed. Each occurrence is tabulated in a matrix (Fig. 1C) in which rows represent stage scores and columns represent the number of consecutive epochs. Each row in the matrix can be plotted as a frequency distribution representing all of the occurrences of a single sleep stage for the entire study period. Frequency distributions (Fig. 1D) are plotted in log-log coordinates because of the large range in values.

When two or more records are analyzed together, the analysis is performed for equal periods of time. The group data presented in this chapter were tabulated for the shortest time in bed with lights out (406 min) for any subject in either condition. In this way the opportunity to engage in sleep was equated for each night, allowing a comparison between subjects and conditions on the frequencies of occurrence of consecutive epochs of sleep. All of the FACE plots in this

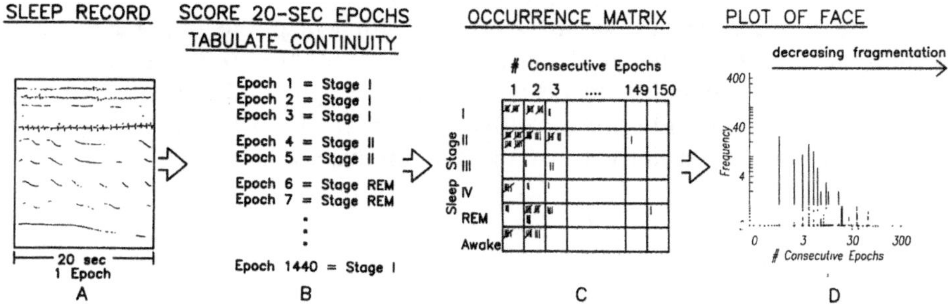

Fig. 1 A-D. Frequency analysis of consecutive epochs (FACE). **A** A page from a manually scored sleep record with an epoch length of 20 s. **B** List of scores for the entire record which are analyzed as occurrences of consecutive epochs of similar stage at every stage change. Each occurrence is tabulated in a computer matrix (**C**) by the number of consecutive epochs. At the end of the tabulation of all stages of sleep, each row of the matrix represents all of the occurrences of one stage. Each row of the matrix is then plotted as a frequency histogram (**D**)

chapter represent group data for seven subjects with OSAS who were studied with and without nCPAP. The frequency distributions for each condition were formed by summing the frequency distributions for each of the seven subjects in the group. Thus, every frequency for every stage of sleep in the group distributions represents the sum of the number of times that duration of stage occurred for each of the seven subjects.

Differences between pairs of frequency distributions were analyzed by forming cumulative relative frequency distributions for each frequency distribution (see Fig. 4) and applying the Kolmogorov-Smirnov (K-S) test for two distributions to the pair [17, 18].

Results

Elimination of Apneas

Treatment with nCPAP produced the expected reduction in obstructive apneas. On night 1 (without treatment) the mean apnea index was 74.2 per h (SEM 6.5). On night 2 (with nCPAP treatment) the mean apnea index was significantly reduced to 8.2 per h (SEM 3.0; $p < 0.001$). The mean lowest SaO_2 on night 1 was 47.3% (SEM 10.5%); on night 2 the mean lowest SaO_2 was significantly increased to 87.3% (SEM 1.5%; $p < 0.05$). The elimination of apneas on night 2 was also reflected in significantly decreased movement time and number of body movements, as shown in Table 1.

Conventional Summary of Sleep Structure

In addition to the changes in movement-related variables that resulted from the elimination of apneas (Table 1) there were several significant changes in overall

Table 1. Effect of nCPAP treatment on sleep structure

		Without treatment (SEM)		With treatment (SEM)	
Total sleep time	(min)	306.7	(23.1)	333.5	(14.4)
Awake	(min)	46.0	(15.9)	45.3	(8.6)
stage NREM-1	(min)	61.0	(8.8)	29.3	(5.8)*
stage NREM-2	(min)	210.4	(19.9)	148.5	(26.6)
stage NREM-3	(min)	6.8	(2.5)	34.9	(10.5)*
stage NREM-4	(min)	0.5	(0.4)	27.0	(9.6)*
REM sleep	(min)	28.0	(5.9)	93.9	(12.2.)***
Movement time	(min)	44.5	(7.0)	9.5	(4.6)**
Number of body movements		423.1	(60.1)	75.0	(18.4)***
Number of stage changes		523.0	(52.1)	225.7	(34.4)***

*Significance of paired t-test: * $p < 0.05$; ** $p < 0.01$; *** $p < 0.001$

sleep structure. Total minutes spent in stage NREM-1 decreased, while total minutes of stage NREM-3 and -4 an REM sleep increased. Although there were no differences in TST or stage NREM-2, the decrease in the total number of stage changes was highly significant.

Frequency Analysis of Consecutive Epochs

The exact nature of the changes in sleep structure after the elimination of apneas is made clearer by examining the frequency distributions for the occurrences of each sleep stage. Figure 2 shows that the decrease in time spent in stage NREM-1

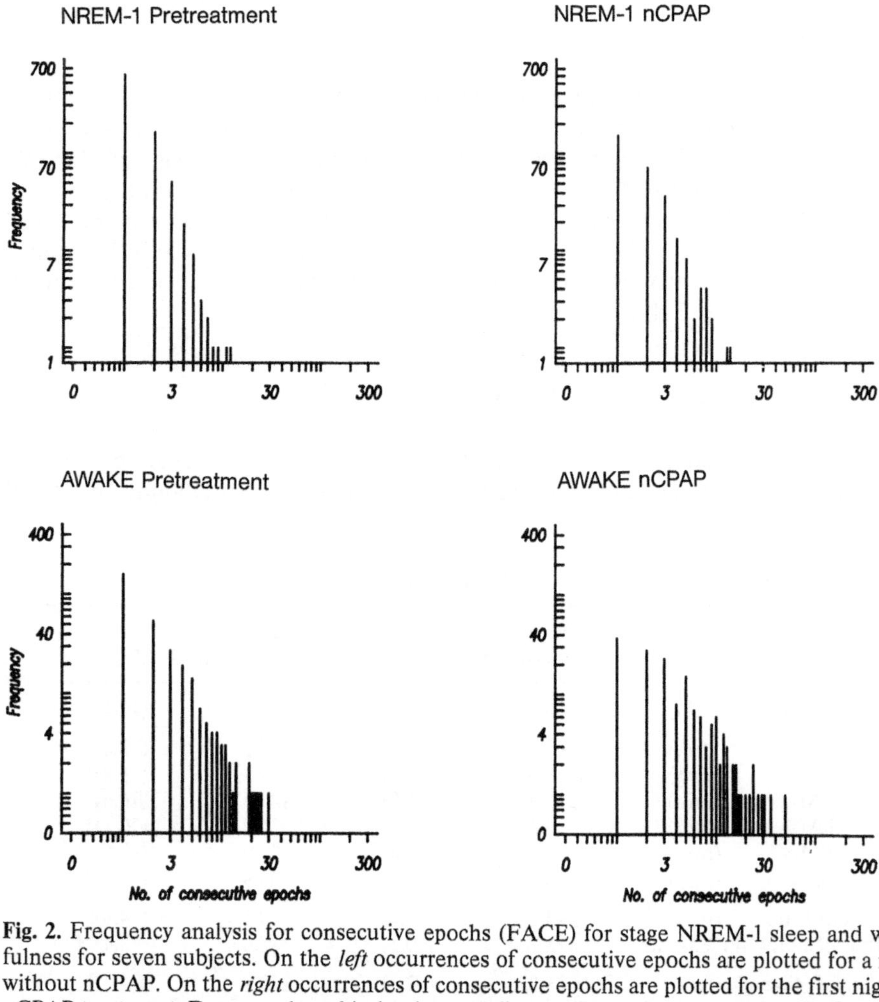

Fig. 2. Frequency analysis for consecutive epochs (FACE) for stage NREM-1 sleep and wakefulness for seven subjects. On the *left* occurrences of consecutive epochs are plotted for a night without nCPAP. On the *right* occurrences of consecutive epochs are plotted for the first night of nCPAP treatment. Data are plotted in log-log coordinates. Epoch length is 20 s, therefore three consecutive epochs equals 1 min of uninterrupted sleep

was predominantly a decrease in episodes of one epoch duration, from 609 occurrences without nCPAP treatment to 152 with nCPAP. Although there was no difference in the number of minutes of time awake with and without nCPAP, there is a difference in the distribution of consecutive epochs. This is due both to a decrease in the number of brief occurrences of time awake because of the elimination of apneas and to an increase in the number of longer awake periods because of adjustments to the nasal mask on the first night of use.

The distributions of stages NREM-3 and -4 (Fig. 3) reveal the large increase in time spent in these stages and show clearly that on the pretreatment night all of the slow-wave sleep occurred in episodes of 1 min or less. During treatment with nCPAP, in addition to short episodes of slow-wave sleep, there were many occurrences several minutes in length and longer.

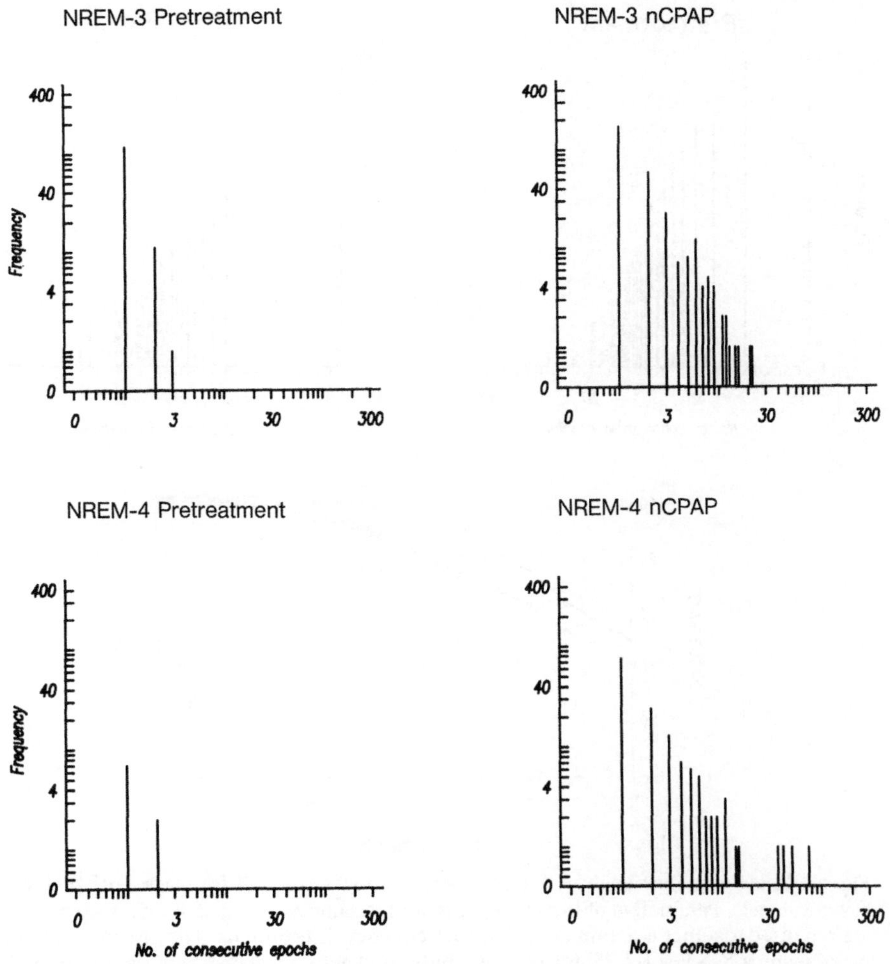

Fig. 3. Frequency analysis for consecutive epochs (FACE) for stage NREM-3 and -4 sleep for seven subjects. Parameters of the histograms are the same as in Fig. 2

Analysis of stage NREM-2 is especially interesting in these subjects because there was no difference in the total amount of this stage with and without nCPAP (Table 1). However, Fig. 4a shows substantial differences in the distribution of consecutive epochs. There was a decrease in the number of occurrences of 1 min or less from 1045 to 268. In addition, there were 8 occurrences of 10 min or longer before treatment and 28 with treatment. When the two frequency distributions in Fig. 4a were plotted as cumulative frequency distributions in Fig. 4b, a Kolmogorov-Smirnov (K-S) test confirmed the significant difference ($p < 0.01$) between the two conditions.

Although the total minutes of stage REM in the two treatment conditions were significantly different in the conventional analysis, the changes in continuity were not readily apparent. Not only was there more REM sleep, but it occurred in longer continuous episodes and fewer fragmented episodes in the

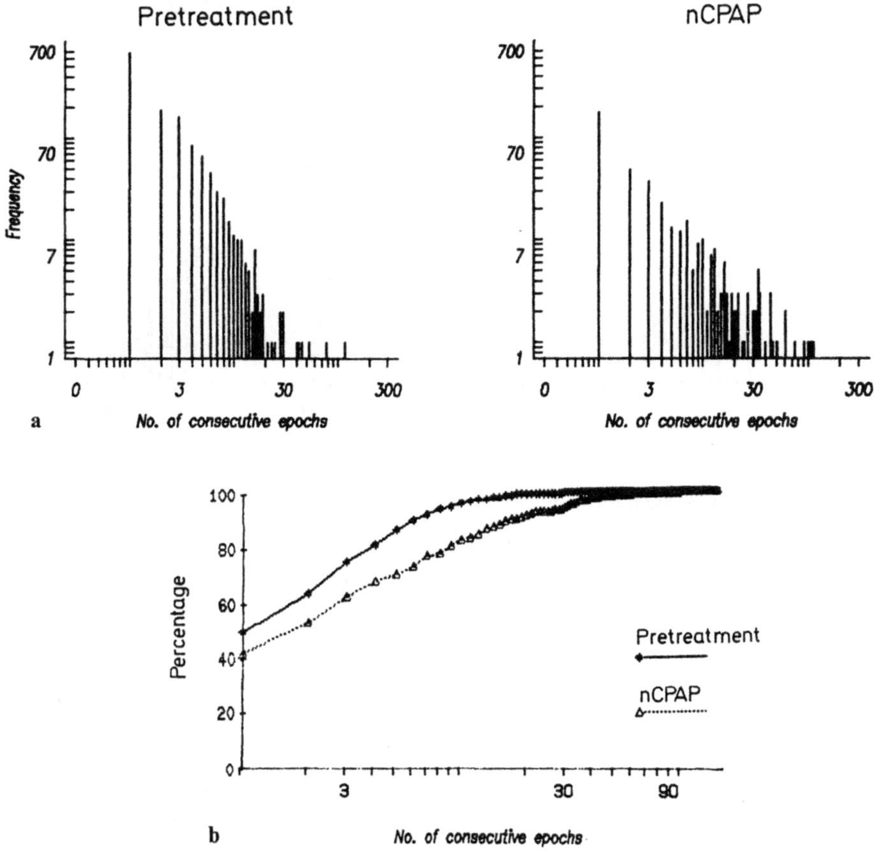

Fig. 4a, b. a Frequency analysis for consecutive epochs (FACE) for stage NREM-2 sleep for seven subjects. Parameters of the histograms are the same as in Fig. 2. **b** The histograms from **a** are replotted together as cumulative relative frequency distributions. The distributions are compared using a K-S test [17, 18] for two distributions. There is a statistically significant difference between the pretreatment *(closed diamonds)* condition and the nCPAP condition *(open triangles)* ($p < 0.01$)

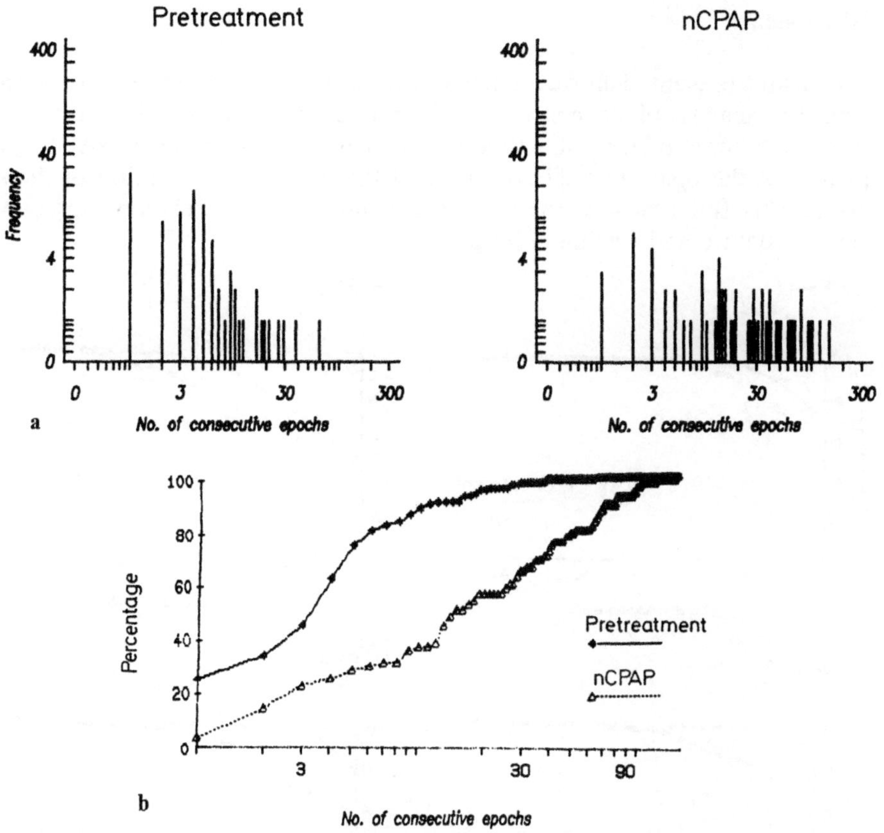

Fig. 5a, b. a Frequency analysis for consecutive epochs (FACE) for REM sleep for seven subjects. Parameters of the histograms are the same as in Fig. 2. **b** The histograms from **a** are replotted as described in Fig. 4. The difference between the pretreatment distribution *(closed diamonds)* and the nCPAP distribution *(open triangles) was significant* ($p < 0.01$) by K-S test [17, 18]

nCPAP condition than in the pretreatment condition (Fig. 5a). The difference between the two conditions is seen strikingly clearly in the cumulative distributions (K-S test; $p < 0.01$) in Fig. 5b.

The changes in sleep fragmentation before and during treatment are summarized in Fig. 6. In each stage there is a higher percentage of occurrences of short fragmented lengths in the pretreatment condition compared with the nCPAP condition. The differences are significant for each stage except stage NREM-4, which did not have enough pretreatment occurrences to make a statistical comparison possible. Although the total amount of movement time was significantly decreased during nCPAP treatment, movement time was not included in this analysis because its distribution was the same in both conditions.

Discussion

The results presented above are illustrative of the information that can be gained from the analysis of sleep structure. Combined with an analysis of the conventional measures of the total time spent in the stages of sleep, FACE gives a picture of the distributional changes and the degree of disruption of the sleep cycle. This fuller picture may be helpful in explaining relationships between sleep structure and waking behavior.

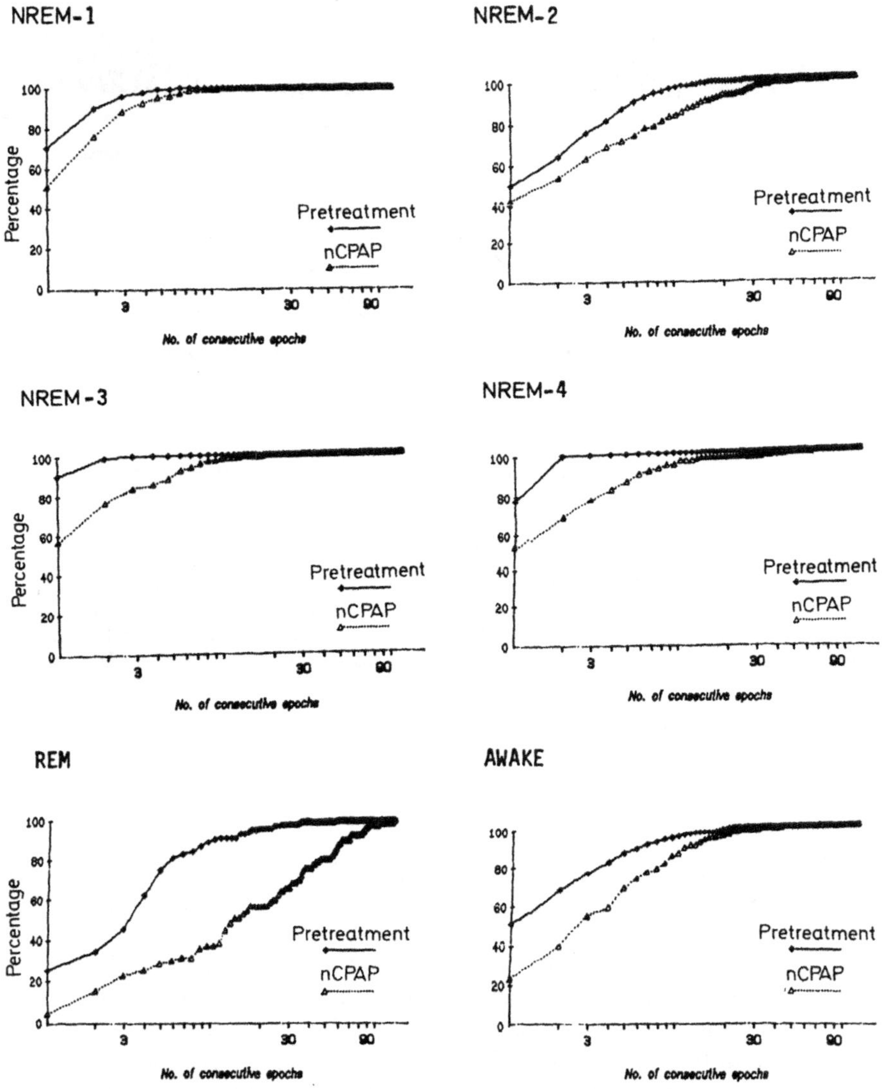

Fig. 6. Frequency analysis of consecutive epochs (FACE) for six stages of sleep for seven subjects. A pretreatment condition *(diamonds)* and nCPAP conditions *(triangles)* are plotted on each graph. Statistical significance of differences between distributions except for stage NREM-4, were significant ($p < 0.01$) by K-S test [17, 18]

Three major changes occur in sleep structure on the first night of nCPAP treatment in OSAS which result from the elimination of apneas:

1. an increase in the amount of time spent in slow-wave sleep,
2. an increase in the amount of time spent in REM sleep, and
3. an improvement in sleep continuity (or a decrease in sleep fragmentation).

One may speculate that of these three changes, it is the last which is most closely associated with improvement in daytime behavior. Some circumstantial evidence supporting this idea comes from Williams et al. [19] and Feinberg [20]. These authors found that some individuals in early middle age (the same age range as many of the subjects in this study) had little measurable slow-wave sleep yet did not report daytime problems or sleepiness. Although the evidence is far less straightforward, REM sleep can be reduced substantially by some antidepressant drugs with a concomitant improvement in mood and without daytime sleepiness [21]. On the other hand, whether sleep fragmentation occurs because of a sleep disorder [2, 3, 6] or through experimental manipulation [4, 5], the result is usually an increase in sleepiness and change in mood.

In a recent study Bonnet et al. [22] divided patients with sleep apnea into three groups according to the number of apneas observed. There were no differences in total minutes of sleep stages and no correlation between the apnea index and sleepiness ratings among the groups, despite the differences in numbers of apneas. However, they observed that sleepiness as rated by the subjects was negatively correlated with the longest uninterrupted periods of sleep. They concluded that in order to understand daytime sleepiness it may be more important to record the longest periods of unfragmented sleep rather than simply the total number of interruptions during the sleep period. The idea that reversal of sleepiness may require some minimum period of sleep continuity has also been suggested recently by Stepanski et al. [3].

It appears that changes in the quantity of specific stages of sleep are not necessarily associated with changes in daytime behavior, while changes in the fragmentation of sleep are almost always associated with them. This may reflect an inherent difference in tolerance for changes in total amounts of sleep or sleep stages as compared to tolerance for changes in sleep continuity.

The results in this study and the others mentioned above support the idea that examining the continuity or fragmentation of sleep is important for understanding sleep physiology and the relationship of sleep to waking behavior. Issues like the effect of repeated interruptions on the function of the sleep process and the possible role of a minimum period of sleep continuity need further explanation. The frequency analysis of consecutive epochs is a method for describing the continuity of each occurrence of each stage of sleep in both graphic and statistical terms. The method may be used with any set of conventions for parceling sleep into a set of classes useful for testing hypotheses.

Acknowledgements. The author is indebted to Drs. DM Rapoport, CS Hollander and RM Goldring for their contributions to this work. Financial support was provided by the National Institutes of Health, Division of Research Resources, Grant RR96.

References

1. Roth T, Hartse KM, Zorick FJ, Conway W (1980) Multiple naps and the evaluation of daytime sleepiness in patients with upper airway sleep apnea. Sleep 3:425–439
2. Rosenthal L, Roehrs T, Sickesteel J, Zorick F, Wittig R, Roth T (1984) Periodic movements during sleep, sleep fragmentation, and sleep-wake complaints. Sleep 7:326–330
3. Stepanski E, Lamphere J, Badia P, Zorick F, Roth (1984) Sleep fragmentation and daytime sleepiness. Sleep 7:18–26
4. Badia P, Harsh J, Balkan T, O'Rourke D, Burton S (1985) Behavioral control of respiration in sleep and sleepiness due to signal-induced sleep fragmentation. Psychophysiology 22:517–524
5. Bonnet MH (1985) Effect of sleep disruption on sleep, performance, and mood. Sleep 8:11–19
6. Gastaut H, Tassinari CA, Duron B (1966) Polygraphic study of the episodic diurnal and nocturnal (hypnic and respiratory) manifestations of the Pickwick syndrome. Brain Res 1:167–186
7. Guilleminault C, Tilkian A, Dement WC (1976) The sleep apnea syndromes. Annu Rev Med 27:465–484
8. Sullivan CE, Issa FG, Berthon-Jones M, Eves L (1981) Reversal of obstructive sleep apnoea by continuous positive airway pressure applied through the nares. Lancet I:862–865
9. Rapoport DM, Sorkin B, Garay SM, Goldring RM (1982) Reversal of the "Pickwickian syndrome" by long-term use of nocturnal nasal-airway pressure. N Engl J Med 307:931–993
10. Rothenberg SA, Rapoport DM (1985) Sleep architecture in the obstructive sleep apnea syndrome (OSAS) with and without nasal continuous positive airway pressure (nCPAP) treatment. Fed Proc 44:836
11. Rothenberg SA, Rapoport DM (1985) Recovery from sleep deprivation in the obstructive sleep apnea syndrome (OSAS) treated with nasal continuous positive airway pressure (nCPAP). Sleep Res 14:204
12. Holzer BC, Pressman MR, Fry JM (1985) REM sleep and slow wave sleep (SWS) rebound with nasal CPAP treatment of sleep apnea. Sleep Res 14:165
13. Issa FG, Sullivan CE (1986) The immediate effects of nasal continuous positive airway pressure treatment on sleep pattern in patients with obstructive sleep apnea syndrome. Electroencephalogr Clin Neurophysiol 63:10–17
14. Weitzman ED, Kahn E, Pollak CP (1980) Quantitative analysis of sleep and sleep apnea before and after tracheostomy in patients with hypersomnia-sleep apnea syndrome. Sleep 3:407–423
15. McEvoy RD, Thornton AT (1984) Treatment of obstructive sleep apnea syndrome with nasal continuous positive airway pressure. Sleep 7:313–325
16. Rechtschaffen A, Kales A (eds) (1968) A manual of standardized terminology techniques and scoring system for sleep stages of human subjects. Public health service publication no 204 US Government Printing Office, Washington DC
17. Smirnov N (1948) Table for estimating the goodness of fit of empirical distributions. Ann Math Stat 19:280–281
18. Massey FJ Jr (1952) Distribution table for the deviation between two sample cumulatives. Ann Math Stat 23:435–441
19. Williams RL, Karacan I, Hursch CJ (1974) Electroencephalography (EEG) of human sleep:clinical application. Wiley, New York
20. Feinberg I (1974) Changes in sleep cycle patterns with age. J Psychiatr Res 10:283–306
21. Vogel GW (1983) REM sleep deprivation and depression. In: Chase M, Weitzman ED (eds) Sleep disorders: basic and clinical research. Spectrum, New York, pp 393–400 (Advances in sleep research, vol 8)
22. Bonnet MH, Downey R, Wilms D, Dexter J (1986) Sleep continuity theory as a predictor of EDS in sleep apneics. Sleep Res 15:105

Paroxysmal Awakenings from Sleep – A Model of Sleep Fragmentation Causing Excessive Daytime Sleepiness

R. PELED

Introduction

Excessive daytime sleepiness and hypersomnia are common complaints. In most cases, daytime hypersomnia is the result of disrupted nighttime sleep. For example, in the sleep apnea syndrome, disturbed breathing disrupts sleep by many arousals and awakenings, causing severe sleep fragmentation (Fig. 1). The same is true for periodic leg movements in sleep (nocturnal myoclonus) where arousals follow the abnormal movements in the lower extremities.

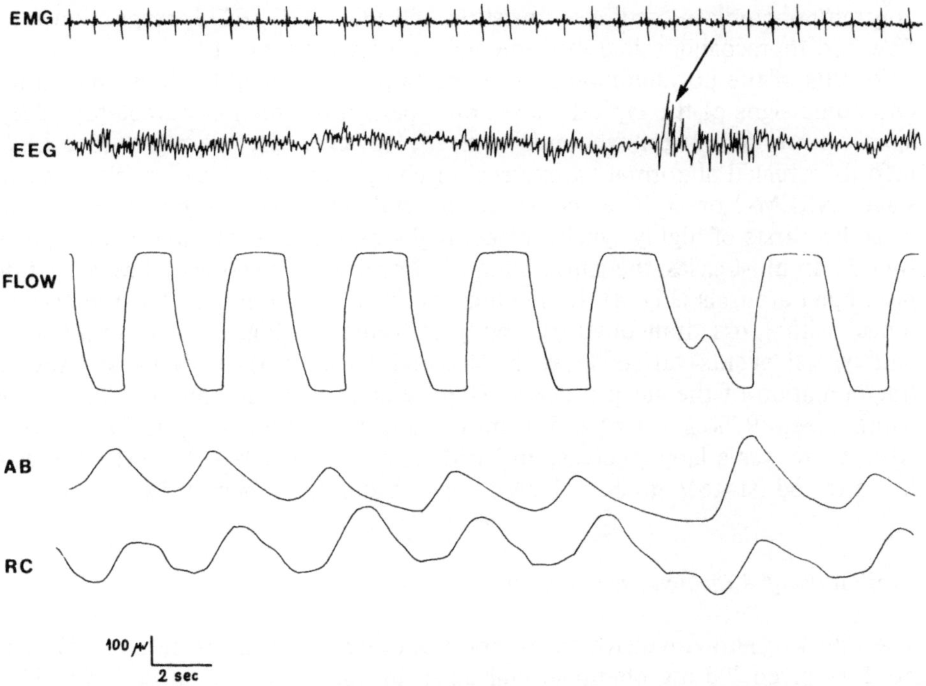

Fig. 1. Polysomnogram of a patient with sleep apnea syndrome showing hypopnea associated with an arousal (K-complex) *(arrow)*. *AB*, abdominal; *RC*, rib cage

The relationship between sleep and epileptic seizures has been known for years. In some epileptic patients seizures occur more or less exclusively during sleep, and the term "sleep epilepsy" has been applied to this kind of convulsive disorder. In spite of the wealth of clinical data, the question of whether epilepsy per se may lead to a sleep disorder is still controversial [1]. The *New Nosology of Sleep Disorders,* published by the Association of Sleep Disorder Centers [2], classified nocturnal seizures as a dysfunction associated with sleep (D4b) or a parasomnia, rather than a sleep–wake disorder associated with insomnia or hypersomnia. We describe here a group of patients who manifested atypical polysomnographic findings (seizure activity in sleep associated with brief arousals) and suffered from hypersomnia. We believe that the abnormal electroencephalographic activity, which may be a special form of nocturnal epilepsy, constitutes the major cause of the excessive somnolence in these patients.

Patients and Methods

Seven males (aged 17–42 years) and seven females (aged 17–59 years) were referred to the Technion Sleep Laboratory because of complaints of chronic fatigue, mild to severe daytime sleepiness, and morning headaches. Some also complained about restless sleep. In the majority of patients, the duration of the complaints extended over 1 year. None of them had any abnormal waking EEG findings or a history of epileptic fits. All patients underwent 1–2 whole-night polysomnographic recordings consisting of EEG, EOG, ECG, respiration (airflow and thoracoabdominal movements), and leg movements.

Results of the polysomnographs of the 14 patients failed to show any pathognomonic signs of the typical causes of hypersomnia such as narcolepsy, sleep apnea, or periodic leg movements in sleep. However, the overnight sleep EEG records revealed abnormal paroxysmal discharges appearing exlusively in sleep stages NREM-2 or -3. They consisted of "epileptic K-complexes" (Fig. 2) and episodic bursts of highly synchronized, high-amplitude, sharp waves and spikes (Fig. 3). In most cases, the paroxysmal EEG events were associated with brief or prolonged arousals (Fig. 4). In some cases these were followed by true awakenings, with gross, nonconvulsive body movements (Fig. 5). The number of paroxysmal events varied between 28 and 181 (Table 1). They caused severe fragmentation of the sleep process. There was an increased amount of waking within sleep (9.1% ± 12.0%) and of movement time within sleep (5.7% ± 5.4%). Also, there was a large decrease in REM sleep (12.9 ± 5.3%); NREM sleep was less affected (stage 2, 48.1% ± 14.9%; stages 3 and 4, 19.3% ± 10.3%).

Evaluation of Anticonvulsive Therapy

The effect of anticonvulsive treatment was evaluated in three patients. Patient no. 2 received 100 mg phenobarbital taken in one daily dose at bedtime. This resulted in an immediate and dramatic improvement of her daytime symptoms (decreased daytime sleepiness and less fatigue). Two other patients, nos. 13 and

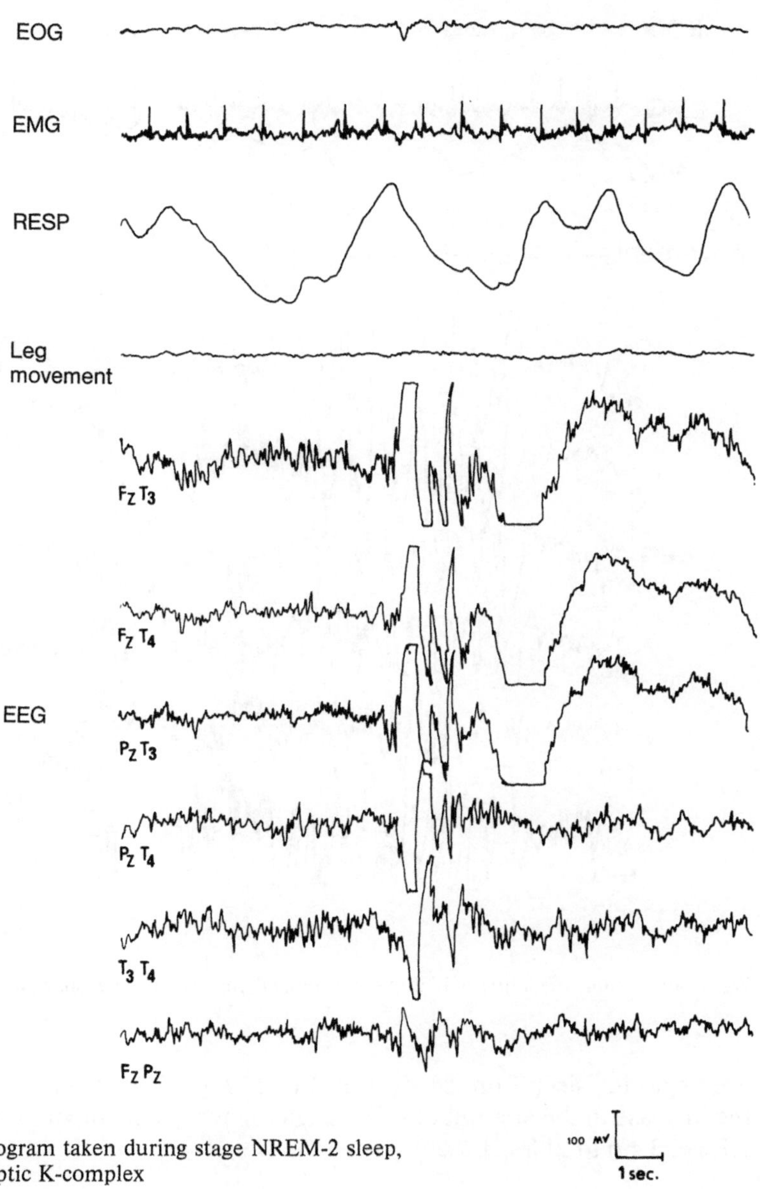

Fig. 2. Polysomnogram taken during stage NREM-2 sleep, showing an epileptic K-complex

14, received treatment with clonazepam (2 mg and 3 mg, respectively) taken at bedtime. Both benefited from the treatment and reported an improved night's sleep with a nearly complete disappearance of their daytime symptoms. In all three posttreatment sleep recordings there was an increase in sleep efficiency from 60% ± 4% to 85% ± 8% and a marked decrease in the number of paroxysmal

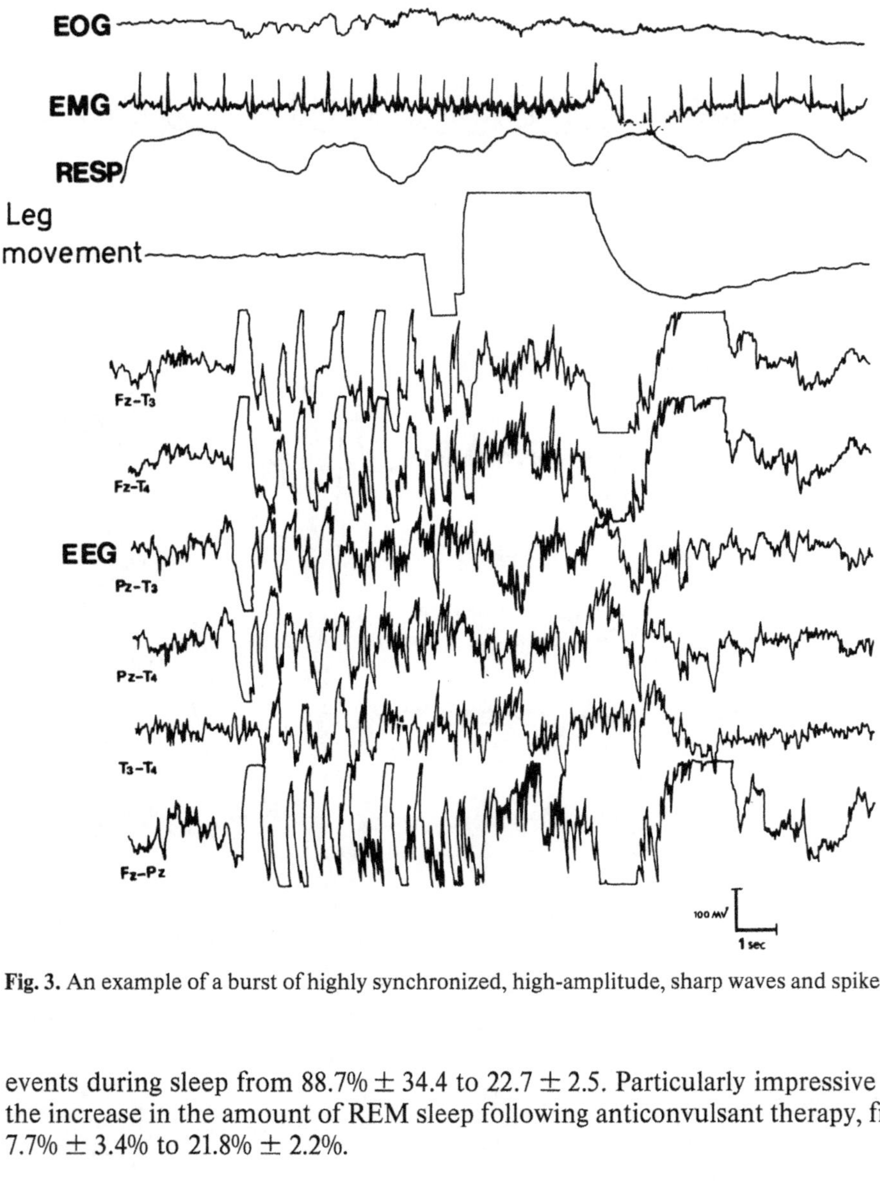

Fig. 3. An example of a burst of highly synchronized, high-amplitude, sharp waves and spikes

events during sleep from 88.7% ± 34.4 to 22.7 ± 2.5. Particularly impressive was the increase in the amount of REM sleep following anticonvulsant therapy, from 7.7% ± 3.4% to 21.8% ± 2.2%.

Discussion

Excessive daytime sleepiness (EDS) is a prevalent complaint: recent studies estimated that about 4% of the adult population complain of EDS [3, 4]. In the majority, sleep recordings revealed sleep apnea, periodic movements in sleep, or narcolepsy. Although all the patients we described here were referred to the Technion Sleep Laboratory because of severe EDS, none had any of the usual causes of EDS. The common finding was abnormal epileptic EEG activity asso-

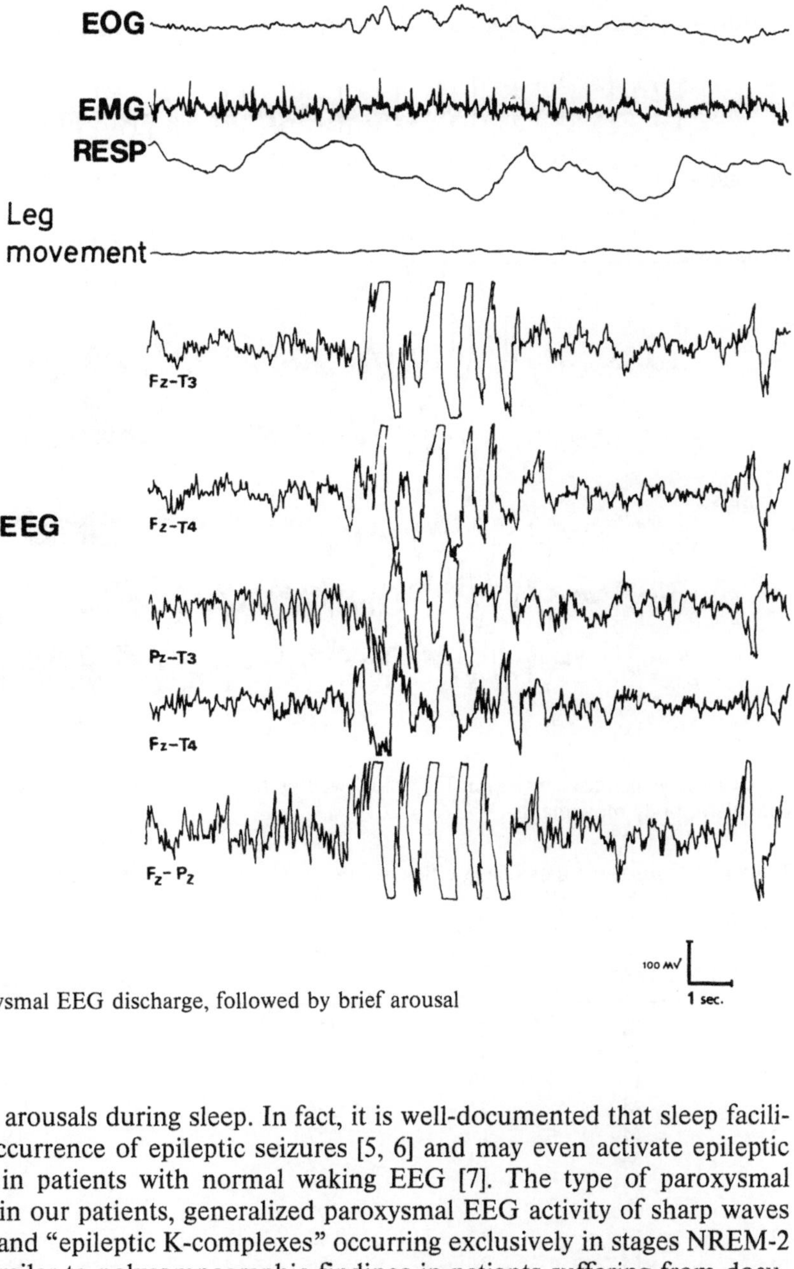

Fig. 4. Paroxysmal EEG discharge, followed by brief arousal

ciated with arousals during sleep. In fact, it is well-documented that sleep facilitates the occurrence of epileptic seizures [5, 6] and may even activate epileptic discharges in patients with normal waking EEG [7]. The type of paroxysmal discharges in our patients, generalized paroxysmal EEG activity of sharp waves and spikes and "epileptic K-complexes" occurring exclusively in stages NREM-2 and 3, is similar to polysomnographic findings in patients suffering from documented generalized epilepsy. In epileptic patients generalized epileptic discharges, with or without accompanying seizures, are activated in NREM sleep and are diminished or totally suppressed in REM sleep [1, 5, 6, 8–11]. We therefore believe that our findings represent a unique form of epileptic attacks during sleep causing paroxysmal arousals and awakenings. The resulting sleep fragmentation is manifested in daytime hypersomnia.

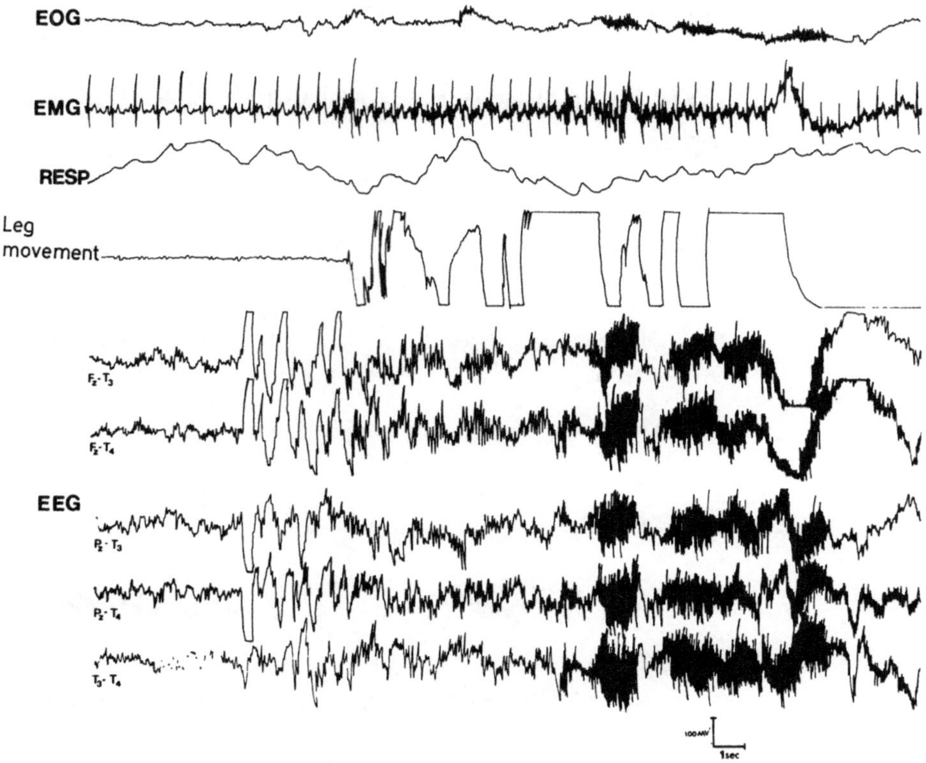

Fig. 5. Paroxysmal discharge as in Fig. 3 followed by full awakening response with gross, non-convulsive body movements

Table 1. Patients sleep data (sleep efficiency indexratio of total sleep time to time in bed)

Patient	Sex	Age (years)	Brief arousals	Arousals with gross movements	Sleep Efficiency Index
1	M	25	110	71	0.80
2	F	43	89	27	0.58
3	F	30	65	13	0.86
4	M	37	94	28	0.75
5	M	17	57	19	0.93
6	M	20	99	26	0.70
7	F	43	57	5	0.85
8	F	59	99	14	0.71
9	M	42	96	15	0.80
10	M	21	85	9	0.83
11	M	25	24	4	0.78
12	F	48	31	9	0.65
13	F	30	80	20	0.65
14	F	58	43	7	0.58
Mean		35.57	73.5	19.07	0.747
SD		13.71	27.42	16.96	0.106

As previously mentioned, the question of whether epilepsy may cause sleep disorders is still controversial [1]. Many epileptics complain about decreased vitality and subnormal daytime performance. These complaints are frequently attributed to the primary disease, psychological reasons, or the anticonvulsant treatment, rather than to sleep disturbances. However, careful review of the literature reveals that severe daytime fatigue and true hypersomnia, the two most preponderant complaints of the patients under study here, have been documented in epileptic patients previously. In Gibbs' et al. [12] description of epileptic patients we find: "Hypersomnia was common, and in *10 patients it was of such degree as to resemble narcolepsy"* (our italics). The fact that epileptic seizures may disrupt sleep organization has also been documented [11, 13]. The most extreme examples are nocturnal seizures during sleep in the Lennox-Gastaut syndrome that "disrupt the sleep structure, producing sleep deprivation, analogous to that produced by arousals of obstructive sleep apnea, with daytime somnolence" [14]. In general, epileptics have the tendency to sleep more superficially and to awake from sleep more often than normal people [15]; they have reduced NREM-4 and infrequent and irregular REM periods [16]. The patients described in our series also showed a marked decrease in REM sleep, and in this respect too, their disorder resembles nocturnal epilepsy.

A consistent finding in our patients, which is of great interest, are the paroxysmal EEG discharges of spikes and sharp waves associated with K-complexes. Such activity was termed by Passouant "complexe K-epileptique" [17], and "dyshormia" by Niedermeyer [18]. In normal people, K-complexes, usually followed by sleep spindles, appear spontaneously or in response to sudden stimuli during stage NREM-2 [19, 20]. The spontaneous K-complexes are considered to be EEG arousal responses to interceptive stimuli, such as respiratory changes [21]. Since it has been shown that a K-complex with superimposed faster rhythms has a more pronounced arousing effect than normal K-complexes, these may be partially responsible for the sleep fragmentation [22, 23]. It is possible that in epileptic patients in general, as well as in the patients described here, there is an elevated state of cortical excitability during stage NREM-2 sleep. Therefore, these K-complexes are associated with brief arousal responses rather than being aborted as in normal sleep, and give rise to prolonged awakenings. Daytime fatigue is the immediate result of the nocturnal sleep fragmentation. In this respect it resembles other sleep disorders such as sleep apnea syndrome and periodic leg movements during sleep.

Our hypothesis that these patients suffer from a form of nocturnal epilepsy is clearly supported by the preliminary results of the anticonvulsant treatment. All three patients treated with anticonvulsant medications so far have reported a marked improvement in their daytime symptoms. Sleep recordings demonstrated a marked increase in sleep efficiency and in REM sleep. Furthermore, there was an impressive decrease in the number of abnormal paroxysmal discharges associated with arousals.

In conclusion, our present results suggest that the possibility of paroxysmal discharges during sleep associated with arousals should be taken into consideration in the clinical evaluation of patients complaining of EDS. This should be considered particularly when all other causes of EDS are excluded by laboratory recordings during sleep. In these cases careful evaluation of the EEG is essential for a proper diagnosis.

References

1. Passouant P (1982) Historical views on sleep and epilepsy. In: Sterman MB, Shouse MN, Passount P (eds) Sleep and epilepsy. Academic, New York, pp 1–6
2. Diagnostic classification of sleep and arousal disorders (1979) Sleep 1:106–108
3. Bixler ED, Kales A, Sodatos CR, Kales JC, Healey S (1979) Prevalence of sleep disorder in the Los Angeles metropolitan area. Am J Psychiatry 136:1257–1262
4. Lavie P (1981) Sleep habits and sleep disturbances in industrial workers in Israel: main findings and some characteristics of workers complaining of excessive daytime sleepiness. Sleep 4:147–158
5. Janz D (1974) Epilepsy and the sleeping waking cycle. In: Vinken PJ, Bruyn GH (eds) Handbook of clinical neurology, vol 15. Elsevier, Amsterdam, pp 457–490
6. Gibberd FB, Bateson MC (1974) Sleep epilepsy: its patterns and prognosis. Br Med J 2:403–405
7. Gibbs EL, Gibbs FA (1974) Diagnostic and localizing value of electroencephalographic studies in sleep. Assoc Res Nerv Ment Dis 26:366–376
8. Delange M, Baldy M, Cadilhac J, Passouant P (1964) Study of epilepsies with bilateral EEG discharges. The influence of night sleep on the attacks and the discharges. Electroencephalogr Clin Neurophysiol 17:476
9. Delange M, Cadilhac JC, El Kassabgui M, Cadilhac J, Passouant P (1967) Electroencephalogr Clin Neurophysiol 23:219
10. Gastaut H, Broughton R (1965) A clinical and polygraphic study of episodic phenomena during sleep. Recent Adv Biol Psychiatry 7:197–221
11. Broughton R (1972) Sleep and clinical pathological states. In: Chase MH (ed) The sleeping brain. Brain Research Institute, University of California, pp 363–446
12. Gibbs EL, Fuster B, Gibbs FA (1948) Peculiar low temporal localization of sleep induced seizure discharge of psychomotor type. Arch Neurol Psychiatry 60:95–97
13. Passouant P, Besset A, Carriere A, Billiard M (1974) Night sleep and generalized epilepsies. In: Levin P, Koella WP (eds) Sleep 1974. Karger, Basel, pp 185–186
14. Ferriss G (1984) Sleep disorders. In: Greon JB (ed) Neurologic clinics: borderland between neurology and psychiatry, vol 1. Saunders, Philadelphia, pp 51–69
15. Declerck AC (1983) Interaction epilepsy-sleep-antiepileptics. Thesis, State University Limburgh. Swets and Zeitlinger, Lissethe, p 19
16. Bordas FM, Talairach J, Bancaud J (1966) Incidence d'accès sur l'organisation du sommeil de nuit des épileptiques. Rev Neurol 115:556–561
17. Passouant P, Cadilhac J, Latour H (1951) Renseignements apportés par la stimulation auditive au cours du sommeil des épileptiques. Rev Neurol 84:619–623
18. Niedermeyer E (1982) Petit mal, primary generalized epilepsy and sleep. In: Sterman MB, Shouse MM, Passouant P (eds) Sleep and epilepsy. Academic, New York, pp 191–207
19. Davis H, Davis PA, Loomis AL, Harvery EM, Hobart F (1939) Electrical reactions of the human brain to auditory stimulation during sleep. Neurophysiology 2:500–514
20. Roth M, Shaw J, Green J (1956) The form voltage distribution and physiological significance of the K-complex. Eletroencephalogr Clin Neurophysiol 8:385–402
21. Lavie P (1983) Nasal breathing during sleep. In: Guilleminault C, Lugaresi E (eds) Sleep/wake disorders, epidemiology and long term evaluation. Raven, New York, pp 151–162
22. Kellaway P, Fox BJ (1952) Electroencephalographic diagnosis of cerebral pathology in infants during sleep. J Pediatr 41:262–287
23. Hess R, Urech E, Wieser HG (1962) Arousal patterns in depth recordings from epileptics. In: Sterman MB, Shouse MM, Passouant P (eds) Sleep and epilepsy. Academic, New York, pp 209–217

Various Components of Respiratory Control During Sleep, Rest, and Strain

F. Raschke

Processes that control respiration are not stationary. They vary with the level of consciousness and the functional state. Internal and external exertion determine for example, neural respiratory rhythm generation, timing of respiratory phases, magnitude of tidal volume, and functional residual capacity (FRC) level. The various components contributing to respiratory control are separated in this paper into three levels with graded priority:

1. metabolic and humoral control (O_2-supply, CO_2-removal, acid-base status),
2. respiratory cycle synchronous reflexes (inflation and deflation reflex, mucosal receptors keeping airways patent), and
3. intrarespiratory cycle nonspecific afferents (cardiovascular system, sensory system, voluntary and behavioral control).

These levels change from rather tonic to distinctly phasic in terms of control modalities. The same applies for external load conditions, e.g., physical work. Long-lasting (tonic) stressors require metabolic control of respiratory pattern with changes in frequency and amplitude. On the other hand short-term efficiency is necessary for impulse or force-developing movements, realized by strict phase coordination between respiratory and motor action.

Thus exogenous stimuli modulate respiratory times and tidal volume on the metabolic level, trigger the respiratory rhythm on the reflex level, and coordinate respiratory phases on the autonomic (even behavioral) level [11]. An outline of endogenous and exogenous factors is given in Fig. 1.

The following paper is restricted to recent sleep investigations concerning very slow, modulating (first level), and fast-phase entraining (third level) input variables.

Slow Modulation of Respiratory Control

Chemosensitivity during sleep changes with the sleep stage as has been shown in humans during hypercapnic [2], hypoxic [4], and unloaded respiration [5]. According to these investigations minute ventilation or ventilatory response decreases from wakefulness, through light and deep sleep, to REM sleep. Arousal on the other hand enhances respiratory response, as has been emphasized by Phillipson and Sullivan [8]. Thus a modulation of respiratory drive will occur

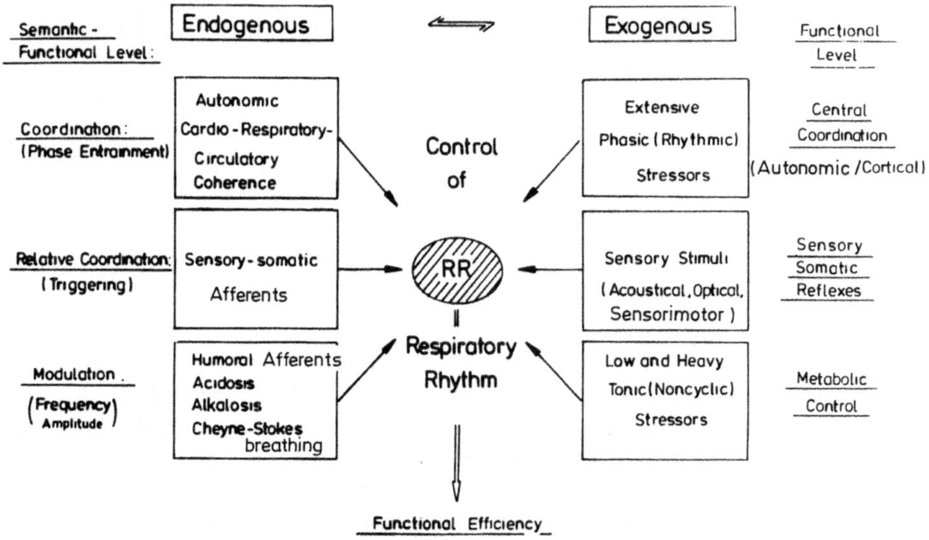

Fig. 1. Outline of three levels of control of respiratory rhythm under endogenous *(left)* and exogenous *(right)* conditions

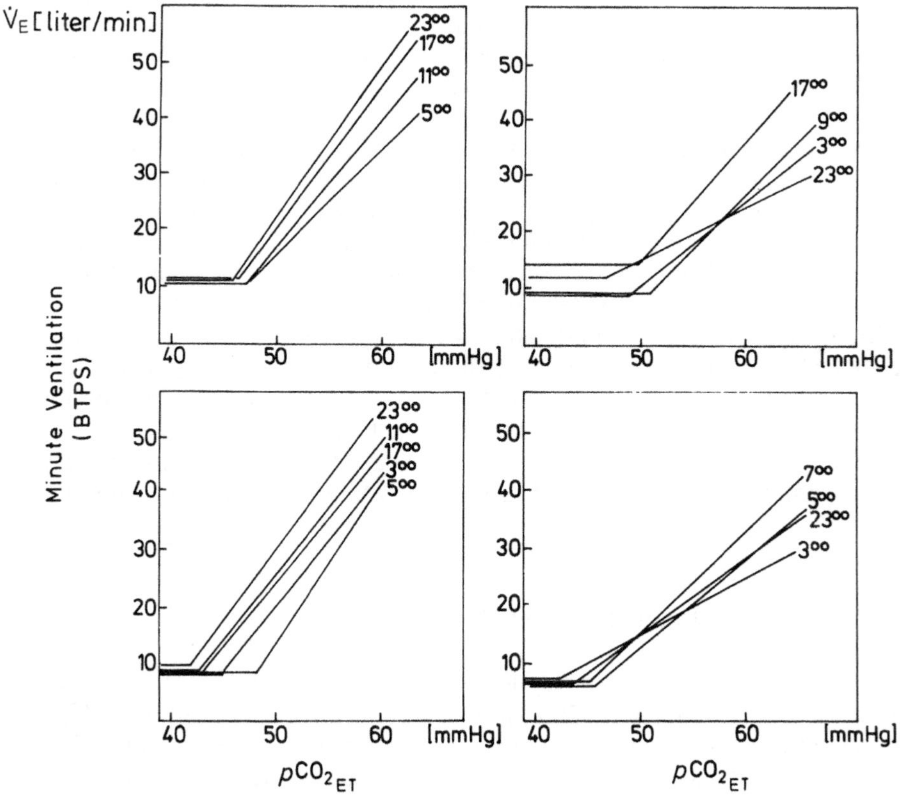

Fig. 2. Linear regression lines from hyperoxic progressive hypercapnic rebreathing maneuver in four healthy male subjects at different times of day. *BTPS*, body temperature pressure saturated

with ultradian cycles. To test the basic chemosensitivity in the 24-h cycle, we investigated nine healthy male subjects in collaboration with Möller. The subjects were kept under constant environmental conditions: bed rest for 24 h, room temperature 18° C, 55% relative humidity, isocaloric low protein diet. They were tested by 13 experiments every 2 h using rebreathing (6 liters) during hyperoxic progressive hypercapnia and isocapnic progressive hypoxia. The start of the experiment was randomized during the day.

In Fig. 2 regression lines from the hypercapnic response in four subjects are given. Changes in the slope and intercept reveal circadian variation with nocturnal minima.

Most of the subjects (six) showed a dominant shift in intercept. We therefore took the center of gravity of the pooled minute ventilation data (10 for each 2-h measurement) of each subject, and calculated the change in intercept from this 24-h mean. The result is given in Fig. 3. The mean intercept of the CO_2 response curve varies with an amplitude of about ± 3 mmHg during the 24-h run. The absolute minimum is found at 5:00 a.m., which is the farthest shift to the right.

These results show that in addition to the sleep cycle and arousal variations of metabolic respiratory drive, a circadian modulation is superimposed, resulting in a complex basic pattern of respiratory control.

Phase Entrainment (Coordination) of Respiratory Rhythm Generation

In contrast to those basic changes in chemosensitivity acting mainly on a tonic level, short-term phasic events such as from the cardiovascular system are capable of triggering the onset of inspiratory and expiratory phases. This pheno-

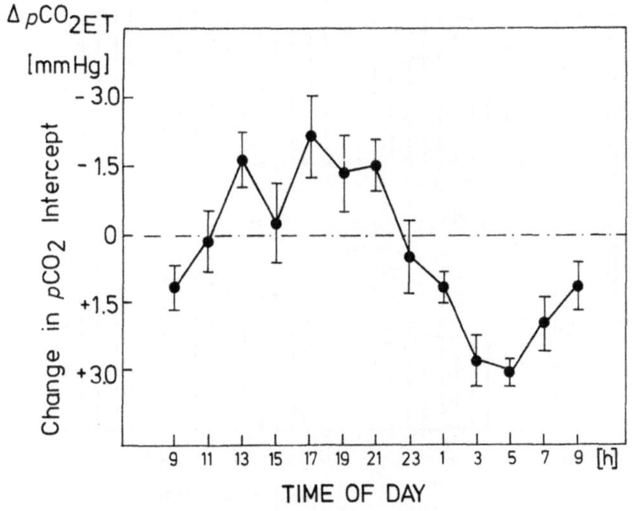

Fig. 3. Change of the end tidal partial CO_2 pressure (pCO_{2ET}) from the individual 24-h mean intercept. Pooled data of nine healthy male subjects ($\bar{x} \pm$ SEM). Hyperoxic CO_2 rebreathing maneuver applied every 2 h under constant environmental and nutritional conditions

menon was first found by Schoenlein [13] in fish and subsequently studied by Bucher and coworkers in the rabbit [1] during numerous investigations. In humans the studies from Hildebrandt (this volume) showed cardiorespiratory phase coordination during sleep with whole number ratios between the cardiac and respiratory cycle lengths at night. Raschke [11] examined this phenomenom during various sleep stages, wakefulness, and physical and psychovegetative strain. This led to the conclusion that cardiorespiratory phase coordination only occurs during resting conditions, being intensified during sleep. The slightest stressor caused the coherence to break down completely. During sensorimotor load, however, the onset of the expiratory phase was preferentially coupled to the push button movement in a reaction time task [10], or inspiration coincides with the onset of the stance phase while walking or trotting [12]. Thus the interactant in respiratory phase coordination switches from the cardiovascular system during rest to distinct sensorimotor or locomotive system phases (Fig. 1.).

Since cardiorespiratory phase coordination has not yet been investigated during periodic breathing with intermittent mixed apneas, the following study was carried out. In collaboration with the Department of Internal Medicine, University of Marburg, we examined three male patients who were developing excessive mixed apneas (apnea indices: 48, 74, and 69).

Figure 4 gives six histograms of inspiratory onset with respect to the cardiac cycle. Inspiratory onsets from nasal thermistors were determined with the aid of a computerized pattern recognition method with cardiac tracheal artefact

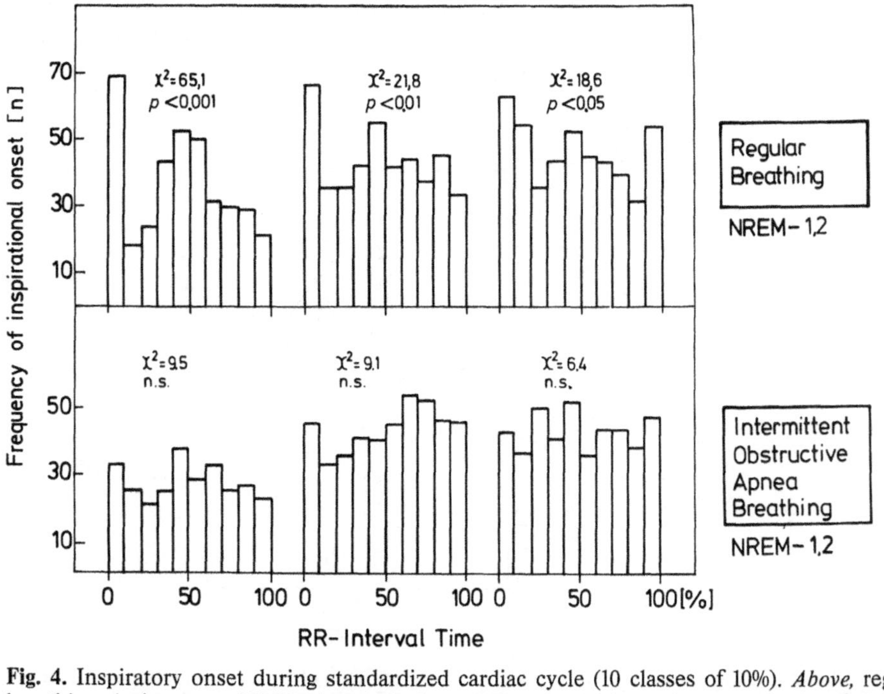

Fig. 4. Inspiratory onset during standardized cardiac cycle (10 classes of 10%). *Above,* regular breathing during stage NREM-1 and -2 sleep. *Below,* intermittent hyperventilation following obstructive sleep apneas (identical sleep stages). From *left to right,* three different patients

removal [9]. The x-axis gives the standardized cardiac cycle length (RR), divided into 10 classes of 10%. For the three patients, 280, 320, and 350 inspiratory onsets were counted respectively in the upper and lower rows. The histograms above are taken from regular breathing during sleep stages NREM-1 and 2, and those below from intermittent hyperventilation breathing. χ^2-values indicate the deviation from an even distribution and thus signify cardiac-inspiratory phase coordination. Preferred systolic coupling (peaks in the first class) during regular breathing is just comparable to our previous results in healthy young males [9]. However, during intermittent hyperventilation cardiorespiratory coherence is inhibited completely.

Discussion

We have found circadian variations of the pCO_2 intercept, with lowest sensitivity during the night. The slopes of the response curves change in a similar direction, but the amount was less pronounced. Previously observed sleep stage variations are superimposed and promote additional oscillations of respiratory drive. The reduction of chemical stimuli effectiveness with sleep onset therefore is only one part of a complex threshold dynamic which leads one to expect Cheyne-Stokes breathing pattern during sleep [3] or even central sleep apnea under the relative lack of chemical drive.

Our results from cardiovascular-respiratory coordination, which appears to be a very prominent characteristic of NREM sleep in normal subjects, demonstrate that this phenomenon is present even in patients with sleep apnea syndrome, but only during regular breathing. The centrally induced, phase-coherent action of the cardiovascular and respiratory systems is inhibited during hyperventilation. We suggest that in this case the control is changed to modulating metabolic demands as seen during wakefulness and under external load (Fig. 1). Arousal reactions which typically terminate obstructive apnea breathing [6, 7] support this hypothesis. In consequence a mere phasic or a mere tonic dominance of regulation seems to be realized alternately during periodic breathing when mixed apneas are intermittent.

Acknowledgement. The author gratefully thanks the members of the working group, Time series analysis and internal medicine, from the Department of Internal Medicine, University of Marburg, for generous support and cooperation.

References

1. Bucher K, Schwitter H, Hool-Zulauf B, Batschelet E (1972) Links between cardiac and respiratory rhythmicity. Res Exp Med (Berl) 157:281–288
2. Bülow K (1963) Respiration and wakefulness in man. Acta Physiol Scand [Suppl] 209:1–110
3. Cherniack NS, von Euler C, Homma I, Kao FF (1979) Experimentally induced Cheyne-Stokes breathing. Respir Physiol 37:185–200
4. Douglas NJ, White DP, Weil JV (1982) Hypoxic ventilatory response decreases during sleep in man. Am Rev Respir Dis 125:286–289

5. Douglas NJ, White DP, Pickett CK, Weil JV, Zwillich CW (1982) Respiration during sleep in normal man. Thorax 37:840–844
6. Martin RJ, Pennock BE, Orr WC, Sanders ME, Rogers RM (1980) Respiratory mechanics and timing during sleep in occlusive sleep apnea. J Appl Physiol 48:432–437
7. Peter JH (1984) Klinik der Hypersomnien. Internist 25:547–551
8. Phillipson EA, Sullivan CE (1978) Arousal: the forgotten response to respiratory stimuli. Am Rev Respir Dis 118:807–809
9. Raschke F (1982) Automatic pattern recognition of the onset of respiratory phases using thermistor techniques. In: Stott FD, Raftery EB, Clement DL, Wright SL (eds) Proceedings of the fourth international symposium on ambulatory monitoring, Gent 1981. Academic, London, p 349
10. Raschke F (1985) Preferred phases of coordination between respiratory and sensorimotor movements. Pflugers Arch 405:R67
11. Raschke F (1986) The hierarchical order of cardiorespiratory coupling. In: Grossmann P., Janssen K, Vaitl D (eds) Cardiorespiratory and cardiosomatic psychophysiology. Plenum, New York, p 207
12. Raschke F, Delles H (1985) Phase-coordination of locomotion, respiration, and heart beat in trained and untrained humans. Pflugers Arch 403:R70
13. Schoenlein K (1895) Beobachtungen über Blutkreislauf und Respiration bei einigen Fischen. Z Biol 32:511–547

Interindividual Differences in Sleep Patterns During Night and Shift Work

R. Moog

Sleep, which appears to be a critical component of circadian rhythms, is as a rule impaired by shift work. The sleep-wake cycle and other parts of the circadian system show interaction. There are differences in tolerance to shift work among subjects, depending, for example, upon the circadian phase structure, as in so-called morning and evening types.

Individual differences in sleeping behavior may thus be expected as well, when adaptations to altered time regimens are required.

In order to study the behavior of the circadian system as subjects are exposed to different shift systems, healthy subjects with different circadian phase positions were required to work 6 weeks in shift systems where rotation speeds were experimentally varied.

Admittedly, spontaneous sleeping behavior may not be observable when a subject is forced to work at night and to sleep during the day; here we have to anticipate masking effects in sleep behavior, at least in those subjects not adapted to the given routine. But sleep is not the only domain where masking is likely to occur. In fact, even the circadian course of core temperature is subject to such masking, namely, by activity [3, 5].

In order to minimize the biases in question we employed a system of "control days". That is, subjects were kept on bedrest for 24 h and on a low-protein diet, sleeping at their convenience. Sleep was monitored by means of EEG recordings and other standard procedures. Subjects were observed on these control days before the experiment as well as on the 3rd and 7th day of each week.

On shift days subjects were given work assignments in the institute laboratory but spent their leisure time as they wished and slept at home. Thus their frame of reference remained within social and geophysiological periodicities to which they were accustomed.

On the actual shift days, onset and termination of sleep were recorded through self-reports. The correlation between reported sleeping times on control days, and sleeping times as determined by means of EEG recordings consistently exceeded $r = 0.9$ in all experimental groups.

Differences in adaptation among subjects with circadian system variances are to be expected in that shift work is necessarily accompanied by disturbances of those circadian systems. Differences in tolerance to night and shift work, especially between subjects with dissimilar circadian phases (morning and evening types; see the survey by [2]) have been reported in various contexts [1, 4, 6, 7].

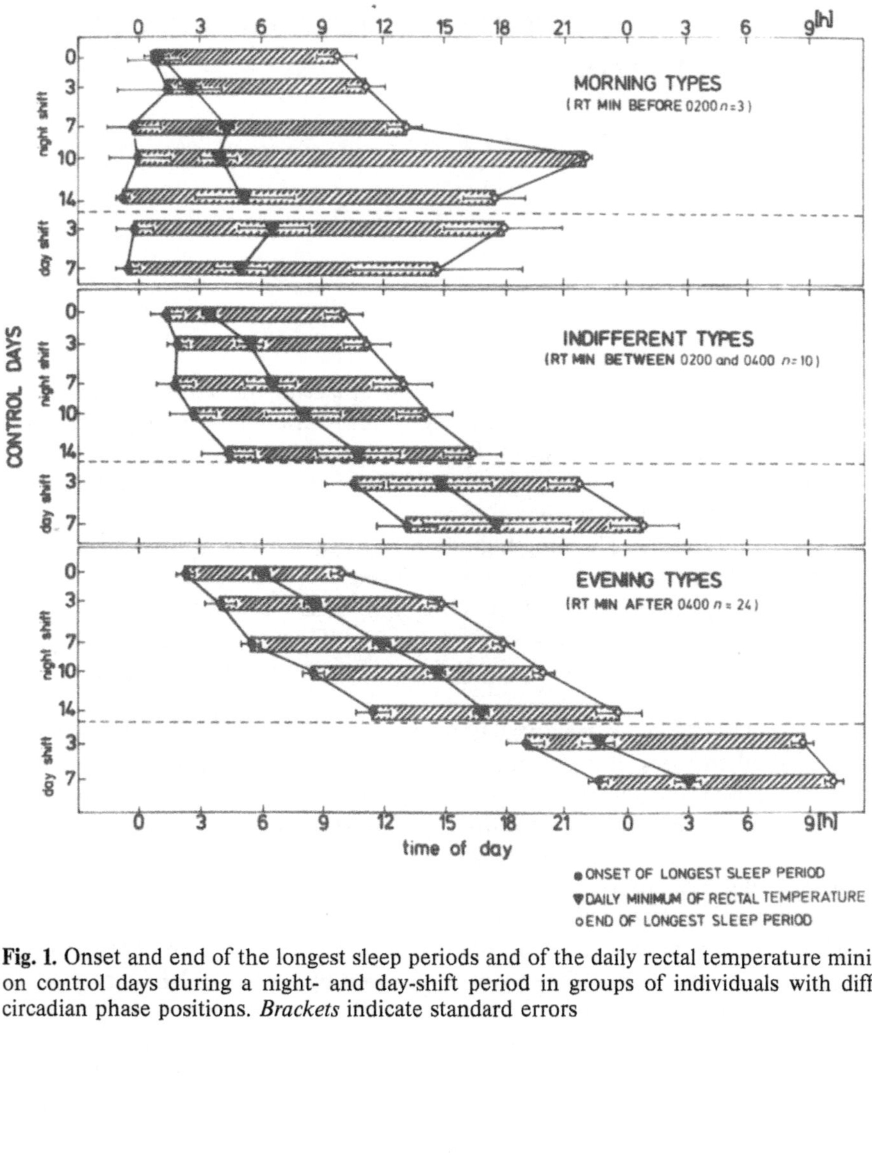

Fig. 1. Onset and end of the longest sleep periods and of the daily rectal temperature minimum on control days during a night- and day-shift period in groups of individuals with different circadian phase positions. *Brackets* indicate standard errors

As a first step we observed the onset and termination of the main sleep periods as well as the circadian minimum of rectal temperature in subjects exhibiting diverse circadian phase positions. Figure 1 shows the patterns for the longest sleep periods on control days, and the phase of the rectal temperature rhythm as indicated by the daily minimum. The earlier the individual phase position, the more marginal the adaptation to the shift regimen with respect to the onset and termination of the longest sleep period, as well as to the 24-h temperature minimum on control days.

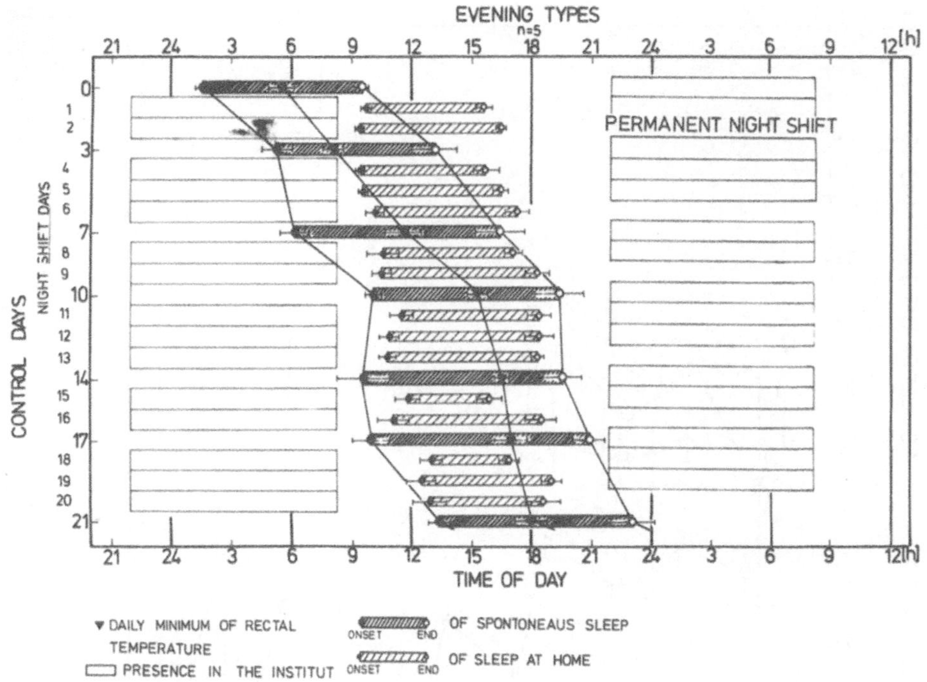

Fig. 2. Onset and end of the longest sleep periods on control days and at home. In addition, the daily minimum rectal temperature on control days during a night-shift period in a group of evening-type individuals is displayed. *Brackets* indicate standard errors

As one would expect, home sleep was not in phase with the spontaneous sleep on control days until the subjects were rather well-adapted to the night shifts. Figure 2 shows the rectal temperature minimum as well as the main sleep periods for the evening-type group, who worked 21 days on night shifts. Differences between sleeping times at home on shift days and spontaneous sleep times on control days therefore indicate the extent of the subjects' ability actually to sleep on shift days when they were physiologically ready.

As shown in Fig. 3, however, the earlier the circadian phase position, the larger were those differences. This effect vanished in the course of adaption to the night-shift routine, especially in the evening-type group. Morning-type individuals particularly seemed to be unable to sleep when they were physiologically ready for sleep on shift days. This is presumably due to their lag of circadian adaptation to night shifts.

This may also be the cause for the shorter sleep duration on shift days in morning-type individuals as displayed in Fig. 4. Sleep duration on control days on the other hand was found to be longer in morning-type individuals. The earlier the phase position of the subjects, the longer the main sleep periods. Possibly, this might indicate something like an index of recovery needs.

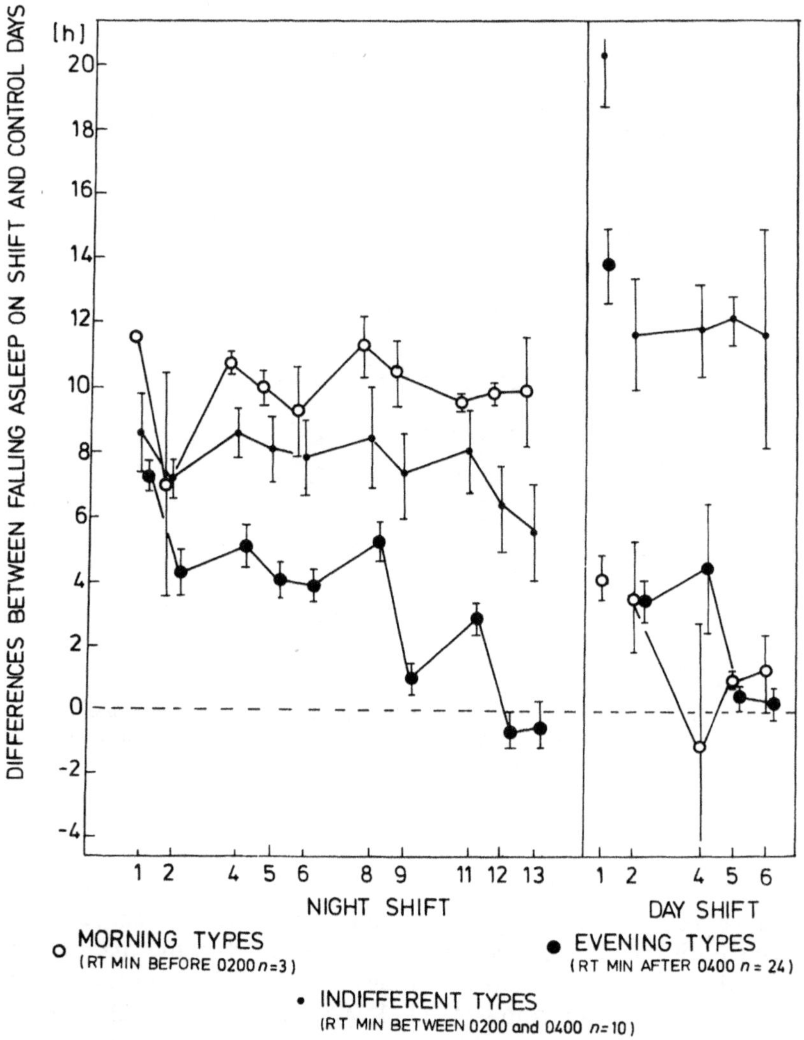

Fig. 3. Masking effects of sleep onsets depending on the individual circadian phase position (differences between the onsets of the longest spontaneous sleep period on control days and the onsets of sleep on the immediately preceding or following shift day). *Brackets* indicate standard errors

Further variations between evening- and morning-type individuals are found between the state of the circadian rectal temperature rhythm and onset of sleep (Fig. 5). Evening-type subjects are able to fall asleep even when the rectal temperature is rising or around the maximum. As a result they are able to compensate sleep deficits more easily than subjects with earlier circadian phase position, especially by taking naps.

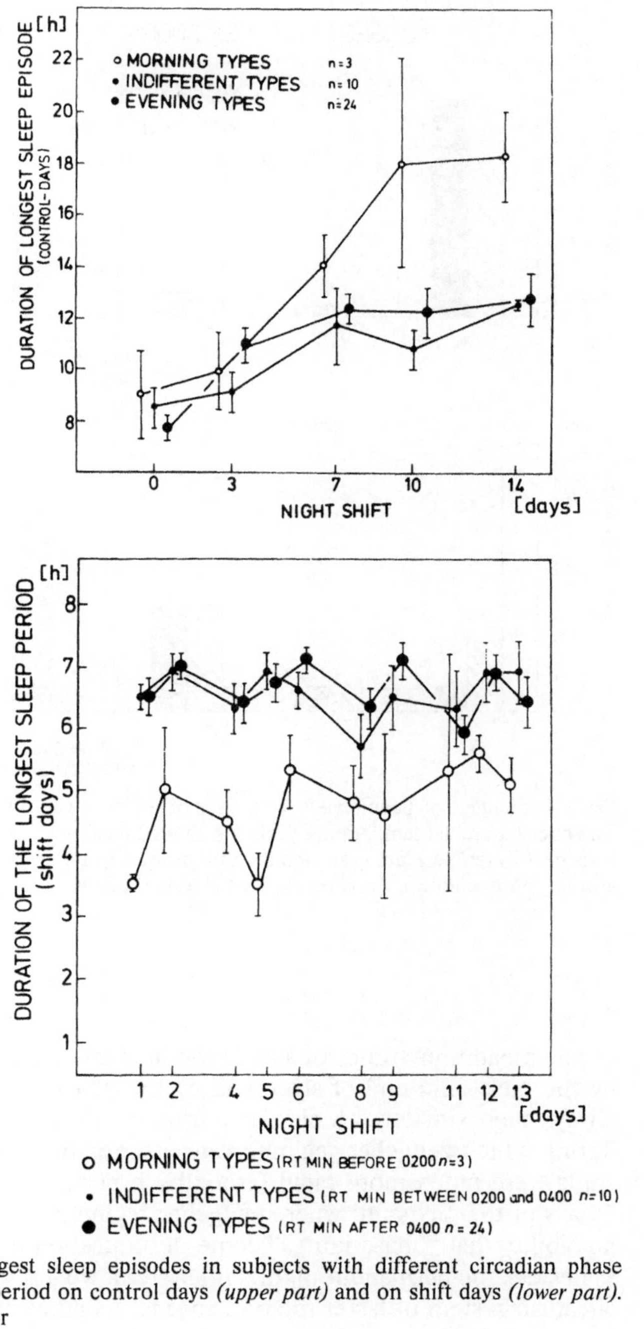

Fig. 4. Mean duration of longest sleep episodes in subjects with different circadian phase positions during a night-shift period on control days *(upper part)* and on shift days *(lower part)*. *Brackets* indicate standard error

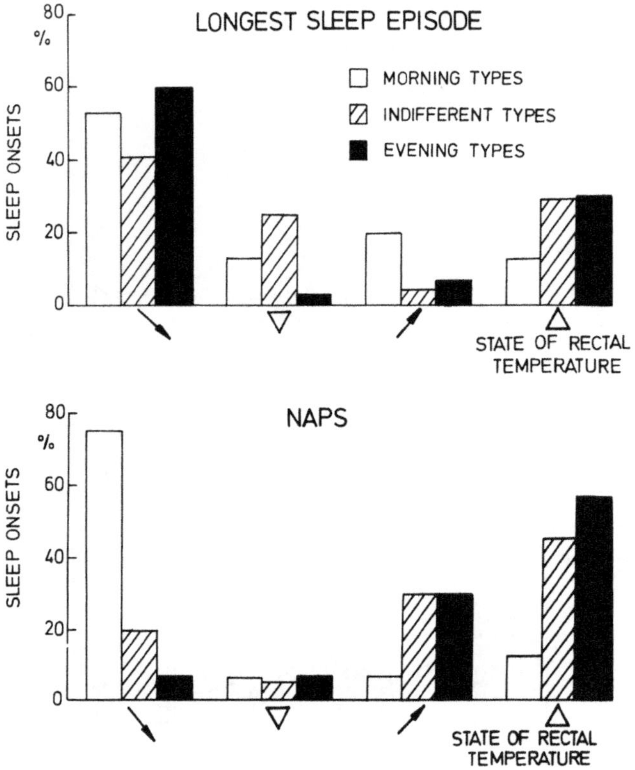

Fig. 5. Percentage of sleep onsets for groups of subjects with different circadian phase positions. The circadian rectal temperature period is divided into four classes, as follows: (↗) temperature is rising, (▽) temperature is around the minimum, (↘) temperature is falling, (△) temperature is around the maximum. *Brackets* indicate standard errors

The mean time trends of adaptation in evening-type individuals - as indicated by the onset and end of sleep and by the phases of rectal temperature - were always approximately 1 h per day during the first 10 days on night shift, a period during which zeitgeber regimens are essentially incoherent. In contrast, phase shifts were much more rapid (around 2 h per day, on average) during the first 3 days of the day shift, where zeitgeber regimens are more coherent; there is a possibility that "phase jumps" come into question in these instances.

Besides the permanent night-shift system, we also observed the effects on the circadian system of faster rotation speeds. As an example, Fig. 6 shows that the three evening-type subjects tracked the 8-h shifts of work onset every 7 days almost completely, once again by phase shifts of approximately 1 h per day as far as both timing of sleep and rectal temperature minima were concerned whereas (Fig. 7) indifferent-type individuals were not able to follow even this slowly rotating system.

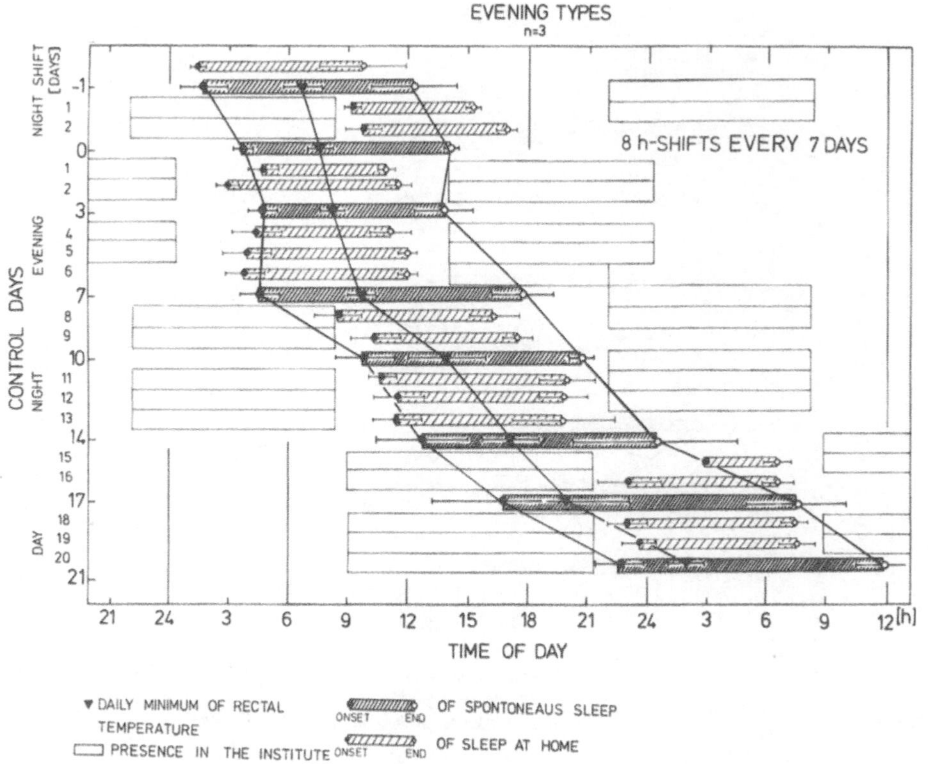

Fig. 6. Onset and end of main sleep periods and mean course of the circadian rectal temperature minimum on control days, compared with the sleeping periods on shift days at home in evening-type individuals. Duty hours were shifted 8 h every 7 days. *Brackets* indicate standard error

Comparisons between different systems with respect to differences in timing of sleep at home and on control days are given in Fig. 8. Phase differences between sleeping times at home on shift days and spontaneous sleep on control days thus may indicate the degree of ability of the subjects to sleep on shift days when they were physiologically ready for sleep (compare Fig. 3). It is clear that the faster the shift rotation, the larger the phase differences; likewise, the earlier the circadian phase of the subject, the larger are these differences.

As shown in Fig. 9, if subjects were able to adapt to a shift system, they always adapted to the incoherent zeitgeber regimens at approximately 1 h per day. This was true not only for rectal temperature phases but also for timing of sleep. For example (Fig. 10) six evening-type subjects were able to follow a 25-h sliding system, whereby they would begin work 1 h later each day. In this experiment subjects followed this regimen in respect to timing of sleep at home as well. This would indicate that these subjects were able to follow or track a shift system (at least under these experimental conditions) which imitated, in approximation, the free-running circadian period.

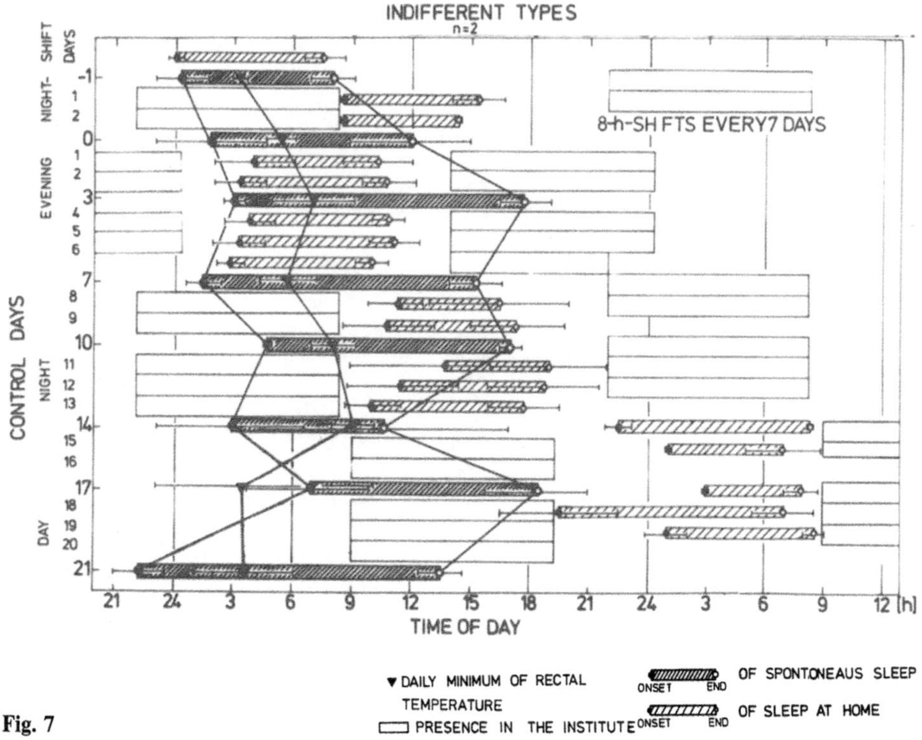
INDIFFERENT TYPES
n=2
NIGHT- SHIFT DAYS
CONTROL DAYS
EVENING
NIGHT
DAY
8-h-SHIFTS EVERY 7 DAYS
TIME OF DAY
▼ DAILY MINIMUM OF RECTAL TEMPERATURE
PRESENCE IN THE INSTITUTE
ONSET END OF SPONTONEAUS SLEEP
ONSET END OF SLEEP AT HOME

Fig. 7

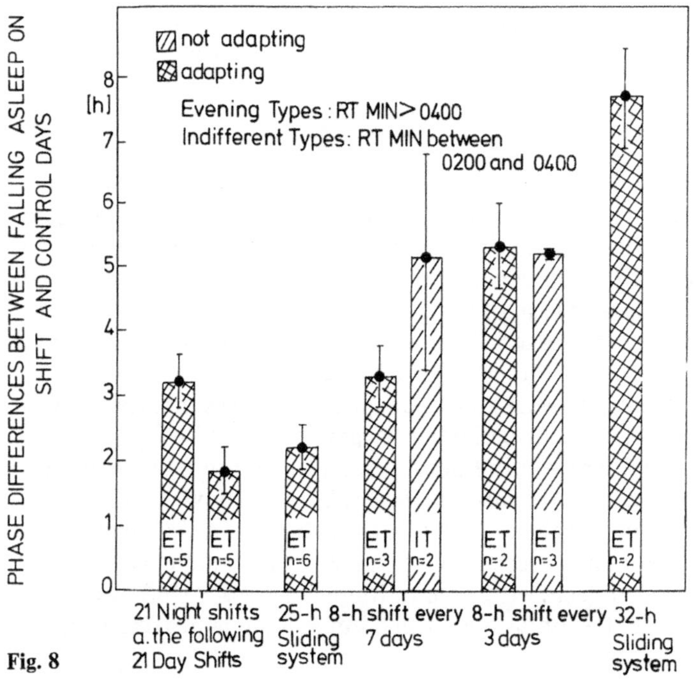
PHASE DIFFERENCES BETWEEN FALLING ASLEEP ON SHIFT AND CONTROL DAYS
[h]
not adapting
adapting
Evening Types : RT MIN > 0400
Indifferent Types: RT MIN between 0200 and 0400
ET n=5
ET n=5
ET n=6
ET n=3
IT n=2
ET n=2
ET n=3
ET n=2
21 Night shifts a. the following 21 Day Shifts
25-h Sliding system
8-h shift every 7 days
8-h shift every 3 days
32-h Sliding system

Fig. 8

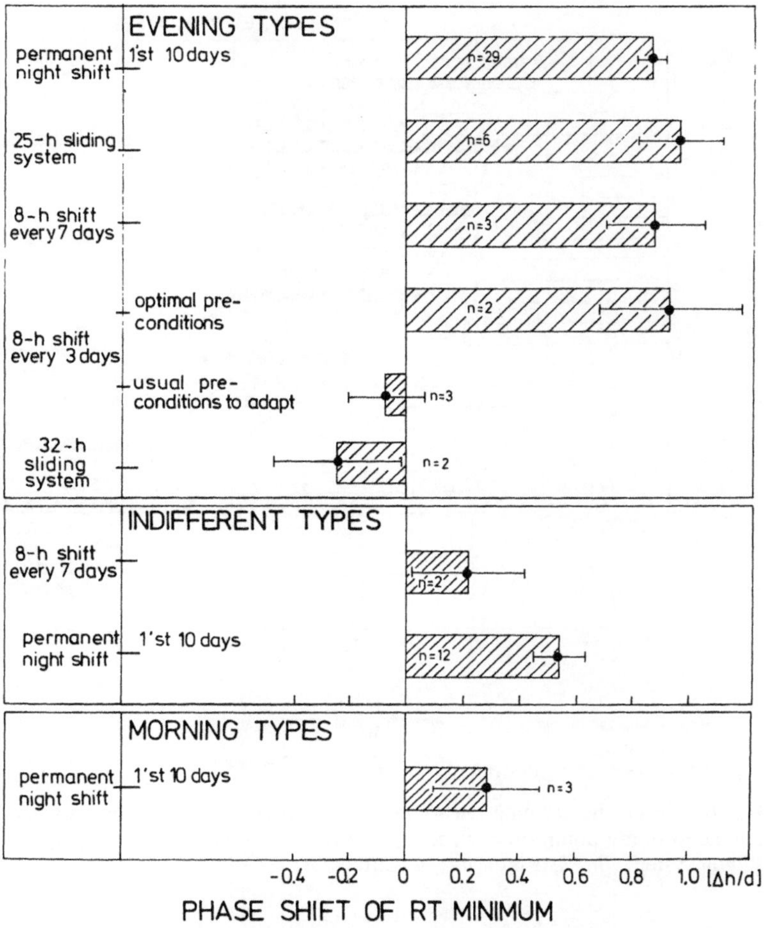

Fig. 9. Circadian phase shifts of the daily rectal temperature minimum in several groups of subjects who successfully adapted or failed to adapt to different shift systems. *Brackets* indicate standard error

---

Fig. 7. Mean courses of onset and end of main sleep periods and mean course of the circadian rectal temperature minimum on control days as compared with the sleeping periods on shift days at home in indifferent-tpye Subjects. Duty hours were shifted 8 h every 7 days. *Brackets* indicate standard error

Fig. 8. Mean masking effects of sleep onset depending on rotation speed and the individual circadian phase position (differences between the onset of the longest spontaneous sleep period on control days and the onset of sleep on the immediately preceding or following shift day). *Brackets* indicate standard errors

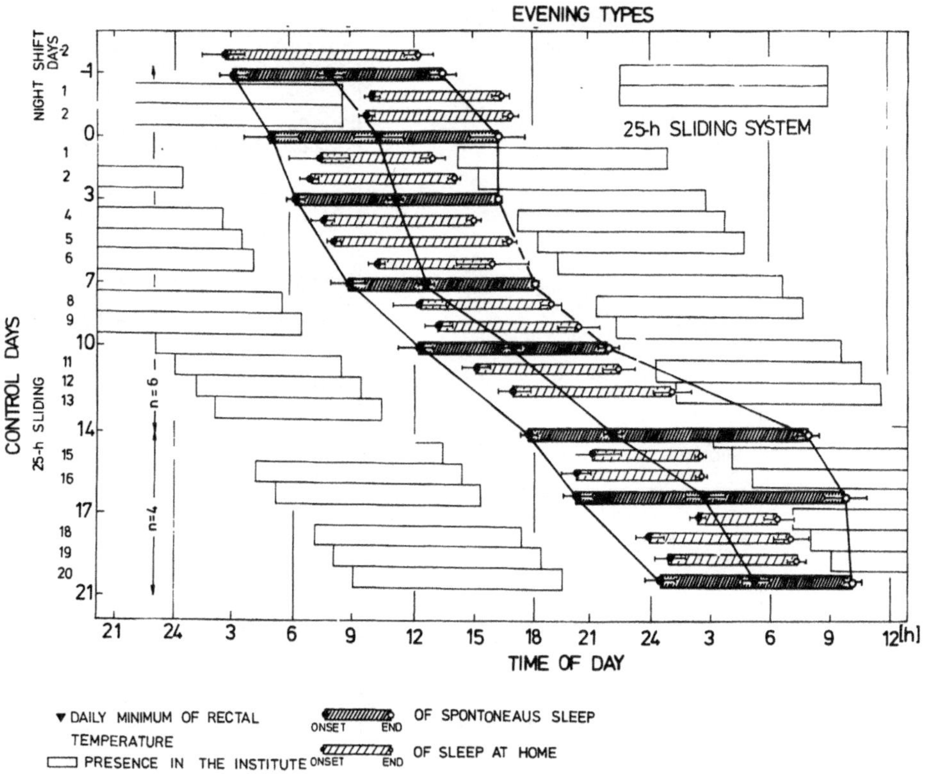

Fig. 10. Onset and termination of main sleep periods, and mean course of circadian rectal temperature minimum on control days, as compared with home sleep on shift days, in a 25-h sliding system. *Brackets* indicate standard error

Conclusions

Even the Evening-type individuals, who presumably have the most favorable preconditions for successful circadian-phase adaptation to night work, exhibit increasing difficulties when required to adjust to shift systems involving faster rotation schedules.

Where adaptation to incoherent zeitgeber regimens does occur, as in selected classes of shift work, the mean speed of phase delays amounted to about 1 h per day. This was not only true in respect to the timing to spontaneous sleep, (and by the way, in urine-excretion phasings, subjective variables like well-being also. This may indicate a free-running state. Accordingly circadian adaptation to incoherent zeitgeber regimens may not depend primarily upon the ability to respond to a set of zeitgebers which have already shifted their phases, but rather upon the ability to neglect the zeitgebers associated to the geophysical day.

References

1. Hildebrandt G (1985) Individual differences in susceptibility to night and shift work. In: Haider M, Koller M, Cervinka R (eds) Night an shift work: longterm effects and their prevention. Lang, Frankfurt
2. Kerkhof GA (1985) Interindividual differences in the human circadian System. A review. Biol Psychol 20:83–11
3. Minors DS, Waterhouse JM (1985) The use of constant routines in unmasking the endogenous component of human circadian rhythms. Chron Intern 16:205–216
4. Moog R (1981) Morning-evening-types and shift work. A questionnaire study. In: Reinberg A, Vieux N, Andlauer P (eds) Night and shift work: biological and social and aspects. Pergamon, Frankfurt, pp 481–488
5. Moog R, Hildebrandt G (1985) Comparisons of different causes of masking effects. In: Haider M, Koller M, Cervinka R (eds) Night and shift work: longterm effects and their prevention. Lang, Frankfurt
6. Ross WD (1956) Practical psychiatry for industrial physicians. Thomas, Springfield
7. Torsvall L, Akerstedt T (1980) A diurnal type scale. Construction, consistency and validation in shift work. Scand J Work Environ Health 8:283–290

The Application of Time-Series Analysis to the Diagnosis of Complex Internal Disorders: Sleep Apnea

T. PENZEL, and J. H. PETER

Introduction

Clinical pictures in internal medicine are usually defined in terms of threshold values of certain specific parameters. Hypertension, for instance, is defined as a systolic arterial blood pressure in excess of 140 mmHg or a diastolic reading of more than 95 mmHg. Complex clinical pictures such as sleep apnea cannot be adequately described in this way, however, as they involve a large variety of interrelated parameters whose development has to be evaluated over a longer period of time. As far as ECG parameters are concerned, such monitoring has long been practised in intensive care units. In complex disorders, though, parameters of a widely different nature have to be taken into account and interpreted in a comprehensive approach. A systematic comparison of, for example, ECG, EEG, blood pressure, and various respiratory parameters is not easily accomplished. It is here that the methods of time-series analysis become indispensable [1].

Prerequisites

As a prerequisite for analysis, several conditions have to be fulfilled at the stage of data acquisition. First of all, the recordings must be made in such a way that complete or selective reproduction is possible without any information being lost in the process. If the recordings are to be computer evaluated, it is desirable that they should be made directly in digital form [6]. In cooperation with the Central Laboratories for Electronic Development (Marburg), we have devised a recording method which meets these requirements. (The details and principles involved are reported in the chapter by T. Penzel, K. Meinzer and J. H. Peter in this volume.)

Figure 1 shows an example of such a recording which includes EEG, EOG, respiratory parameters, integrated mental EMG, partial arterial oxygen tension, pulmonary artery blood pressure, integrated snoring amplitude (microphone recording), and continuous computed beat-to-beat calculation of heart rate. The first striking feature in the apnea picture is the periodic behavior of respiratory activity and of heart rate. One of the first tasks of time-series analysis is to describe and quantify such behavior [8].

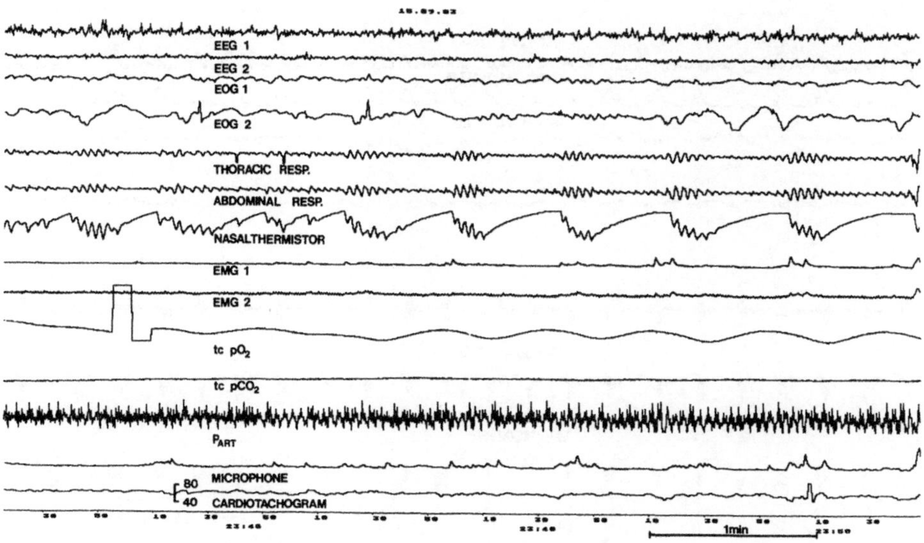

Fig. 1. Digital recording of regular obstructive sleep apnea

Evaluation of Heart Rate and Respiration

An initial evaluation of heart rate and respiratory activity can be accomplished with easy-to-use methods by calculating the mean rates over a gliding time window, the size of which will have a decisive effect on the results obtained. By using gliding means and integrating the curves (see Appendix), we can calculate an integrated respiratory activity from the respiratory excursion curves. This is basically a gliding determination of variance, which can then be correlated with the beat-to-beat heart rate curve.

The coefficient of correlation in its temporal development is shown in the third curve from the top in Fig. 2. Its value is close to +0.5. This result reflects the link between the two parameters but does not yet provide any information on the causal relationship. A series of evaluations has shown that this coefficient of correlation is always high in cases of regularly compensated apnea, i.e. in cases of apnea in which the drop in partial arterial oxygen tension caused by hypoventilation or apnea is compensated by subsequent hyperventilation. During irregular or uncompensated apnea, the coefficient approximates zero, as it does during periods of undisturbed respiration. Readings of the coefficient close to zero therefore have a limited use as an indicative value. But correlation analyses are also a valuable means in the determination of time shifts between the individual parameters in order to ascertain the actual sequence of events and changes, e.g. if an increase in heart rate precedes the resumption of respiration after apnea (which seems to be the case), or vice versa.

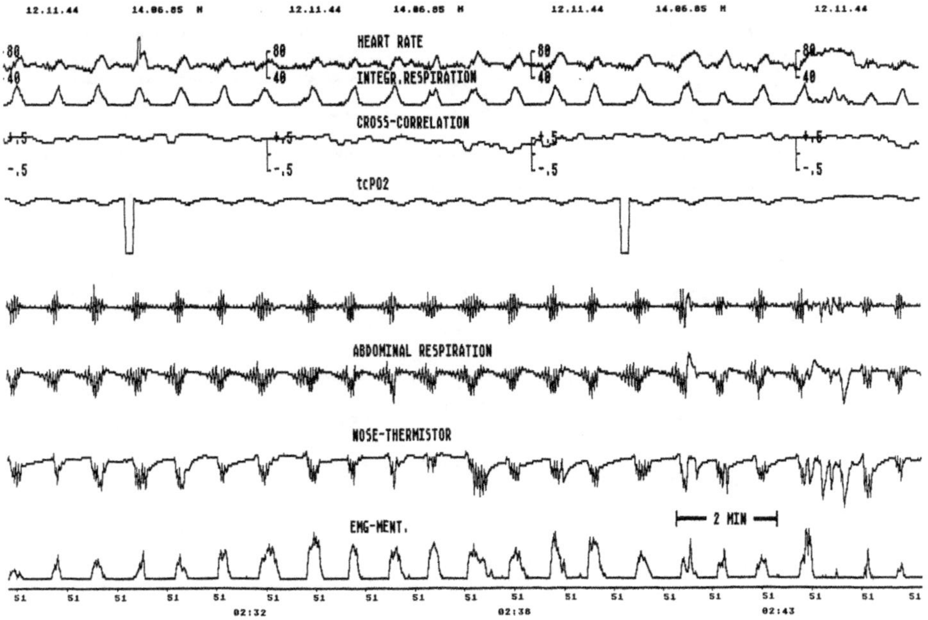

Fig. 2. Regular compensated apnea. From the top: heart rate, integrated thoracic respiratory activity, cross-correlation computed on a gliding scale of heart rate/integrated respiratory activity, partial arterial oxygen tension (transcutaneously), thoracic respiratory activity (inductive plethysmography), abdominal respiratory activity (inductive plethysmography), respiratory flow (nasal thermistor), integrated activity of a mental EMG

EEG Evaluations

Different methods of time-series analysis are required for EEG evaluation. The EEG provides a vast amount of data, making successful data reduction a necessity in the course of the evaluation. Data reduction must always ensure that all relevant data are recognized among the incoming signals, and only redundant data are discarded. Data reduction on the time axis, for example, i.e., the rejection of data pertaining to particular points or sections of the temporal course of the recording, would diminish the usefulness of the EEG as a basis for evaluative judgments. But here time-series analysis offers solutions in the form of transformations. Fourier transform seems to be particularly suited for EEG evaluation.

Figure 3 provides a continuous representation of the EEG power spectra of a patient with sleep apnea while falling asleep. A condensed plot of respiratory activity as recorded with the aid of a nasal thermistor has been added. A great proportion of EEG activity in the α-range (8–13 Hz) is clearly visible in the foreground. As the patient falls asleep, α-activity decreases, and the first apneas appear. The intermittent bursts of α-activity which can be observed in the power spectra represent arousals following the termination of the apnea episodes.

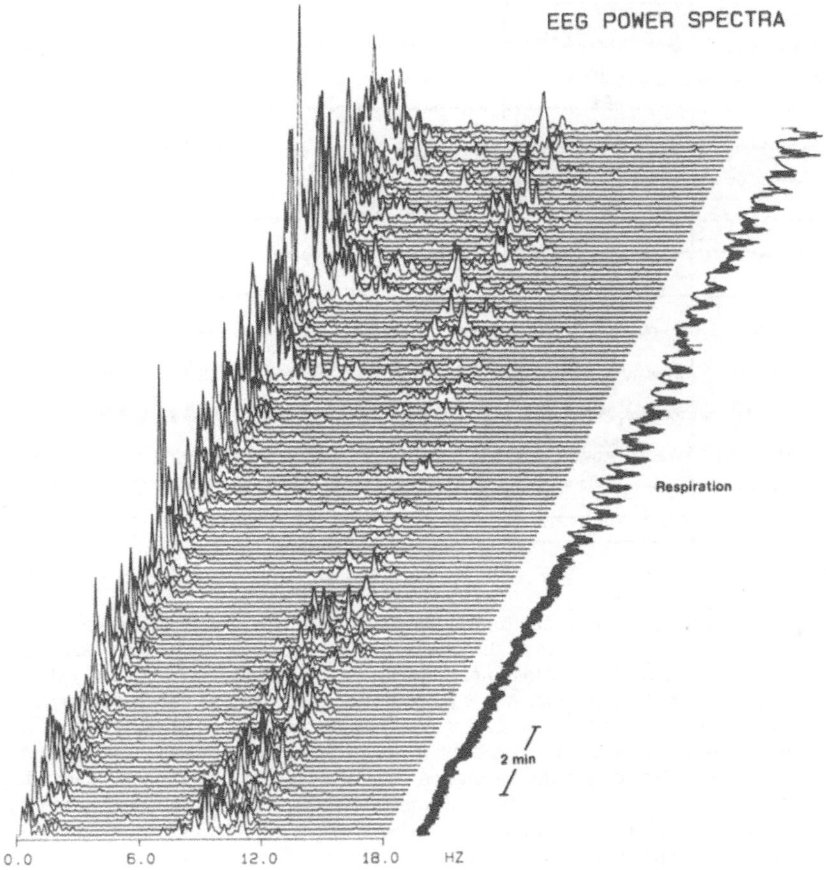

Fig. 3. EEG power spectra of a patient falling asleep. With the onset of sleep, α-activity gives way to low-frequency ϑ-activity. Apneas are recognizable in the condensed plot of the respiration curve *(right)* and by intermittent bursts of α-activity in the EEG. Recorded over 20 min

Transformations are in fact not a form of data reduction, but rather a means of presenting data differently. The temporal development of the EEG power spectra will therefore have to be represented in a suitably reduced form in order to facilitate a systematic comparison with other physiological parameters and to permit adequate calculation routines.

Data Reduction of the EEG

A simple form of data reduction can be achieved by extracting physiologically relevant frequency bands from the power spectra [3]. In the following, we have calculated the intensities in the α-band, indicative of alertness, and the ϑ-band (3–5 Hz), which is characteristic of sleep. These activities have been rendered in a

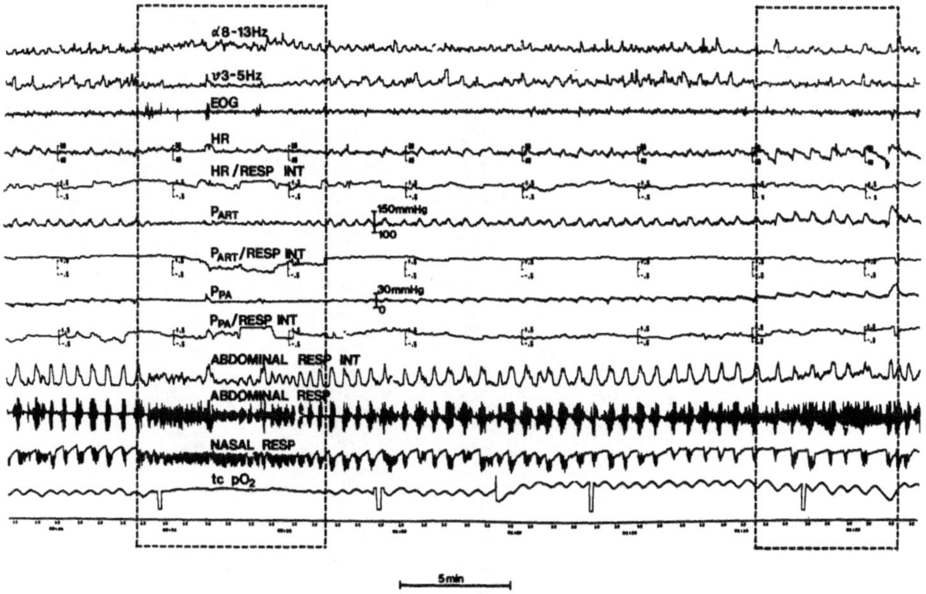

Fig. 4. Continuous 40-min recording, illustrating various methods of time-series analysis. Two sections *(boxed)* are discussed in the text: apnea disappears as the patient wakes up *(left)*, and a series of prolonged apneas leads to pathological blood pressure readings and extreme bradycardia *(right)*. From the top: α-activity, ϑ-activity (frequency bands extracted from the EEG power spectra), EOG, heart rate (beat-to-beat continuous computation), coefficient of correlation of heart rate/integrated respiratory activity, mean arterial blood pressure, coefficient of correlation of mean arterial blood pressure/integrated respiratory activity, mean pulmonary artery pressure, coefficient of correlation of mean pulmonary artery pressure/integrated respiratory activity, integrated abdominal respiratory activity (basis of the correlations shown above), abdominal respiration (inductive plethysmography), respiratory flow (nasal thermistor), partial arterial oxygen tension (transcutaneously)

form representing their continuous development in time and have been juxtaposed with other parameters. Figure 4 shows a section of such a comprehensive recording, involving data reduction and illustrating the multiparameter approach. The upper two curves in this figure show the α- and ϑ-activities, which, in their alternation, give an indication of the arousals terminating each apnea episode. These indications can be compared with the synchronous development of the curves describing the respiratory activity (abdominal respiration, recorded by means of inductive plethysmography; integrated respiratory activity computed on the basis of the original recording; and airflow, measured by means of a nasal thermistor). The figure shows that the apneas cease after about 7 min of the recording section, and respiration returns to normal. At the same time, ϑ-activity drops completely, α-activity increases, and eye movements are recorded by the EOG: the patient has woken up. He remains awake for a couple of minutes, falls asleep again, and the apneas reappear.

In the section indicated on the far right of the figure, one can clearly discern a series of particularly long apnea episodes which coincide with distinct hypoxemia and extreme bradycardia. Mean arterial blood pressure can be seen to rise to pathological values (around 150 mmHg) as these episodes terminated. The figure also shows the moving calculation of the coefficients of correlation between integrated respiratory activity and heart rate, mean systemic arterial blood pressure, and mean pulmonary artery blood pressure. These parameters are closely linked during apnea, as expressed by a high coefficient of correlation. This tie is resolved during the period of wakefulness.

While this figure illustrates the complicated interaction of different parameters during the regulatory dysfunctions which characterise sleep apnea, it also illustrates the limits of such an elaborate approach. A synopsis of the frequency bands of the EEG and other parameters can only be an intermediary stage. The ultimate aim in the application of time-series analysis to the investigation of a complex disease such as sleep apnea will be the on-line classification of sleep and vigilance stages as well as the assessment of apnea, that is, a mode of representation of the recorded data which incorporates the appropriate criteria of interpretation, and thus permits a diagnostic assessment.

Classification and Assessment

One of the aims of time-series analysis is to reduce data in a way which will permit interpretation combined with classification. This approach is here discussed, taking the EEG as an example again. EEG classification was "taught" to the computer by feeding in the results of a competent classification of the EEG. The teacher classified the original EEG, which was split into 2-s segments, according to Loomis [5] and modified according to Fruhstorfer and Bergström [2], as these classification criteria are more suitable for the dynamic course of changes in vigilance than the Rechtschaffen and Kales classification [4, 9], which employs rigid 30-s windows and uses specific events as criteria (K-complexes, sleep spindles). We then tried to select as few parameters as possible from the Fourier spectra of the EEG which would permit an adequate discrimination of vigilance stages. The efficiency of two parameters is illustrated by Fig. 5, in which "ν (.7)" represents frequency and wavenorm ("Norm") was used as an amplitude (or rather total power) criterion (see Appendix).

The figure shows the discrimination of vigilance stages which was a result of the computed evaluation of 40 tests of 2-s segments of the EEG, composed of unambiguous specimens of the various stages as classified by hand. The mean values and standard deviations of the individual stages are indicated and the areas in which the respective segments were found are mapped out. We paid particular attention to the overlapping areas, which represent segments of the test set which could not be unambiguously defined by means of the two criteria employed. These segments were found, in a comparison with the manual assessment, to be either true transitional segments between two vigilance stages, or had previously been classified not by virtue of their own characteristics alone, but by taking the time environment (preceding and subsequent segment) or a

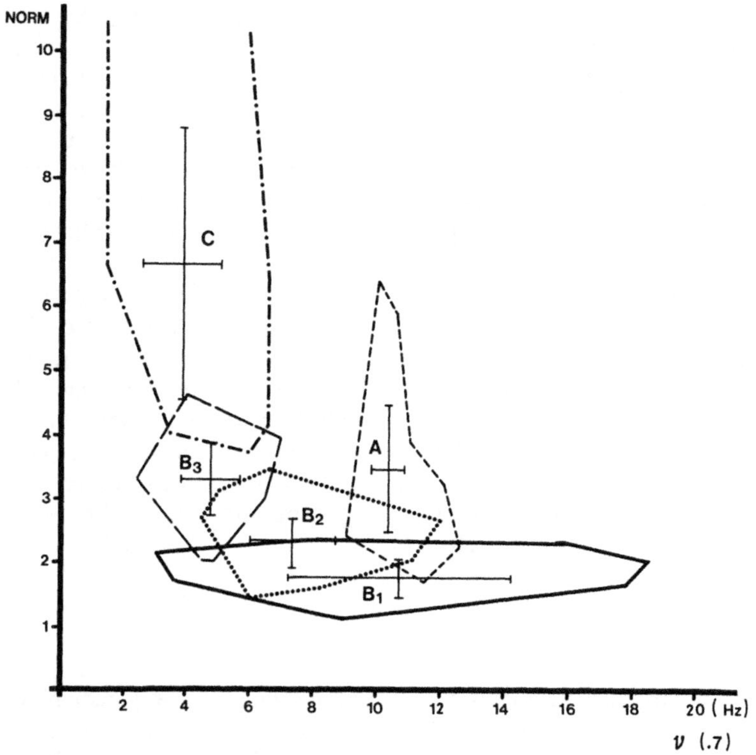

Fig. 5. Computed separation of EEG vigilance stages; 440 results from a 2-dimensional parameter field evaluation of 2-s EEG segments. Mean values and standard deviation indicated. For the definition of parameters, see Appendix

second EEG lead (C_z-O_2) into account. It is evident, though, that despite the unusually high resolution of the evaluation, two appropriately chosen criteria can be sufficient for a fairly clear discrimination of vigilance stages. The inclusion of additional parameters would no doubt further improve the results, but would also tend to defeat the aim of data reduction.

Pattern Analysis and Recognition

The recognition and analysis of characteristic patterns constitutes a particular challenge to time-series analysis. Such methods are nowadays incorporated in long-term ECG instruments for the recognition of ventricular extrasystoles. Similar methods are important for the analysis of sleep apnea [7]. Figure 6 shows a pattern which can be observed in cases of prolonged apnea. The acceleration of the cardiac rhythm, which usually appears at the termination of the apnea episode, is here repeated several times while apnea continues. After several pro-

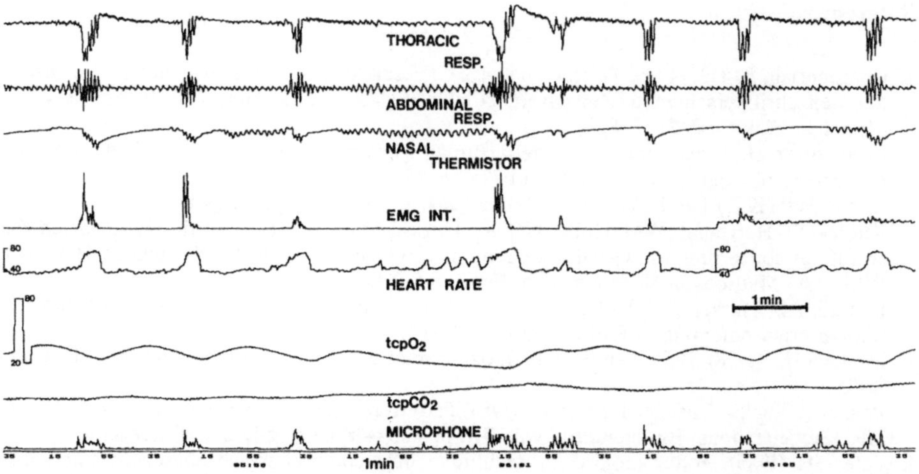

Fig. 6. Recording of a pattern with frustrated increases in heart rate during prolonged apnea and insufficient compensation of hypercapnia and hypoxia

nounced ups and downs of heart rate, extreme hyperventilation sets in but fails to compensate for the severe decrease in arterial oxygen tension which was the consequence of this long apneic period. Hypercapnia persists for some time in this pattern of irregular and uncompensated apnea. The microphone recording shows that the end of this episode is accompanied by exceptionally long and loud snoring. The successful recognition of such patterns with the methods of time-series analysis is an important prerequisite for a detailed interpretation of individual results.

Summary

The problems and examples discussed here clearly show that the methods of time-series analysis are an indispensable aid to the full understanding of the mechanisms underlying such complex clinical pictures as sleep apnea. Time-series analysis has two main functions here: the first is the task of data reduction in a way which selects relevant and discards redundant information; the second is the task of helping to detect, distinguish and interpret physiological and pathophysiological patterns.

Acknowledgement. The authors wish to thank Prof. Dr. Petzold for extensive discussions and many valuable suggestions.

References

1. Chamberlain LJ (1972) Die Zeitreihenanalyse. Dieser Artikel ist in drei Teilen in drei Heften der Zeitschrift erschienen. Zeitschrift: „Elektronik" 21. Jahrg. Heft 7, 8, 9 Franzis-Verlag München Elektronik 21 (7, 8, 9)
2. Fruhstorfer H, Bergstrom RM (1969) Human vigilance and auditory evoked responses. Electroencephalogr Clin Neurophysiol 27:346–355
3. Koella WP (1973) Die Physiologie des Schlafes. Kohlhammer, Stuttgart
4. Kubicki St, Herrmann WM, Höller L (1985) Critical comments on the rules by Rechtschaffen and Kales concerning the visual evaluation of EEG sleep records. In: Kubicki St, Herrmann WM (eds) Methods of sleep research. Fischer, Stuttgart, pp 19–35
5. Loomis AL, Harvey EN, Hobart GA III (1937) Cerebral stages during sleep, as studied by human brain potentials. J Exp Psychol 21:127–144
6. Meinzer K (1978) IPS - eine neue Programmiertechnik für Mikrocomputer, Elektronik 15:35–42
7. Penzel T, Fuchs E, Mayer J, Peter JH (1984) Pattern recognition of sleep apnea. In: Kimmich HP, Klewe HJ (eds) Biotelemetry, vol VIII. pp 435–438 Döring-Druck, Braunschweig
8. Peter JH (1985) Holter monitoring technique in a comprehensive approach: ambulatory monitoring of sleep apnea. In: Hombach V, Hilger HH (eds) Holter monitoring technique. Schattauer, Stuttgart, pp 127–149
9. Rechtschaffen A, Kales A (eds) (1968) A manual of standardized terminology, techniques and scoring system for sleep stages of human subjects. Public Health Service. US Government Printing Office, Washington DC

Appendix

1. Calculation of the integrated respiratory activity, i(t), from original inductive plethysmographic recordings, x(t)

$$i(t) = \frac{1}{\tau_1} \int_{t-\tau_1}^{t} | x(\hat{t}) - m(\hat{t}) | \, d\hat{t}$$

where m(t) is a gliding mean

$$m(t) = \frac{1}{\tau_2} \int_{t-\tau_2}^{t} x(\hat{t}) \, d\hat{t}$$

In order to permit subsequent on-line analysis, the integrals were not calculated symmetrically but recursively. A suitable τ value is of vital importance. Our experience suggests $\tau_1 = 4.26$ s and $\tau_2 = 8.53$ s.

2. Calculation of the criteria $v(\chi)$ and Norm $\|x\|$ for computed assessment of EEG vigilance stages: x(t) is the original EEG curve

$$\| x(t) \| = + \sqrt{\frac{1}{2\tau} \int_{t-\tau}^{t+\tau} | x(\hat{t}) |^2 \, d\hat{t}}$$

The calculation of $v(\chi)$ is somewhat more complicated: the EEG x(t) is thus transformed so that the mean value of the function equals 0.

$$\hat{x}(t) = x(t) - \frac{1}{2\tau} \int_{-\tau}^{\tau} x(t) \, dt$$

A Fourier transformation is then applied, and the power spectrum $\rho^2(\nu)$ is computed:

$$\rho^2(\nu) = \int_{-\tau}^{\tau} \hat{x}(t)e^{-2\pi i\nu t}dt \int_{-\tau}^{\tau} \hat{x}(t)e^{2\pi i\nu t}dt$$

On this basis we calculate the power distribution function with the range 0–30 Hz. Relevant power proportions in excess of 30 Hz are not to be expected:

$$\chi(\nu) = \frac{\int_0^{\nu} \rho^2(\tilde{\nu})\,d\tilde{\nu}}{\int_0^{30} \rho^2(\tilde{\nu})\,d\tilde{\nu}}$$

This makes $\chi(0) = 0$ and $\chi(30) = 1$. In addition, $\chi(\nu)$ shows a steady increase. The reversible function is formed, and cuts are set at fixed values of χ.

$$\nu(.7) = \nu(\chi = .7)$$

In this case we chose $\tau = 1$ s, thus calculating segments of 2 s each.

Techniques to Construct Respiratory Waveforms from VCG/ECG*

F. Pinciroli, R. Rossi, and L. Vergani

Introduction

It is by now an accepted fact that diagnostics relies more and more on information obtained by instrumental analysis. Such analysis is mostly performed with instruments that can be considered novel for different reasons [1]. Some relevant examples are a new type of transducer [2], the integration of several features hitherto on different devices into one instrument [3], and the use of specific signal processing techniques to extract new information from signals that are commonly and widely used in clinical practice [4].

Although instrumental analysis of respiratory function has significantly progressed in the last few years [5], no important advance has been recorded in long-term ambulatory monitoring of the cycle-by-cycle waveforms derived from respiratory values, in such a way that the patient can still lead a normal life [6]. For instance, instrument bulkiness and possible invasiveness of the technique are still unresolved issues.

When the direct transducing of any physical value becomes especially difficult, one is led to search for other, indirect procedures. In the case of ambulatory monitoring of these waveforms, the search should investigate those biological signals which, although chiefly describing the activity of other than the respiratory system, are nevertheless affected by it. It stands to reason that this approach will pose intricate problems of signal analysis: however, any success would more than make up for the effort.

The electrocardiogram (ECG) undoubtedly is a biological signal that, although not directly describing the respiratory system, is at times significantly affected by it (Fig. 1a). Unfortunately this is not always true; however, the ECG is so easy to obtain that it ought to be the first to be investigated among other possible signals.

This paper deals with some techniques for drawing respiratory waveforms from ECG signals and illustrates some of the results obtained. These techniques are partly new and were first tested by us [7, 8].

* This research has been supported by CNR contributions 83.00946.07/84.02096.07 and contract 85.02689.07

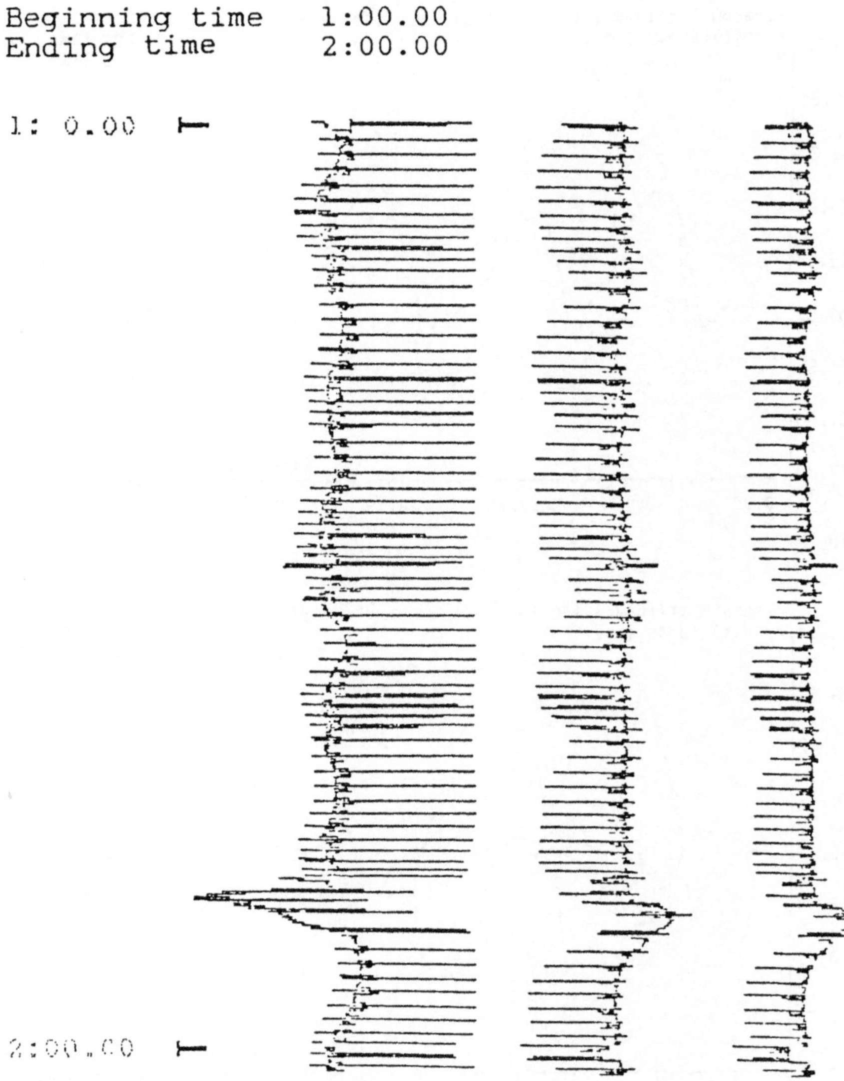

Fig. 1a-e. ECG and some respiratory waveforms reconstruction. **a** It is evident that the AmPP modulation follows respiratory rhythms. **b–e** Various angles for defining AsEC

Materials and Methods

An ECG consists of a set of electrical voltages varying with time, which are read by placing electrodes on the body surface. The ECG originates from the heart's electrical activity and is also affected by the usually neglected influence of the biological tissues lying between the heart and the skin.

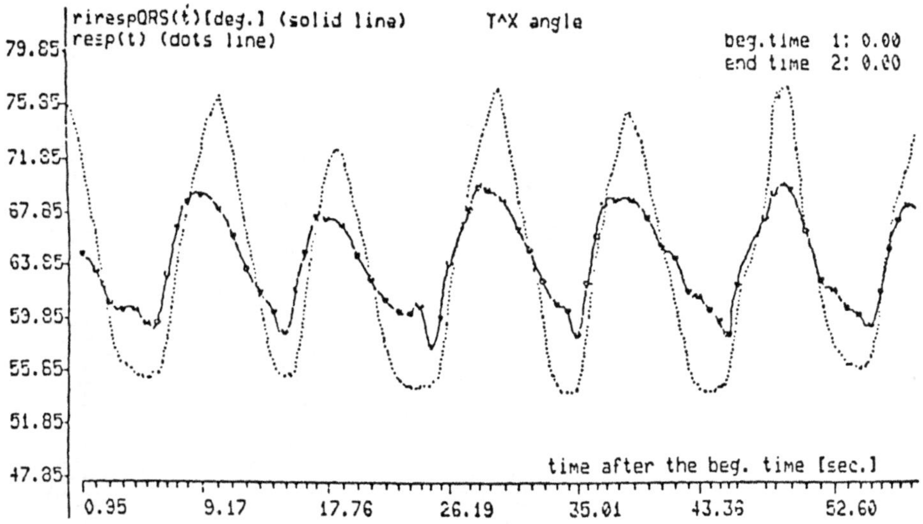

Fig. 1b

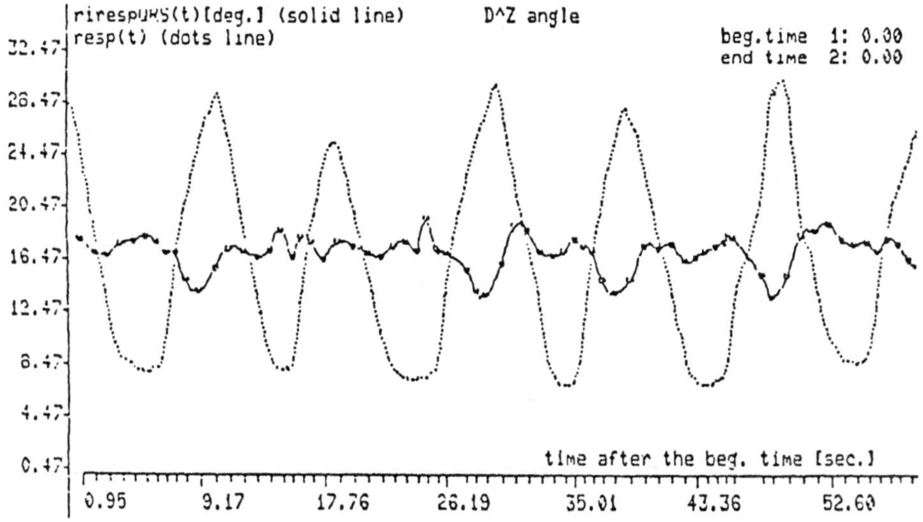

Fig. 1c

The alternation of inspiratory and expiratory stages affects both the total thoracic volume and the pressure applied to the lungs and any other organ contained in the thorax. Thoracic volume and endothoracic pressure can both affect the ECG. It is quite likely, for instance, that a variation of thoracic volume will influence the attenuation of the cardiac electrical activity between the heart and the skin surface. It is also probable that any variation in space distribution of endothoracic pressure will affect the cardiac volume and consequently the density of space distribution of the electric generators within the cardiac volume.

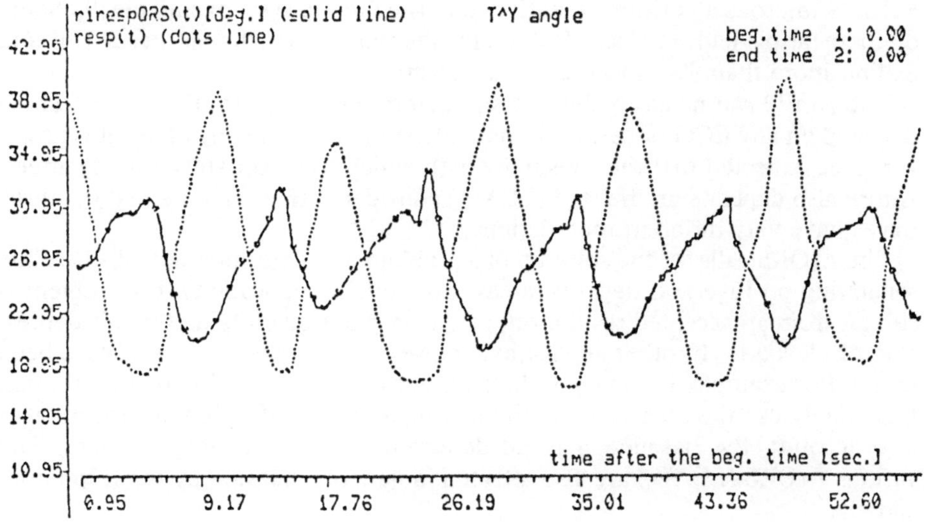

Fig. 1d

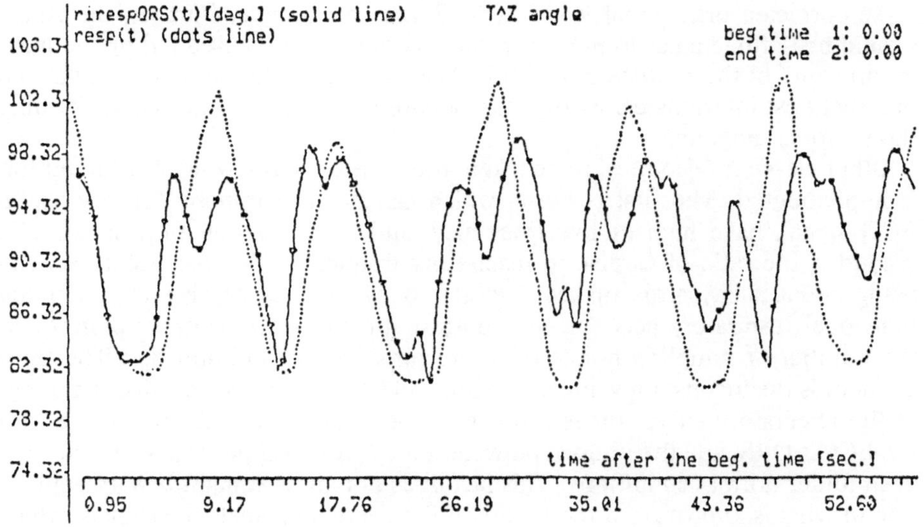

Fig. 1e

These influences should be taken into account when deducing respiratory activity curves from the ECG. It is quite possible, for instance, that the electrical axis of the heart (AsEC) represents the influence of endothoracic pressure. The peak-to-peak amplitude of a cardiac cycle (AmPP) or the area and sign of the QRS (ArQRS) related to the trace of any ECG lead should in turn be significantly affected by the variation of endothoracic volume.

In order to be analyzed on a digital computer, the three techniques mentioned above must have preliminary automatic recognition of the QRS complex on the

ECG. Numerous algorithms mentioned in the literature seem suitable [9]. Some of them also yield very satisfactory results when arrhythmias occur [10] and exhibit more than 99% specificity and sensitivity.

The AmPP can be easily defined and determined. An AmPP ($LEAD_i$) can be detected on any ECG trace considered independently from any other. It is however to be expected that the sensitivity with which the respiratory activity affects AmPP also depends on the lead ($LEAD_i$) considered (Fig. 1a; note that the three traces have very different modulations).

The ArQRS calls for the solution of a problem: the determination of a baseline separating positive and negative areas. For certain applications this problem is still far from an accepted resolution; one example is quantifying the S-T depression or elevation. In other applications however, an answer seems to have been found. For example, in the algorithms for automatic recognition of arrhythmias, that widely use the area as a descriptor, which the classification algorithm takes into account, the baseline may be determined using the P-Q segment. The various ArQRS ($LEAD_i$) are also affected in variable measure by the respiratory activity.

The AsEC is probably the most important value from a calculation viewpoint. To determine it, several traces from an adequate set must be processed. Frank's three corrected orthogonal leads X, Y, Z are an example. Further, the AsEC should be defined so as to prevent problems of the type caused [11] by the maximum value of the vector's magnitude. We feel that it should be defined as the one that best interpolates, by the least square method, the space curve forming the vectorcardiogram.

Other elements also need to be taken into consideration, whichever definition is implemented. The first is noise, which can be superimposed on the useful ECG signal, have high or low frequency, and affect one or more leads. The second is the ratio of cardiac to respiratory frequency. The respiratory activity being equal, tachycardia makes it easier to plot curves capable of describing individual respiratory acts. On the contrary, brachycardia hampers plotting, as the number of sampling points of the respiratory curve diminishes. The third element is the inconstant value of the interval between two successive samplings of the respiratory curve. Indeed, this curve is sampled in correspondence with the ECG's QRS, and the interval between successive QRS peaks is known to vary even under normal conditions. This fact does not allow straightforward application of what is known from the theory of time-sampling analogue signals, which mostly assume the sampling interval to be constant. The fourth element is the selection of the respiratory curves with which to compare the determinations made from the ECG. Although they are not typical of long-term monitoring, it is likely that the respiratory curves to be used for comparison are those of pressure p(t), flow rate f(t), and volume v(t), obtained in a spirometric test.

Results

The results reported in this chapter do not cover the second experimental stage which we have planned and are now carrying out. This second stage differs from

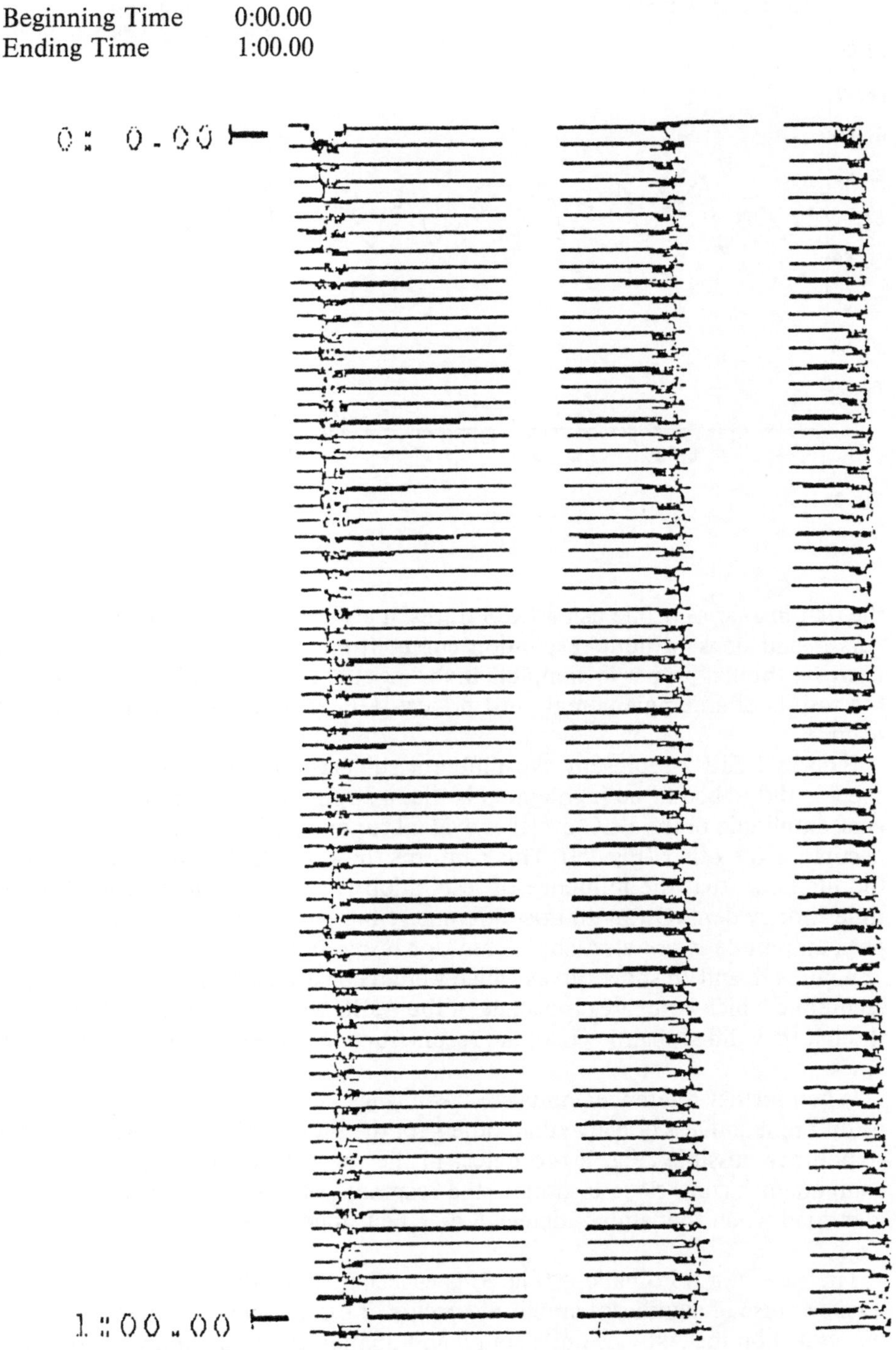

Fig. 2a, b. ECG and some respiratory waveforms reconstruction

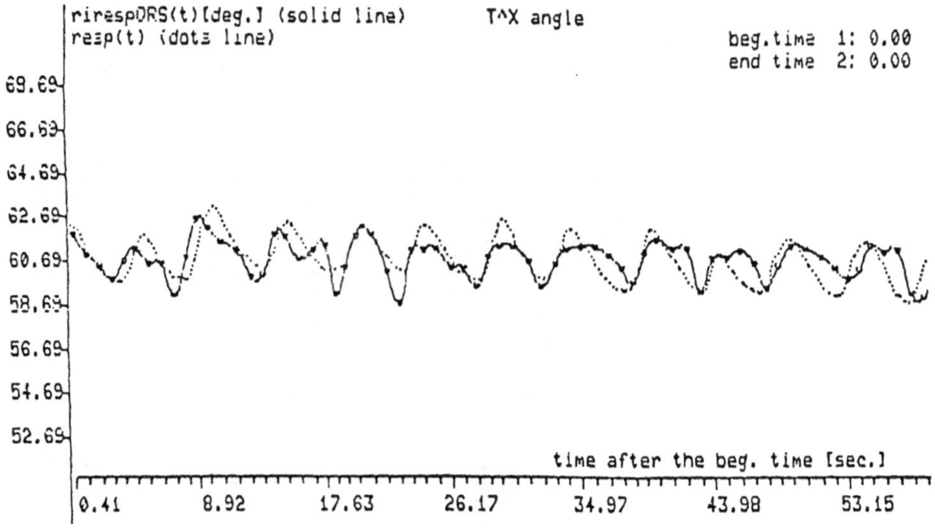

Fig. 2b

the first insofar as, while using ECG traces, it also avails itself of the p(t) and f(t) curves and does without respiration curves from belt impedance meters. We however think it proper to complete the work published earlier [7, 8] and include the results of a complementary test project [12] performed by another research team.

Figures 1 and 2 represent two different subjects who are both normal. The specific difference to be highlighted is that a strong modulation of the peak-to-peak amplitude of the ECG cycles is evident for one patient (Fig. 1a), while none occurs for the other (Fig. 2a). This confirms the hypothesis widely known from the literature that the influence of respiration is at times evident and at other times not evident. Owing to this difference from patient to patient, the peak-to-peak amplitude is not a reliable datum for respiration detection.

Figures 1b and 2b show curves which were reconstructed for both subjects by a technique which compares the angle of the AsEC with a reference direction. Although they differ slightly [7, 8], the reconstruction is clearly satisfactory in both cases.

When further reference points are taken (Figs. 1c, 1d), the reconstruction may be different and less effective than others for the same subject. Nevertheless, it is sometimes possible (Fig. 1e) to detect in the reconstruction the presence of a component having close to double the respiration frequency, which cannot be identified when the latter is detected by a belt impedance meter.

The case of a third patient (Fig. 3) is especially positive: although a high frequency noise of significant amplitude occurs, it can be seen that the reconstruction based on the AsEC is quite sound and unaffected by the unfavorable initial conditions.

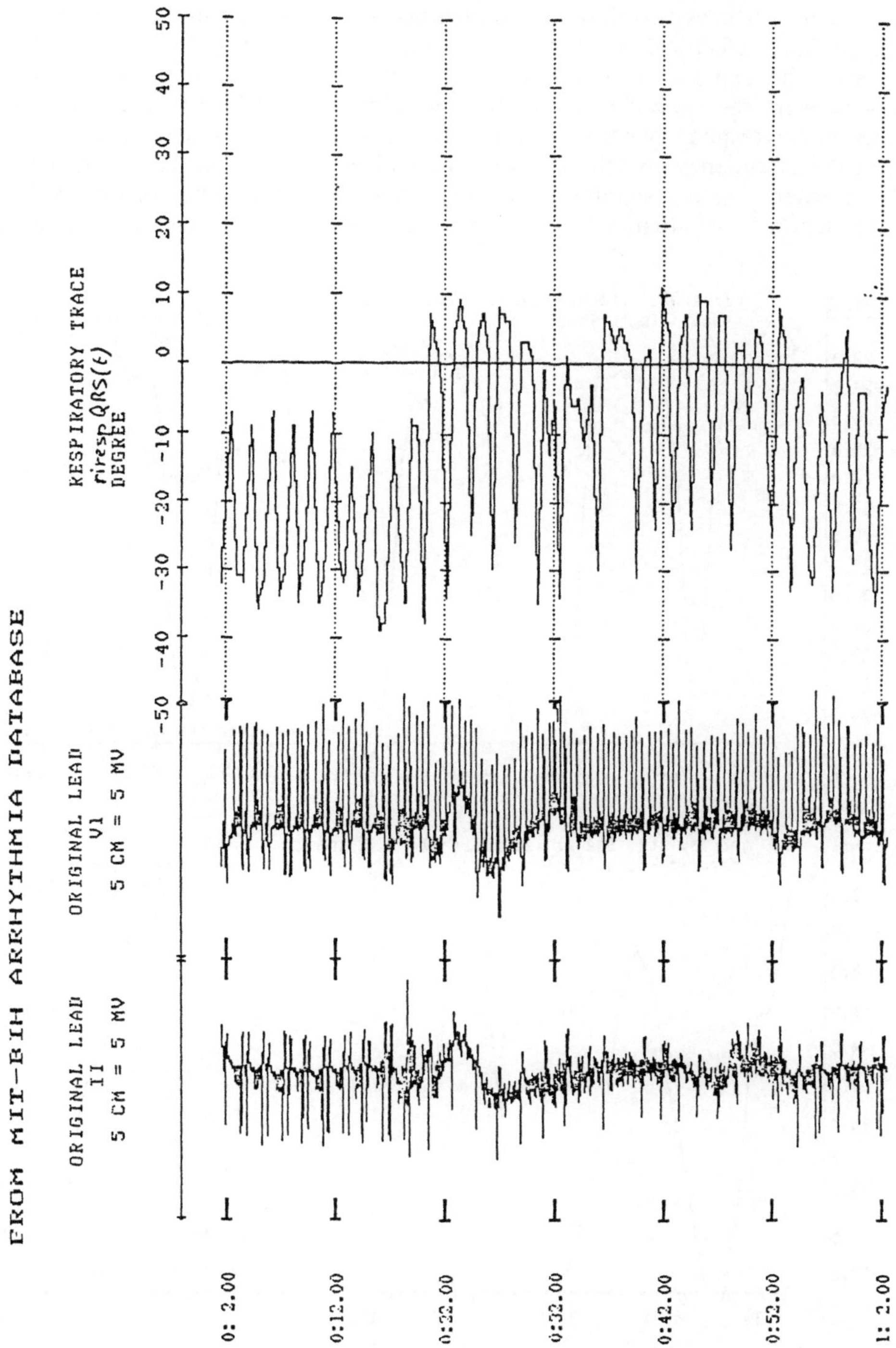

Fig. 3. ECG and AsEC reconstruction of respiratory waveforms; in spite of a high frequency noise on ECG, reconstruction seems to be correct

Figure 4 shows two different reconstructions from the same patient, which differ in the electrical axes considered, namely those of the QRS complex and T wave. This experiment was done because, when the AsEC value is calculated once every cardiac cycle, the number of points may be insufficient to plot an acceptable respiratory curve. There is the risk that this curve may be time-sampled at a frequency insufficient for a reasonable reconstruction. This is especially true when a high respiratory frequency occurs in the presence of low cardiac frequency. This situation should improve when several values are calculated

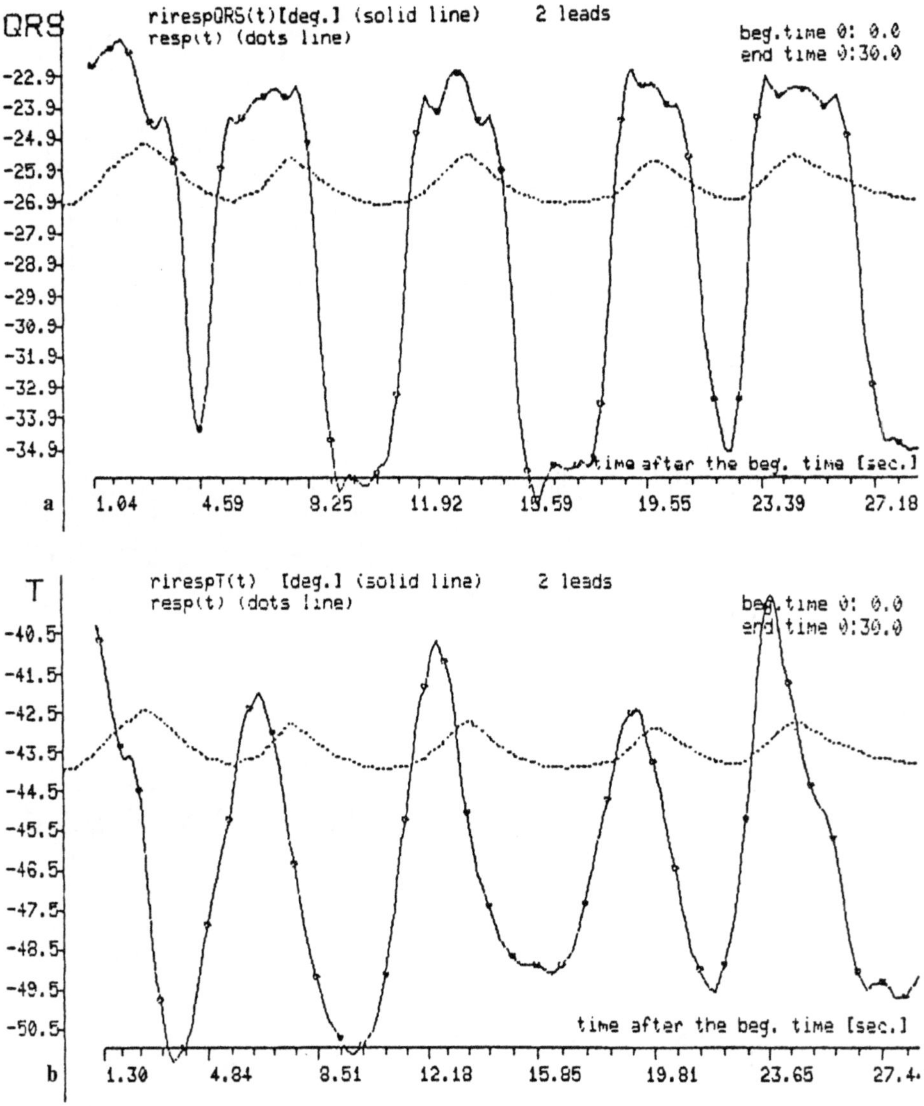

Fig. 4a, b. Two different reconstructions based on AsEC techniques. **a** AsEC is determined on QRS complex; **b** AsEC is determined on T wave

within one cardiac cycle. For us, the first step was to verify whether both reconstructions, separately based on the dominant axes of the QRS-complex and T wave, are reliable. This is proved by Fig. 4. A still unresolved issue is how to facilitate their technically difficult integration.

Another definition was explored by a team with whom we have been collaborating for some time [12]. They started from the ECG traces relative to two orthogonal leads. After subtracting the baseline from each, the area of the QRS for a window of preset duration was determined. The measured area is proportional to the signal's mean amplitude and therefore also to the projection of the mean electrical cardiac vector on the direction determined by the ECG lead. When both leads are orthogonal, the arc tangent of the areas measured in both leads yields the mean axis. Published examples refer to central apnea, obstructive apnea, mixed apnea, and hypopnea, and seem to allow distinctions between them.

Conclusion

It is to be hoped that the development of this research approach will allow reconstruction of the waveform of a respiratory cycle from ECG leads in a fair number of cases. Thus the patient could do without any transducer dedicated to the specific detection of respiratory values. A further possibility is reconstruction on ambulatory patients from Holter's ECG traces. This would also allow better assessment of the onset and interruption of specific arrhythmia, for which the decay of respiratory performance might be the triggering event.

References

1. Manzoni P, Oldano G, Pinciroli F (1982) The electrocardiomultigraphimeter as a basic instrument for developing effective personal computing in cardiology. In: The journal of IEE proceedings 129 (part A; 5):340–351
2. Raciti M, Kraft G, Ruschi S, Marchesi C, De Rossi D, Contini C (1986) A new transducer for breathing rate, cardiac sounds, and apexcardiogram in ambulatory monitoring. In: Proceedings of the 2nd international symposium on Holter monitoring, Jerusalem, March 23–25
3. Pinciroli F, Pellegrini A, Falcetti G, Antognini F (1986) Electrocardiomultigraphimeter on home-computer. (to be published)
4. Pinciroli F (1985) Ratios sequences of close R-R intervals in cardiac arrhythmias. In: Int J Biomed Comput 18:237–271
5. Stott FD, Raftery EB, Clement DL, Wright SL (eds) (1982) ISAM-GENT 1981. Proceedings of the 4th international symposium on ambulatory monitoring and second gent workshop on blood pressure variability. Academic, New York
6. Dal Palu' G, Pessina AC (eds) (1986) ISAM-Gent 1985. Proceedings of the 5th international symposium on ambulatory monitoring. CLUEP, Padova
7. Pinciroli F, Rossi R, Vergani L (1985) Detection of electrical axis variation for the extraction of respiratory information. In: Ripley KL (ed) Proceedings of the 1985 IEEE computers in cardiology. International Conference. Linköping, Sweden, September
8. Pinciroli F, Rossi R, Vergani L, Carnevali P, Mantero S, Parigi O (1986) Remarks and experiments on the construction of respiratory waveform from electrocardiographic tracings. Comput Biomed Res 19:391–409

9. Wolf KH, MacFarlane PW (eds) (1980) Optimization of computer ECG processing. North Holland, Amsterdam
10. AA.VV (1982) Recording and analysis systems: quality control and performance criteria. In: Wenger NK, Mock MB, Ringquist I (eds) Ambulatory electrocardiographic. Year Book Medical, Chicago
11. Pinciroli F, Rossi R, Vergani L (1985) Virtual leads for the ambulatory ECG monitoring: remarks on the persistency of their direction. Comp Biomed Res 18:62–78
12. Moody GB, Mark RG, Zoccola A, Mantero S (1985) Derivation of respiratory signals from multi-lead ECGs. In: Kipley KL (ed) Proceedings of the 1985 IEEE computers in cardiology international Conference. Linköping, Sweden, September, IEEE Computer Society Press

Use of Tracheal Sound Recordings to Monitor Airflow During Sleep

N. MESLIER, and J. L. RACINEUX

Various methods have been used for continuous airflow monitoring during sleep, including the use of oral and nasal thermistors and the face mask pneumotachygraph. Recording of tracheal breath sounds has been proposed by Krumpe [1] and Cummiskey [2] for the detection and quantification of sleep apnea and hypopnea. Tracheal sound recording was compared only with the conventional method of thermistors but not with direct measurements of airflow using a pneumotachygraph.

We simultaneously recorded the tracheal sound and pneumotachygraph signals

a) to analyze tracheal sounds and tidal volume during each sleep stage in healthy patients,
b) to compare these two methods for sleep apnea monitoring, and
c) to assess the usefulness of tracheal sounds for characterizing snores.

Methods

Patients. We studied ten subjects, four of whom were healthy men from our laboratory. None of the volunteers presented evidence of cardiorespiratory disease nor did they report disturbed nocturnal sleep. Four patients were known to have a sleep apnea syndrome. Two patients were snorers.

Polygraphic Recording. Each patient was subjected to an all-night polygraphic recording including sleep parameters, respiratory movements, and oxygen saturation (ear oxymeter: Hewlett-Packard 47 201 A). Respiratory flow rate was measured by a face-mask pneumotachygraph. The tracheal breath sounds were detected by a microphone (Brüel-Kjaer 4144) air-coupled to a stethoscope head (Littman).

Recording Analysis. The all-night recording was scored for sleep stages according to standard criteria [3]. Apnea was defined on the pneumotachygraph recording as a cessation of airflow for at least 10 s and on the sound signal as a complete lack of breath sounds for the same period. An episode of snoring involved snores occurring for at least 10 s. Snores with hypopnea were characterized by an expiratory sound area (Ae) lower than 50% of the wakefulness value and by a difference in phase of thoracic and abdominal signals. We measured, on healthy patient recordings, tidal volume (V_T) and Ae for each respiratory cycle over sample periods from each sleep stage.

Results

Breathing and Tracheal Sound

V_T and Ae were studied during quiet breathing periods in each sleep stage in four healthy patients. Two patients reached rapid eye movement sleep (REM sleep). V_T decreased from wakefulness to REM sleep (Fig. 1). Despite this reduction in V_T we observed an increase in Ae which was greater in all stages of sleep than in wakefulness (Fig. 2). For this reason the ratio of Ae to V_T was larger in all sleep stages than in wakefulness (Fig. 3).

Sensitivity and specificity of the tracheal sound recording for monitoring hypopnea (defined as a reduction of V_T below 50% of the wakefulness value) were 74% and 96%, respectively.

Apnea Monitoring

In the four patients with sleep apnea syndrome the number of apneas recorded by the two methods was the same. The duration of each apnea on the tracheal sound signal was similar to the duration measured on the pneumotachygraph recording. Thus there was a linear correlation between the two methods. For each patient the coefficient of correlation (r) and the slope of regression (A) relating the two values were equal to 1. The intercept (B) which characterizes the mean duration difference expressed in seconds ranged from −0.17 +0.31 (Table 1).

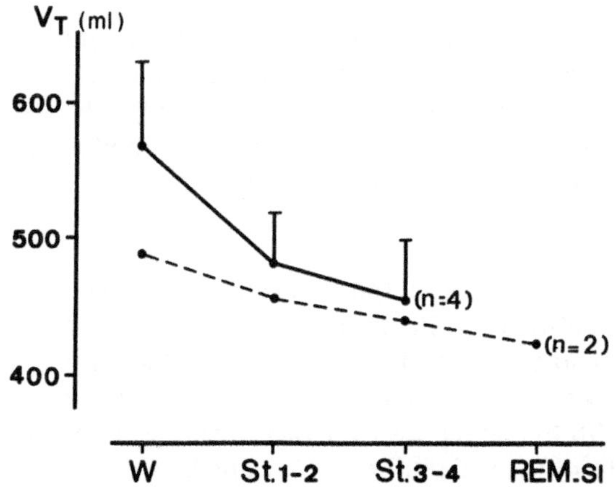

Fig. 1. Tidal volume *(V_T)* changes from wakefulness to REM sleep. The *continuous line* represents mean and standard deviation for the four healthy patients; the *broken line* represents mean for the two patients who reached REM sleep

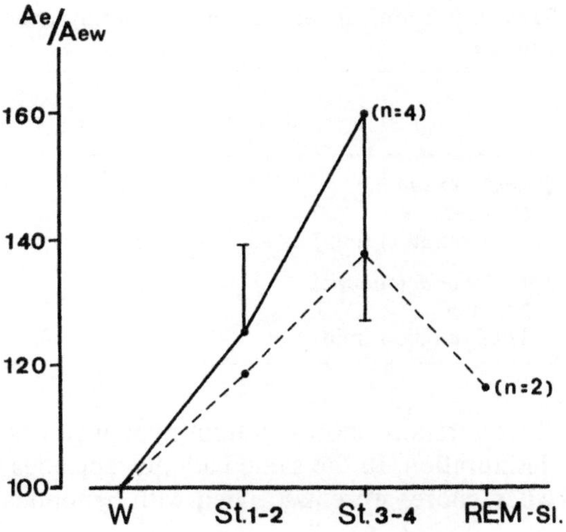

Fig. 2. Expiratory sound area *(Ae)* expressed as a percentage of the wakefulness value *(Aew)* during each sleep stage (same subjects as in Fig. 1)

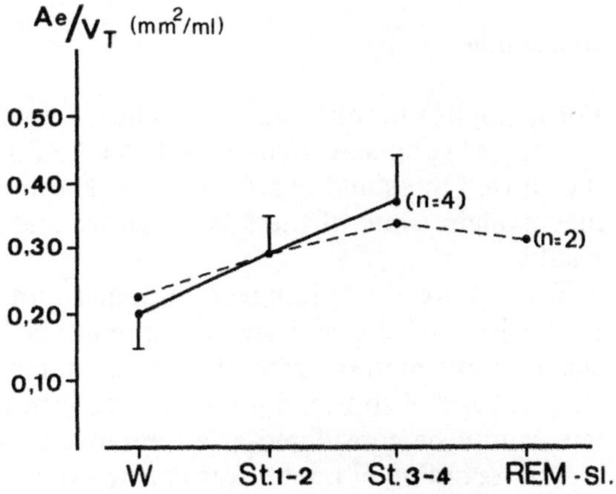

Fig. 3. Ae/V_T from wakefulness to REM sleep (same subjects as in Fig. 1)

Table 1. Apnea quantification by tracheal sound (TS) and pneumotachygraph (P) signals. For each patient the total number of apneas was the same with both methods. Apnea duration is the mean ± SD for all apneas recorded in each patient

Patient	Total number of apneas	Apnea duration (seconds) TS	P
1	147	19.1 ± 7.2	19.2 ± 7.2
2	432	40.3 ± 11.9	40.3 ± 11.9
3	43	23.2 ± 9.7	23.4 ± 9.8
4	659	26.8 ± 16.5	25.7 ± 16.4

Snore Monitoring

In two patients who experienced episodes of snoring, we studied the effects produced by snores with and without hypopnea on oxygen saturation. Whatever

Table 2. Effect of snores without and with hypopnea on oxygen saturation; A, B are the two patients

	Without hypopnea		With hypopnea	
	A	B	A	B
Episodes of snoring				
Number	6	29	43	26
Total duration (min)	6	128	80	14
Episodes of desaturation				
Number	0	1	43	10
Total duration (min)	0	0.45	35	4

their duration, snores without hypopnea were only exceptionally associated with desaturation. In the same patients, episodes of desaturation frequently occurred when snores were associated with hypopnea (Table 2).

Discussion

For hypopnea monitoring the tracheal sound method has high specificity (96%) and rather good sensitivity (74%). As Ae for a given V_T increases during sleep, the chosen threshold of 50% of the wakefulness value is probably too low, which may explain some of the false negative and the small number of false positive results.

There were no differences in apnea number and duration recorded by the tracheal sound method and the pneumotachygraph. When comparing the tracheal sound method with the thermistor method, apneas appear to be more frequent and of shorter duration on the former [2, 4]. Thus the thermistor technique cannot be considered as a reference method for monitoring airflow.

The recording of breath sound is the only method which allows the identification and analysis of snores. Furthermore, we can determine whether snores are associated with partial upper airway occlusion or not. Tracheal breath sound recording is a simple and noninvasive method for monitoring airflow during sleep. It is more accurate and provides more information than the conventional thermistor method.

References

1. Krumpe PE, Cummiskey JM (1980) Use of laryngeal sound recordings to monitor apnea. Am Rev Respir Dis 122:797–801
2. Cummiskey JH, Williams TC, Krumpe PE, Guilleminault C (1982) The detection and quantification of sleep apnea by tracheal sound recordings. Am Rev Respir Dis 126:221–224
3. Rechtschaffen A, Kales AA (1968) Manual of standardized terminology techniques and scoring systems for sleep stages of human subjects. National Institute of Health publication no. 204, Los Angeles
4. Peirick J, Shepard JW (1983) Automated apnoea detection by computer: analysis of tracheal breath sounds. Med Biol Eng Comput 21:632–635

Thoracoabdominal Motion in Health and Disease*

M. J. TOBIN

Investigators have long recognized that examination of chest wall motion provides valuable insights into the activity and coordination of the various respiratory muscles [1]. Over the last century most investigators concentrated on measuring only motion of the ribcage, but Mosso, in 1878, recognized the importance of also studying abdominal motion [2]. However, it was only in the past 20 years, following the landmark study of Konno and Mead [3], that investigators generally began to appreciate the independence and the interrelationship of ribcage-abdominal motion.

Normal Motion of the Ribcage and Abdomen

The primary function of the respiratory muscles is to expand the thoracic cavity, creating a negative intrathoracic pressure and facilitating ventilation. The mechanisms whereby the respiratory muscles increase the thoracic cavity is complex [1, 4, 5]. The diaphragm is the major muscle of respiration and to understand its action fully it is helpful to briefly review the anatomy. The costal fibers of the diaphragm arise from the lowest six ribs, run directly upwards, and are inserted into the central tendinous dome. As the fibers run upwards, they are apposed to the inner surface of the ribcage. This zone of apposition consists of up to one third of the surface area of the ribcage at end expiration, but less on inspiration [6]. With contraction of the diaphragm, the vertical fibers shorten causing the central dome to move down with little change in shape. This lowering of the floor of the thoracic cavity produces a fall in pleural pressure facilitating inspiration. In addition, the associated increase in abdominal pressure causes a visible, outward displacement of the anterior abdominal wall. Since the abdominal contents are basically incompressible (ignoring the 100 to 200 ml of intestinal gas), the diaphragm, abdominal contents, and abdominal wall move as a unit sharing the same volume displacement [7]. However, it is simplistic to consider that abdominal wall motion is quantitatively identical to diaphragmatic displacement as the diaphragm can also expand the ribcage by three different mechanisms. Firstly, the ribs act as if they are hinged to the vertebral column and the sternum, so that upward traction of the costal fibers of the diaphragm produces a

* This work was supported in part by a grant from the American Lung Association of Texas

"bucket handle" movement with lateral expansion and flaring. Secondly, resistance of the abdominal contents to the downward motion of the diaphragm serves as a fulcrum against which the diaphragm contracts with resulting elevation and expansion of the ribcage. Additional ribcage expansion occurs with contraction of the abdominal muscles, which further increase abdominal resistance to diaphragmatic motion. DeTroyer and others [5] have shown the importance of this fulcrum effect; removal of an animal's abdominal viscera changes the result of diaphragmatic contraction from ribcage expansion to a decrease in ribcage size. Finally, the direct transmission of abdominal pressure through the zone of apposition causes expansion of the lower ribcage. Owing to these many effects of the diaphragm on the ribcage, Goldman and Mead [8] hypothesized that the diaphragm was the only significantly active respiratory muscle. Subsequent studies, however, have shown that activation of the intercostal and scalene muscles are necessary for coordinated movement of the chest wall expecially in the erect posture [5]. In the supine position, this coupling relationship is less effective and diaphragmatic action may have little effect on the ribcage; thus, in this position abdominal motion provides a reasonable reflection of diaphragmatic displacement [9].

Important changes occur in the motion of the ribcage and abdomen with variations in body posture (Fig. 1). Ribcage expansion is greatest in the erect posture whereas abdominal expansion predominates when supine [10]. A combination of factors accounts for this postural variation in compartmental contribution

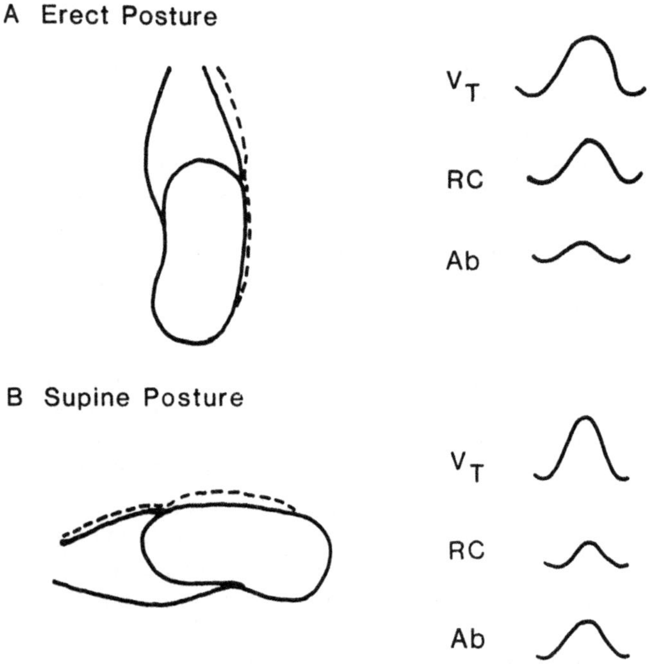

Fig. 1a, b. Ribcage *(RC)* contribution to tidal volume *(V_T)* is greatest in the erect posture whereas abdominal *(Ab)* contribution is greatest in the supine position (reproduced in part with permission from [1])

[1]. Firstly, compliance of the ribcage and abdomen varies with body posture; movement from the upright to the supine position is associated with approximately 40% decrease in ribcage compliance and a fourfold increase in abdominal compliance [11–13]. The reduction in abdominal compliance in the upright position, probably due to passive gravitational changes and active tonic contraction of the abdominal muscles [11, 12], increases the fulcrum effect of the abdominal compartment, thus enhancing the expansive action of the diaphragm on the ribcage and contributing to the greater ribcage movement in this posture. Secondly, the geometric configuration of the internal and external intercostal muscles varies with body posture [14]. In spite of the lower functional residual capacity (FRC) in the supine position, it is considered that the ribcage is more distended at resting end-expiration in the supine posture because gravity causes cephalad displacement of the diaphragm and the abdominal contents. Such ribcage distension stretches the internal (expiratory) intercostal muscles and shortens the external (inspiratory) intercostal muscles. This alteration in respiratory muscle geometry causes the external (inspiratory) intercostal muscle to generate less force for a given contraction since a shortened muscle fiber generates less force. Consequently, outward displacement of the ribcage during inspiration will be less prominent. Therefore, coupling between the diaphragm and the ribcage is less effective in the supine compared to the erect posture. Thirdly, the cephalad motion of the abdominal contents in the supine position due to gravity causes stretching of the diaphragmatic fibers and a reduction in their radius of curvature which, according to the length-tension relationship and Laplace's law, should result in increased diaphragmatic advantage. Finally, Druz and Sharp [15] have demonstrated that the inspiratory muscles which elevate the ribcage, i.e., external intercostal/accessory muscles, display less electromyographic (EMG) activity in the supine compared to the erect position.

Quantitation of Ribcage-Abdominal Motion

Konno and Mead demonstrated that the respiratory system possesses two degrees of freedom of motion, that is the ribcage and abdomen move independently of each other [3]. They also showed that it was possible to obtain indirect measurements of tidal volume with a high degree of accuracy by recording ribcage-abdominal motion using linearized differential transducers [3]. This has subsequently been demonstrated by other investigators using alternative techniques of recording ribcage-abdominal motion, such as magnetometry and inductive plethysmography [1, 16]. Such indirect methods of recording ventilation are especially advantageous in the detailed study of the respiratory cycle [10, 17], since they avoid the spurious alterations in the breathing pattern that inevitably accompany the use of a mouthpiece and noseclip [18, 19]. In their original paper, Konno and Mead also demonstrated the value of displaying the motion of the ribcage and abdomen on an XY plot in order to obtain a better understanding of the mechanisms that determine the pattern of ribcage-abdominal motion [3].

There are three basic types of ribcage-abdominal motion. During normal breathing, both the ribcage and abdomen expand on inspiration and decrease

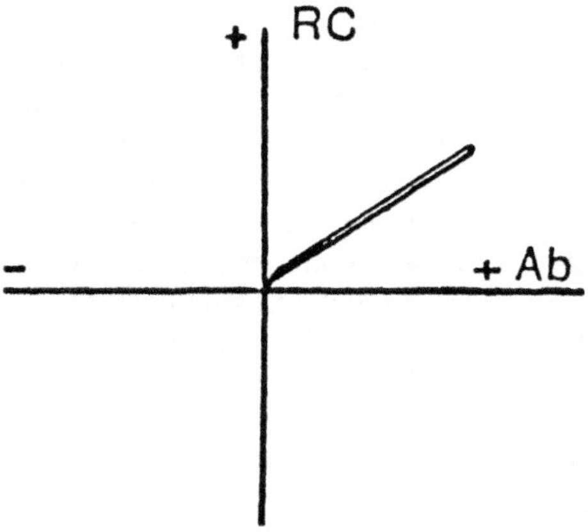

Fig. 2. During normal breathing, the ribcage *(RC)* and abdomen *(Ab)* move at a virtually identical rate, causing the formation of a closed or very slightly open loop when RC expansion is plotted against Ab expansion on an XY plot

back to the resting position during expiration. Since the rate of excursion is virtually the same for the two compartments, an XY plot of ribcage–abdominal motion shows the formation of a closed or a very slightly open loop (Fig. 2.) During asynchronous breathing, the two compartments continue to move in the same direction, but the rate of motion differs, causing an open loop to form on the XY plot. During paradoxical breathing, one compartment moves in an opposite direction to the overall sum or tidal volume signal, causing a portion of the plot of ribcage–abdominal motion to have a negative slope. Using this approach, it is possible to measure the relative contributions of the ribcage and abdomen to tidal volume on a breath-by-breath basis and to determine the phase relationship between motion of the two compartments using a number of indices of asynchrony and paradox.

The degree of asynchrony between ribcage and abdominal motion has been classically quantitated in terms of calculating the phase angle between the two compartments [20]. This computation is based on an analysis of sinusoidal phase shifts; however, it is important to bear in mind that the ribcage and abdomen do not move in a perfect sinusoidal manner. Agostoni and Mognoni [20] calculated the phase angle (Θ) according to the formula $\Theta = \sin^{-1} (m/s)$, where m is the distance between the intercepts of the ribcage–abdominal loop on a line drawn parallel to the X-axis and placed at half the distance between the maximum and minimum ribcage excursion, and s is the maximum excursion of the abdomen (Fig. 3). Asynchrony can also be separated into a component occurring during inspiration and one occurring on expiration. Inspiratory asynchrony can be quantitated by measuring the area enclosed by the inspiratory portion of the loop and a line connecting the commencement and termination of inspiration. Dividing this area by tidal volume normalizes the magnitude of inspiratory asynchrony for the extent of the excursion (Fig. 3). Expiratory asynchrony can be quantitated by a similar manipulation of the expiratory portion of the loop.

Paradoxical motion is found by comparing the direction of compartmental motion against that of the sum (tidal volume) signal. If a compartmental signal is negative (downgoing) when the sum signal is positive (upgoing), motion of that compartment is considered paradoxical at that moment in time (Fig. 3). When

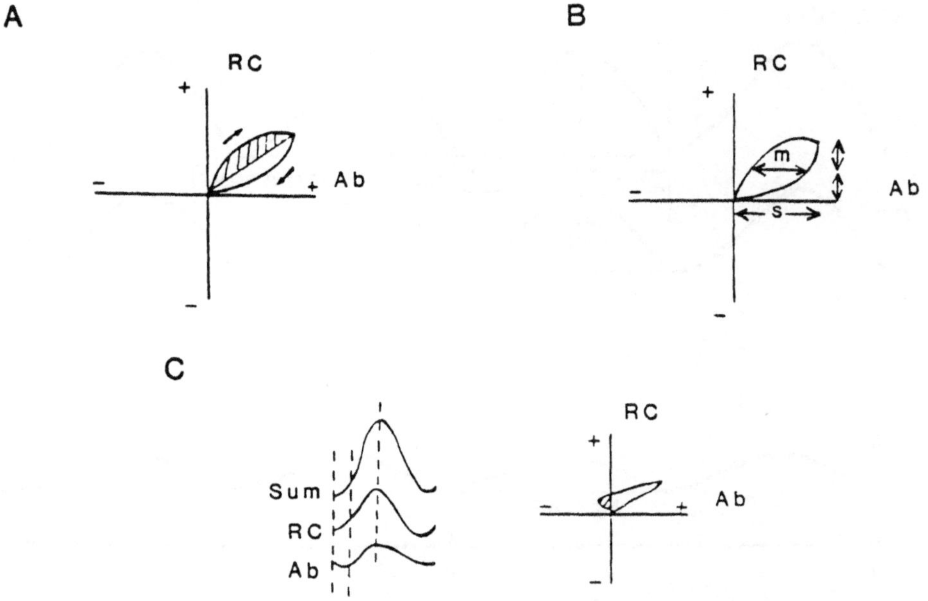

Fig. 3a-c. Derivation of the indices of asynchronous and paradoxical motion of the ribcage *(RC)* and abdomen *(Ab)*. **a** Inspiratory asynchrony is the *shaded area* enclosed by the inspiratory portion of the loop and the straight line connecting the initiation and completion of inspiration; this area is normalized by dividing by tidal volume. **b** Phase angle (Θ) is calculated according to the formula $\Theta = \sin^{-1} (m/s)$. **c** Abdominal paradox is calculated as the percentage of the *Ab* volume signal that is moving in an opposite direction to the sum (tidal volume) signal

displayed on an XY plot, a portion of the loop formed by the ribcage-abdominal excursion will have a negative slope. In order to quantitate the extent of paradoxical motion, the algebraic signs of the derivatives of the ribcage, abdominal, and sum signals are compared. The percentage of compartmental excursion that is out of phase with the sum signal is noted and integrated to obtain the volume. In turn, this volume is normalized for the extent of excursion by dividing by tidal volume. Thus, it is possible to derive four indices of paradoxical volume: inspiratory ribcage, expiratory ribcage, inspiratory abdominal, and expiratory abdominal. Similarly, the percentage of inspiratory and expiratory time that the ribcage and abdomen independently spend in paradoxical motion can be computed.

Another index, termed the maximum compartmental amplitude to tidal volume ratio (MCA/V_T), is a more sensitive but less specific measure of abnormal ribcage-abdominal motion [21]. It measures not only asynchrony but also paradoxical motion of *either* the ribcage or the abdomen. The maximum compartmental amplitude is calculated as the arithmetic sum of the absolute values of ribcage and abdominal excursions irrespective of their phase relationship, whereas the measurement of tidal volume is based on the algebraic sum, which takes into account the phase differences between the two compartments (Fig. 4).

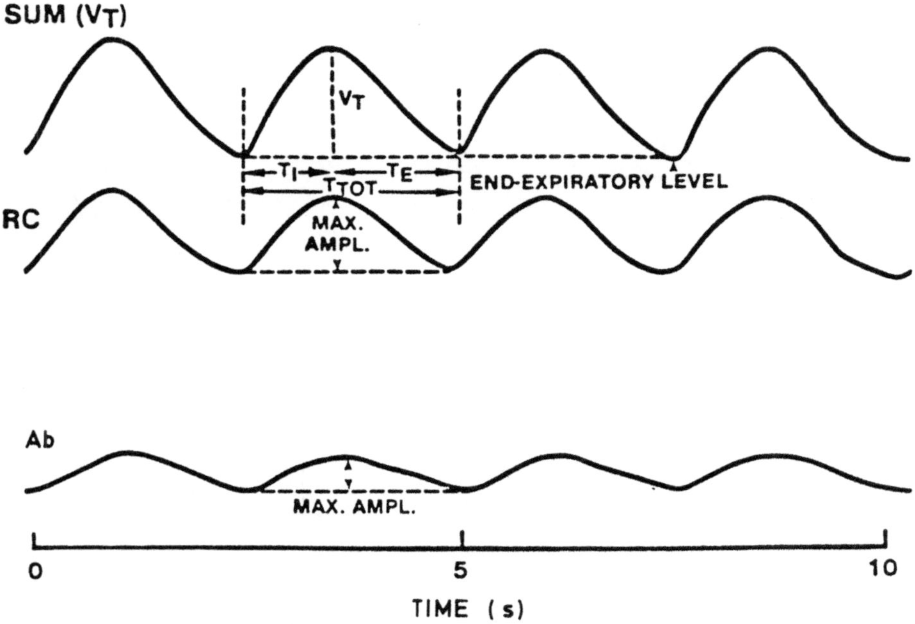

Fig. 4. Schematic recording of the respiratory cycle, depicting the points of reference for calculation of the maximum compartmental amplitude to tidal volume ratio *(MCA/*V_T*)* and other breathing pattern parameters. *MCA* is the arithmetic sum of the maximum amplitudes of ribcage *(RC)* and abdominal *(Ab)* excursions, irrespective of their phase relationship to the algebraic sum signal (*SUM* V_T*)*. When the RC and Ab move in phase with each other, the *MCA/*V_T ratio is equivalent to 1.0. When there is asynchrony or paradoxical motion of the compartments, the *MCA/*V_T ratio is greater than 1.0. T_I is the inspiratory, T_E the expiratory, and T_{TOT} the total breath duration. (Reproduced with permission from [35]).

The MCA/V_T ratio is equivalent to 1.0 when the trough to peak amplitudes of the ribcage and abdominal signals are in phase with the sum signal. When the two compartments display either asynchronous or paradoxical motion, the MCA/V_T ratio exceeds 1.0.

It has been considered that fluctuation between the two major groups of respiratory muscles, the intercostal/accessory muscle group and the diaphragm, may serve as a predictor of respiratory muscle fatigue [22, 23]. Such recruitment and derecruitment of the different muscle groups, which has been termed *respiratory alternans,* can be detected by noting variations in the relative contributions of the ribcage and abdomen to tidal volume. In the original description of this phenomenon [22, 23], the extent of fluctuation was not quantitated. One method of quantitating the breath-to-breath variation in compartmental contribution is to compute the standard deviation of the ribcage to tidal volume ratio over a fixed period of time.

Clinical Significance of Abnormal Ribcage - Abdominal Motion

Calculation of the quantitative indices of abnormal ribcage-abdominal motion, as described in the preceding section, has been obtained in only a few clinical settings [17, 24–26]. However, it is well recognized that patients with cervical cord lesions display severe paradoxical motion of the ribcage, whereas patients with diaphragmatic paralysis display severe abdominal paradox. Recently, there has been considerable interest in the study of ribcage-abdominal motion in patients with diseases of the respiratory system which do not primarily involve the chest wall. Ashutosh, Gilbert, and colleagues [27, 28] noted that patients displaying abnormal motion of the ribcage and abdomen had an increased risk of ventilatory failure necessitating mechanical ventilation [28], and they also had a poor prognosis [27]. Subsequently, Macklem and associates [23, 29, 30] suggested that paradoxical motion of the abdomen could serve as a valuable sign of respiratory muscle fatigue. They state, "This sign is present continuously in diaphragmatic paralysis; but if it develops over a period of minutes or hours, it is virtually pathognomonic of diaphragmatic fatigue" [30]. The rationale behind this proposal is that in the presence of ineffectual diaphragmatic contraction, negative intrathoracic pressure generated by the other respiratory muscles pulls up the diaphragm and causes the anterior abdominal wall to be sucked inwards. Little experimental evidence has been provided to support this reasoning and the interpretation is largely based on a study of patients displaying difficulties during weaning from mechanical ventilation, who demonstrated the combination of abdominal paradox and a shift in the power spectrum of their diaphragmatic electromyogram (EMG) [23]. The authors considered these EMG changes to reflect diaphragmatic fatigue. However, the observation of an association does not necessarily mean a cause and effect relationship. Moreover, a shift in the EMG power spectrum has not been shown to be related to the form of fatigue that is physiologically significant, i.e., low-frequency fatigue [31]. In addition, no attempt was made to separate the effect of abnormal pulmonary mechanics from that of muscle fatigue in the pathogenesis of the abnormal chest wall motion.

We recently addressed this question in two groups of motivated healthy subjects by having them breathe against inspiratory resistive loads [25]. We induced respiratory muscle fatigue by the method of Roussos and Macklem and others [22, 32]. The subjects breathed against an inspiratory resistive load while maintaining 60% of their predetermined maximum mouth pressure in a square-wave fashion. Based on the accepted definition of skeletal muscle fatigue, i.e., the inability to maintain a predetermined load, we considered that all of the respiratory muscles were fatigued at the time when the subject could no longer achieve the target mouth pressure [22, 32]. Quantitative assessment of the extent of ribcage-abdominal asynchrony and paradox was obtained by computing several indices from a series of breaths at fixed time periods from the Konno-Mead plot. The data were obtained using a calibrated respiratory inductive plethysmograph. We reasoned that if muscle fatigue was the primary determinant of abnormal ribcage-abdominal motion, the indices of asynchrony and paradox should be significantly higher during the first few minutes of recovery compared to baseline, because physiologically significant fatigue is known to persist for several

Table 1. Effect of inducing respiratory muscle fatigue on indices of ribcage—abdominal motion

	Baseline	Generating 60% of Pm_{max} First minute	Fatigue point	Recovery
Phase angle (degrees)	8.0 ± 2.0	58 ± 24	71 ± 19	11.0 ± 2.0
RC paradox (% volume)	0.5 ± 0.1	6 ± 3	9 ± 3	0.3 ± 0.2
Ab paradox (% volume)	0.5 ± 0.2	28 ± 14	35 ± 12	4.0 ± 2.0
	└ $p < 0.02$ ┘	└ p NS ┘	└ $p < 0.02$ ┘	

$n = 6$; *RC*, ribcage; *Ab*, abdominal; Pm_{max}, maximal mouth pressure

hours after induction [31]. Also, the values should be greater at the end compared to the beginning of the loaded breathing run, because fatigue is present at the end but not at the beginning of the run, while the level of the respiratory load is the same in the two instances. The results in Table 1 show that the degree of asynchrony (represented by phase angle) and inspiratory paradoxical volume of the ribcage and abdomen increased from baseline during the 1st min of loaded breathing but displayed no further progression from the beginning to the end of the fatigue run. There was an immediate reduction in the extent of asynchrony and paradox upon discontinuation of the load. Breath-to-breath variability in compartmental contribution to tidal volume (*respiratory alternans*) showed a similar response pattern.

In a second experiment the subjects breathed against two levels of load: one was sufficient to require the generation of 30% of maximum mouth pressure (Pm_{max}) and the other was sufficient to require the generation of 60% of Pm_{max}. Comparing the indices during baseline breathing and these two levels of load, we found that the degrees of asynchrony and paradox were significantly related to the level of the load ($p < 0.003$). Of particular importance was the fact that we observed significant asynchrony, paradox, and breath-to-breath variability in compartmental motion in the subjects while generating only 30% of Pm_{max}, a level of mouth pressure that can be sustained indefinitely without fatigue [32]. From these experiments we concluded that asynchronous and paradoxical motion of the ribcage and abdomen are predominantly due to abnormalities in pulmonary mechanics rather than respiratory muscle fatigue.

These findings are more consistent with the traditional rather than the current interpretation of the clinical significance of abdominal paradox. Over 60 years before Hoover's description of lateral ribcage paradox in patients with emphysema [33], Austin Flint [34] wrote, "If the emphysema be accompanied by bronchial obstruction, the lower part of the sternum, the epigastrium, and the inferior part of the chest, laterally, are depressed with inspiration, the natural movements being reversed."

In conclusion, the development of methods to examine ribcage-abdominal motion has yielded important insights into the normal activity of the different respiratory muscle groups in healthy subjects and has also facilitated the study of breathing patterns without requiring instrumentation directly attached to the airway. In addition we are beginning to acquire a better understanding of the pathophysiological basis of abnormal patterns of ribcage-abdominal motion and to develop a clearer appreciation of their clinical significance.

References

1. Tobin MJ (1986) Non-invasive evaluation of respiratory movement. In: Nochomovitz ML, Cherniack NS (eds) Contemporary issues in pulmonary disease: non-invasive respiratory monitoring, vol 4, Churchill-Livingstone, New York, pp 29–57
2. Mosso A (1878) Über die gegenseitigen Beziehungen der Bauch- und Brustatmung. Arch Anat Physiol 5:441–468
3. Konno K, Mead J (1967) Measurement of the separate volume changes of ribcage and abdomen during breathing. J Appl Physiol 22:407–422
4. Sharp JT (1983) The respiratory muscles in emphysema. Clin Chest Med 4:421–432
5. DeTroyer A (1984) Actions of the respiratory muscles on how the chest wall moves in upright man. Bull Eur Physiopathol Respir 20:409–413
6. Mead J (1979) Functional significance of the area of apposition of diaphragm to ribcage. Am Rev Respir Dis 119:31–32
7. Grimby G, Goldman M, Mead J (1976) Respiratory muscle action inferred from ribcage and abdominal v-p partitioning. J Appl Physiol 41:739–751
8. Goldman MD, Mead J (1973) Mechanical interaction between the diaphragm and ribcage. J Appl Physiol 35:197–204
9. Macklem PT (1981) Normal and abnormal function of the diaphragm. Thorax 36:161–163
10. Tobin MJ, Chadha TS, Jenouri G, Birch SJ, Gazeroglu HB, Sackner MA (1983) Breathing patterns: 1. Normal subjects. Chest 84:202–205
11. Konno K, Mead J (1968) Static volume-pressure characteristics of the ribcage and abdomen. J Appl Physiol 24:544–548
12. De Troyer A (1983) Mechanical action of the abdominal muscles. Bull Eur Physiopathol Respir 19:575–581
13. Estenne M, Yernault JC, De Troyer A (1986) Ribcage and diaphragm-abdomen compliance in humans: effects of age and posture. J Appl Physiol 59:1842–1848
14. Gothe B, Bruce EN, Goldman MD (1984) Influence of sleep state on respiratory muscle function. In: Saunders NA, Sullivan CE (eds) Sleep and breathing. Dekker, New York, pp 241–282
15. Druz WS, Sharp JT (1981) Activity of respiratory muscles in upright and recumbent humans. J Appl Physiol 51:1552–1561
16. Mead J, Peterson N, Grimby G, Mead J (1967) Pulmonary ventilation measured from body surface movements. Science 156:1383–1384
17. Tobin MJ, Chadha TS, Jenouri G, Birch SJ, Gazeroglu HB, Sackner MA (1983) Breathing patterns: 2. Diseased subjects. Chest 84:286–294
18. Gilbert R, Auchincloss JH, Brodsky J, Broden W (1972) Changes in tidal volume, frequency, and ventilation induced by their measurement. J Appl Physiol 33:252–254
19. Perez W, Tobin MJ (1985) Separation of factors responsible for change in breathing pattern induced by instrumentation. J Appl Physiol 59:1515–1520
20. Agostoni E, Mognoni P (1966) Deformation of the chest wall during breathing efforts. J Appl Physiol 21:1827–1832
21. Tobin MJ, Jenouri G, Lind B, Watson H, Schneider A, Sackner MA (1983) Validation of the respiratory inductive plethysmograph in patients with pulmonary disease. Chest 83:615–620
22. Roussos C, Fixley M, Gross D; Macklem PT (1979) Fatigue of inspiratory muscles and their synergic behavior. J Appl Physiol 46:897–904
23. Cohen CA, Zagelbaum G, Gross E, Roussos C, Macklem PT (1982) Clinical manifestations of inspiratory muscle fatigue. Am J Med 73:308–316
24. Sackner MA, Gonzalez H, Rodriguez M, Belsito A, Sackner DR, Grenvik S (1984) Assessment of asychronous and paradoxic motion between ribcage and abdomen in normal subjects and in patients with chronic obstructive pulmonary disease. Am Rev Respir Dis 130:588–593

25. Tobin MJ, Perez W, Guenther SM, Lodato RF, Dantzker DR (1987) Does ribcage-abdominal paradox signify respiratory muscle fatigue? J Appl Physiol (to be published)
26. Tobin MJ, Guenther SM, Perez W, Lodato RF, Mador MJ, Allen SJ, Dantzker DR (1987) Konno-Mead analysis of ribcage-abdominal motion during successful and unsuccessful trials of weaning from mechanical ventilation. Am Rev Respir Dis 135:1320–1328
27. Ashutosh K, Gilbert R, Auchincloss JH, Peppi D (1975) Asynchronous breathing movements in patients with chronic obstructive pulmonary disease. Chest 67:553–557
28. Gilbert R, Ashutosh K, Auchincloss JH, et al (1977) Prospective study of controlled oxygen therapy: poor prognosis of patients with asynchronous breathing. Chest 71:456–462
29. Roussos C, Macklem PT (1982) The respiratory muscles. N Engl J Med 307:786–797
30. Grassino A, Macklem PT (1984) Respiratory muscle fatigue and ventilatory failure. Annu Rev Med 35:625–647
31. Moxham J, Edwards HT, Aubier M, DeTroyer A, Farkas G, Macklem PT, Roussos C (1982) Changes in EMG power spectrum (high-to-low) with force fatigue in humans. J Appl Physiol 53:1094–1099
32. Roussos CS, Macklem PT (1977) Diaphragmatic fatigue in man. J Appl Physiol 43:189–197
33. Hoover CF (1920) The diagnostic significance of inspiratory movements of the costal margins. Am J Med Sci 159:633–646
34. Flint A (1856) Physical exploration and diagnosis of diseases affecting the respiratory organs. Blanchard and Lea, Philadelphia
35. Tobin MJ, Jenouri G, Birch S, Lind B, Gonzalez H, Ahmed T, Sackner MA (1983) Effect of positive end expiratory pressure on breathing patterns of normal subjects and intubated patients with respiratory failure. Crit Care Med 11:859–867

Assessment of the Time Structure of Sleep Apneas

F. Raschke, J. Mayer, T. Penzel, J. H. Peter, T. Podszus,
and P. von Wichert

The apnea index serves as a quantitative indication of the seriousness of the disorder [1]. It makes use of the total number of apneic episodes per hour without respect to their duration. However, frequent, long-lasting episodes may lead to a threatening drop in oxygen saturation, eventhough the apnea index will show reduced values. An additional assessment of each apnea length, separated into central, obstructive, or mixed apnea seems invaluable in the differential diagnosis of the pathogenetic components contributing to the sleep apnea syndrome. We therefore developed an automatic procedure which enables, with high accuracy, a computerized evaluation of apnea length.

Methods

Figure 1 gives a pattern of EEG (C_z - O_2), EOG (diagonal), arterial blood pressure (brachial), abdominal respiratory movements (inductive plethysmography), and nasal thermistor recording. The respiratory pattern is characterized by three phases. The first is hyperventilation after preceding obstructive apnea, starting with an inspiratory effort. This phase is typically accompanied [7] by a transient increase in arterial blood pressure and heart rate [4]. The second phase represents central apnea (no flow changes, flat abdominal respiration curve with cardiac artifacts). In the third phase, abdominal movements return, whereas nasal flow still shows little change. The occlusion is terminated during inspiration, initiating another hyperpneic episode. For evaluation of apnea length thermal nasal registration was used, because it produces few artifacts from body movements and transducer displacement.

In Fig. 2 the procedure is developed from top to bottom. The nasal flow curve (A) is recorded with an epoch length of 150 s (1024 data points, sampling rate f_s = 6.8267 Hz). This sequence length turned out to be essential for correct respiratory time estimation, due to the considerable changes in amplitude and shape of the respiratory pattern. In a previously developed pattern recognition procedure [6], we used an epoch length of 18.75 s, which gave the best accuracy for normal breathing during sleep. The entire record of 150 s is derived (B), and the positive changes are used. Squaring, smoothing without phase error, and erasing those values below 2% of the absolute maximum of each record leads to C. This procedure takes into account long-term changes in amplitude, biasing, cardiac arti-

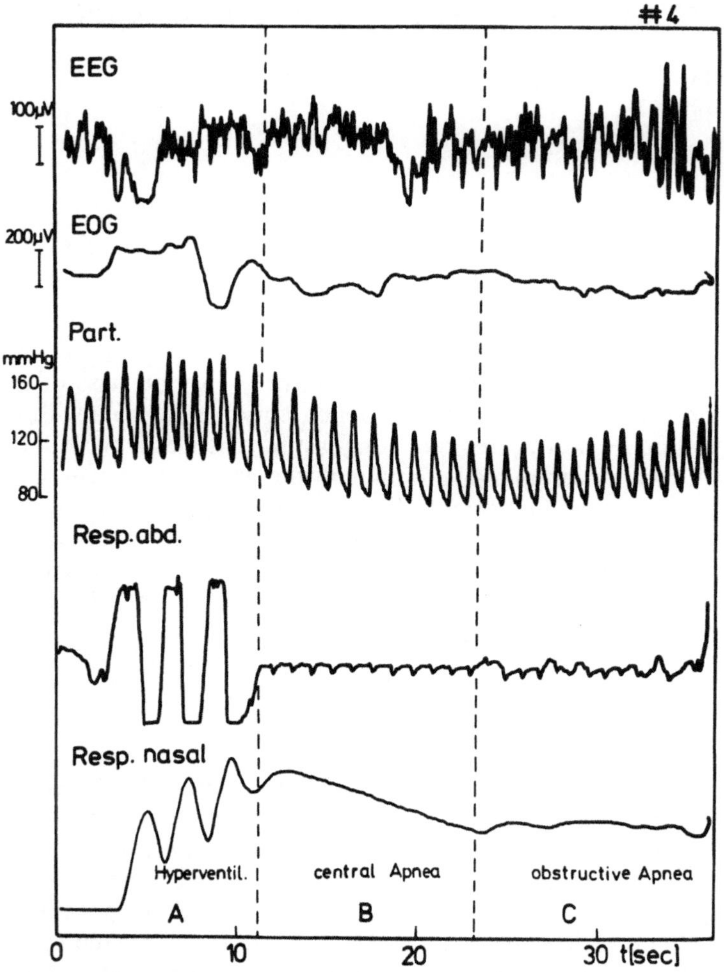

Fig. 1. 35-s record of *EEG, EOG,* brachial artery pressure *(Part.),* abdominal movements *(Resp. abd.),* and nasal flow curve *(Resp. nasal).* Sequences of respiration are separated into: **A,** hyperventilation; **B,** central apnea; and **C,** obstructive apnea

facts, nonbiphasic respiratory cycles, and interindividual differences. From C each onset of positive values is taken as inspiratory onset, whereas the relative maxima in A are taken as expiratory onsets. Magnitude of inspiratory flow ("tidal volume") V_T and respiratory times (T_I) are given in D and E. This pattern analysis yields good accuracy as compared to an analysis by hand (error $< 3\%$).

From total sleep time we analyzed contiguous records of 150 s, and plotted histograms of the interval times between inspiratory onsets.

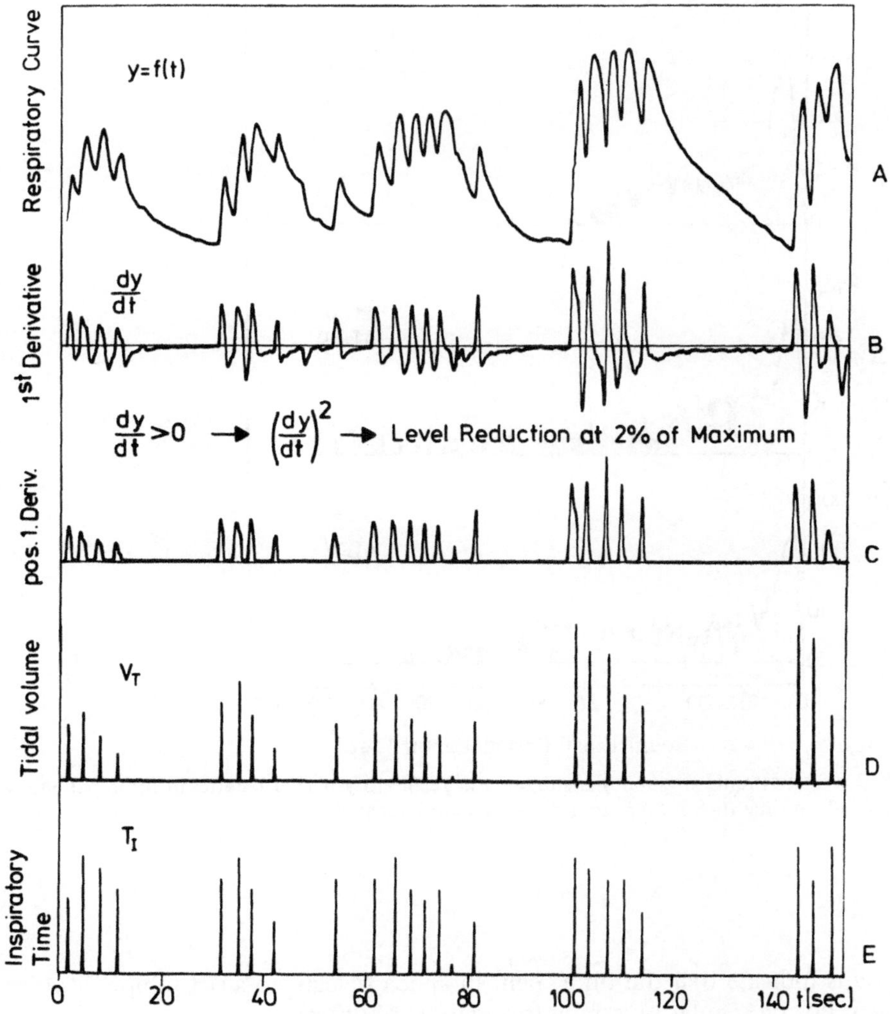

Fig. 2. Automatic procedure for assessment of respiratory times. For details confer text. *pos. 1. Deriv.*, positive first derivative

Results

In Fig. 3 three histograms are given from different patients, whose apnea indices are indicated. The frequency of events is plotted on a logarithmic scale. The histograms reveal on the left side ($\tau < 10$ s) a rather normal distribution of respiratory period length. It is caused by intermittent, regular, hypopneic, or hyperpneic breathing. The broad distribution on the right represents a rather randomized duration of respiratory cycles. These include inspiratory and expiratory times of normal breaths with consecutive mixed apnea duration. These histo-

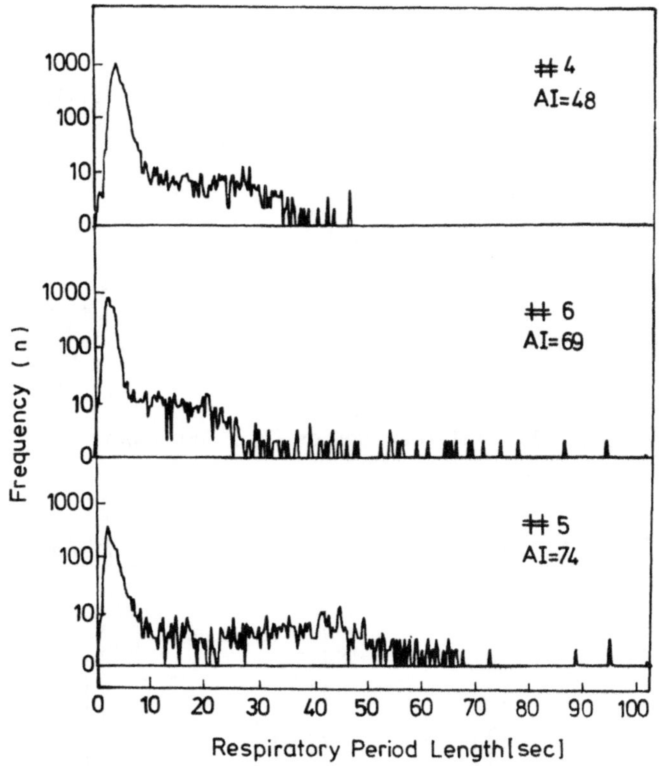

Fig. 3. Logarithmic frequency histograms of respiratory period lengths in three patients over total sleep time (6–8 h). Apnea indices *(AI)* are indicated

grams indicate that the time spent in apnea reveals no strict temporal order as seen during regular breathing (normal distribution).

Discussion

We have developed a procedure enabling an automatic analysis of apnea duration. A broad distribution of apnea length (they can last for 90 s or more) must be related to various components. Although a clearcut separation of central and obstructive apnea length is not possible using only the thermistor records, it is presumed that the random distributions are not related to autonomous control mechanisms. Pure mechanical factors of obstruction may play the main role. Even distinct cycle times of periodic breathing which should lead to bimodal distributions have not been found. Krieger et al. [3] have established histograms of central and obstructive apnea length by hand, and found left-skewed unimodal distributions. They pointed out the high incidence of obstructive apneas which makes these results just comparable to ours, if one considers the logarithmic scale. There is a close relationship between the duration of obstruction and oxygen desaturation on the one hand, and the frequency of obstruction and nocturnal pulmonary [5, 7] and arterial [4] hypertension on the other. The data presented by these authors clearly show that the magnitude of phasic hypertension essentially depends on the duration of obstructive episodes. A combined elaborated index, using number and duration [2] therefore should replace the apnea index, in order to improve the discrimination for seriousness and risk factors of the sleep apnea syndrome. The automatic procedure described here presents an easily programmable approach, enabling further improvements of the criteria describing sleep-related respiratory, cardiovascular, and pulmonary disorders.

References

1. Guilleminault C, von den Hoed J, Mitler MM (1978) Clinical overview of the sleep apnea syndromes. In: Guilleminault C, Dement WC (eds) Sleep apnea syndromes. Liss, New York, pp 1-12
2. Haidmayer R, Pfeiffer KP, Kenner T, Kurz R (1982) Statistical evaluation of respiratory control in infants to assess possible risk for the sudden infant death syndrome (SIDS). Eur J Pediatr 138:145-150
3. Krieger J, Turlot JC, Mangin P, Kurtz D (1983) Breathing during sleep in normal young and elderly subjects: hypopneas, apneas, and correlated factors. Sleep 6:108-120
4. Mayer J, Herres B, Kloss T, Penzel T, Peter JH, von Wichert P (1986) Nocturnal blood pressure behavior in sleep apnea (SA). Sleep Res 15:144
5. Podszus T (1986) Pulmonary arterial and right atrial blood pressure changes during obstructive sleep apnea. Bull Eur Physiopathol Respir 22 [suppl 8]:27
6. Raschke F (1982) Automatic pattern recognition of the onset of respiratory phases using thermistor techniques. In: Stott FD, Raftery EB, Clement DL, Wright SL (eds) ISAM - Gent - 1982. Academic, London, pp 349-358
7. Schroeder JS, Motta J, Guilleminault C (1978) Hemodynamic studies in sleep apnea. In: Guilleminault C, Dement WC (eds) Sleep apnea syndromes. Liss, New York, pp 177-196

An Apnea-Monitoring Device Based on Variation of Heart Rate and Snoring*

J. H PETER, E. FUCHS, M. HÜGENS, U. KOEHLER, K. MEINZER, U. MÜLLER, P. VON WICHERT, and M. ZAHORKA

Introduction

Sleep apnea syndromes are complex clinical pictures. The underlying sleep-induced disturbance of the respiratory regulation causes periodic nocturnal haltings of breathing which are defined as apneas when they last longer than 10 s. The therapeutic reduction of sleep apnea activity (SAA) leads to a reversal of the accompanying symptoms and findings if the disease is recognized and treated during its early stages.

The chief symptoms of sleep apnea syndromes (SAS) affect the patients' psychophysical well-being via deterioration in performance, depressions, and hypersomnia (especially excessive daytime sleepiness, EDS) as well as insomnia during the night. On the other hand, the cardiovascular and cardiopulmonary systems are affected: cardiac insufficiency is one of the key symptoms. Clinical findings in SAS include reduced sleep latency in the EEG, loud and irregular snoring, nocturnal cardiac arrhythmias, systemic and pulmonary arterial hypertension, polyglobulism, adiposis, and metabolic disorders.

The pathological link between sleep or vigilance regulation on the one hand and respiratory control on the other, which is found in patients with SA, explains the wide variety of symptoms and signs. The picture of SAS is a result of the disturbance of the physiological sleep structure by fragmentation and of sleep deprivation. Hypoxia, hypercapnia, acidosis, intrathoracic pressure changes during apnea, and increased catecholamine release during the intermittent activations of the central nervous system in response to apnea contribute to a medium-term severe functional impairment in the cardiocirculatory system. SAS are a frequent cause for sudden nocturnal death. Middle-aged men are especially affected.

The life-threatening dimension of SAS and the possibility of reversing later damage only when the disease is found in time present a challenge to develop an economical procedure of early SAA diagnosis. The high prevalence of the disease strengthens this necessity. Until now, there has been no sufficiently reliable diagnostic procedure which would at the same time be inexpensive and easy to apply. The compact 4-channel unit which we developed earlier for the simul-

* This project was supported by a grant "Meßtechnik in der Medizin" from GSF, Munich, Federal Ministery of Research and Technology, Bonn.

taneous recordings of ECG, 2-channel inductive plethysmography, and transcutaneous partial oxygen tension (pO_2tc) [1] is certainly reliable and valuable in research projects. It is, however, believed to be too complicated for series production and routine use. Still, we have been able in 5 years of research activity to conduct more than 3000 ambulatory measurements with this system,. and we have used it side by side with polysomnographic studies in the sleep laboratory in more than 150 cases. While searching for a reliable and easy-to-use diagnostic unit for general aplications, we have concentrated on the development of a device based on snoring patterns and heart rate behavior.

Methods

By combining ambulatory and stationary diagnostics, we were able to test the suitability and accuracy of many individual parameters in patients with SAA of all degrees and intensities, particularly with regard to the diagnostical cost and effect. We could not find any individual parameter which alone could serve as a simple and reliable indicator of SAA.

Selection of the ECG Criterion

The ECG can be easily applied and works with a minimum of technical apparatus. Heart rate can be continuously calculated from beat to beat. The heart rate pattern which is typical for sleep apnea is the so-called „cyclical variation of the heart rate" (CVHR) [2, 3]. This is characterized by falling heart rate during apnea, and heart-rate accelerations coinciding with apnea-terminating hyperventilation. As a consequence, patients with SAS exhibit a significantly higher variation of the heart rate values during periods of maximum SAA than in periods without or with very low SAA [4]. The variance of the heart rate values in terms of sinus arrhythmia is, however, subject to extreme interindividual differences. Therefore the criterion of "variance" was found to be not very helpful as an absolute figure. Moreover, sinus arrhythmia decreases with age, and is also greatly diminished with increasing damage to the heart. This again would defeat the purpose of the criterion in apnea screening, as diagnosing older men, who frequently suffer from SAA in combination with cardiac impairments, would be especially difficult on the basis of this parameter.

Interindividual differences can be eliminated when not the variance of the heart rate values but their deviation from the values obtained during periods of stable heart rate is used as a criterion for the determination of cyclical variation. By taking the temporal course of heart rate behavior into consideration, intraindividual periods of extreme heart rate variation can be determined. This is accomplished by calculating the heart rate over a moving window of 5 min, determining the moving average value, and indicating those points of time where the actual heart rate shows a deviation $> 20\%$ from the moving average. The period between any two of such time marks is rated as a period of constant heart rate. In a comparison of 12 patients with pronounced SAA ($\geqq 10$ episodes/h sleep) and 12 subjects with low SAA (< 5 episodes/h sleep) we found that periods of constant heart rate lasting only 21–40 s were significantly more frequent in patients with SAA. The heart rate behavior of people without SAA is characterized in contrast by comparatively long periods of constant heart rate.

Selection of the Snoring Parameter

As the criterion "heart rate stability" - or rather "significant deviation from constant heart rate" - loses much of its discriminating value in older patients (as these deviations become less pronounced with the general decrease in heart rate variability with advancing age) we looked for a second parameter which would not have this disadvantage and could serve as a supplementary indicator to the analysis of heart rate in apnea screening. Snoring fulfills these requirements. As opposed to cyclical variation of the heart rate, snoring increases with age. The reduction of cyclical variation is compensated by the amplification of snoring, so that in any age group sufficiently clear results can be obtained. Snoring is also highly specific for SAA: all patients with SAS snore loudly and irregularly. In addition, the recording and evaluation of snoring sounds is technically simple and can be accomplished without invasive methods.

In order to extract from the electroacoustic sound recording a parameter suitable for investigation, we first used a Fourier analysis.

Figure 1 shows a typical power spectrum of snoring noises in apnea patients. Snoring is characterized by high power in the low-frequency range, whereas normal inspiratory and expiratory sounds are reflected by greater intensities of higher frequencies. Figure 2 shows a typical snoring pattern recorded by a laryngeal microphone in combination with respiratory parameters. Having established the existence of apnea-specific snoring events, we constructed a miniaturized filter bank which can be easily fitted into a portable recording unit. This filter bank permits a continuous analysis of snoring noises on the basis of preselected specific frequencies. A detailed description of this method is now being prepared by one of the authors, T. Penzel.

Results

The validity and reliability of the criteria "deviation from constant heart rate" and "snoring frequencies in breathing sounds" were tested in the sleep laboratory. Both are reliable indicators of sleep apnea, the heart rate criterion working better in younger patients and the snoring sound recording in older patients. In middle-aged patients, both worked equally well, as the sample recording shown in Fig. 3 indicates.

Based upon preparatory work in the sleep laboratory, we were able to develop a simple portable device for apnea screening. It includes parameters taken from the ECG beat-to-beat registration and the continuous recording of apnea-specific snoring noise. Figure 4 shows a scheme of the device with a laryngeal micro-

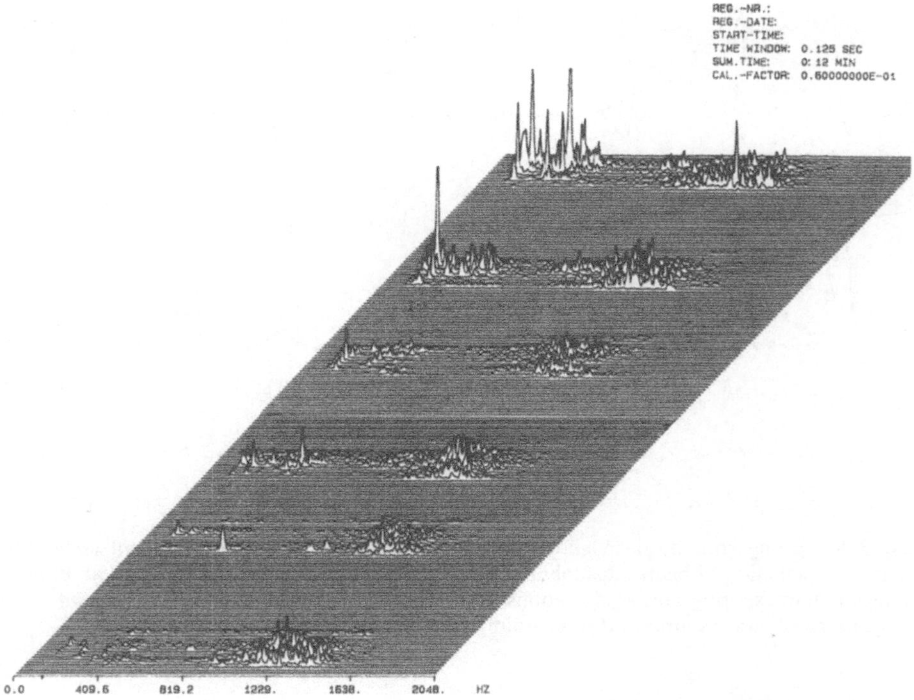

Fig. 1. Power spectra of breathing sounds, calculated once every 0.125 s. The peak intensities in the lower frequency range *(left)* are typical of snoring

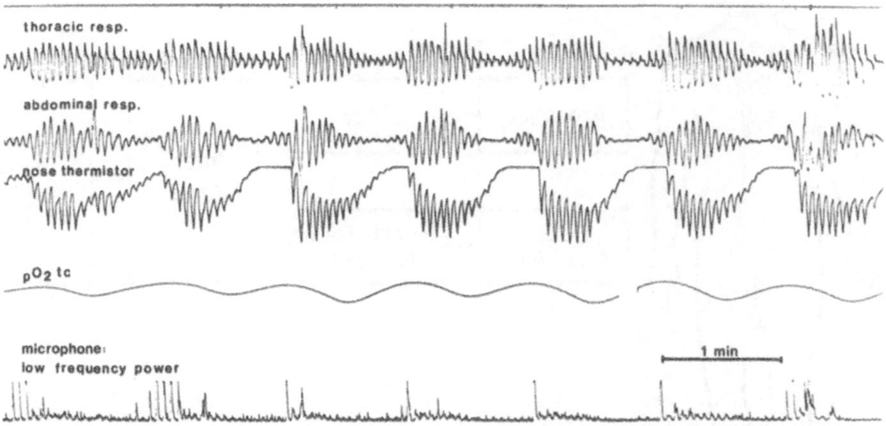

Fig. 2. Apnea recording, including low frequency power of breathing sounds recorded with a laryngeal microphone. Apneas are indicated in the recordings of thoracic and abdominal respirations (inductive plethysmography) and respiratory flow (nasal thermistor) as well as partial arterial oxygen tension. The termination of the apnea episodes is reflected by high power in the sound recording

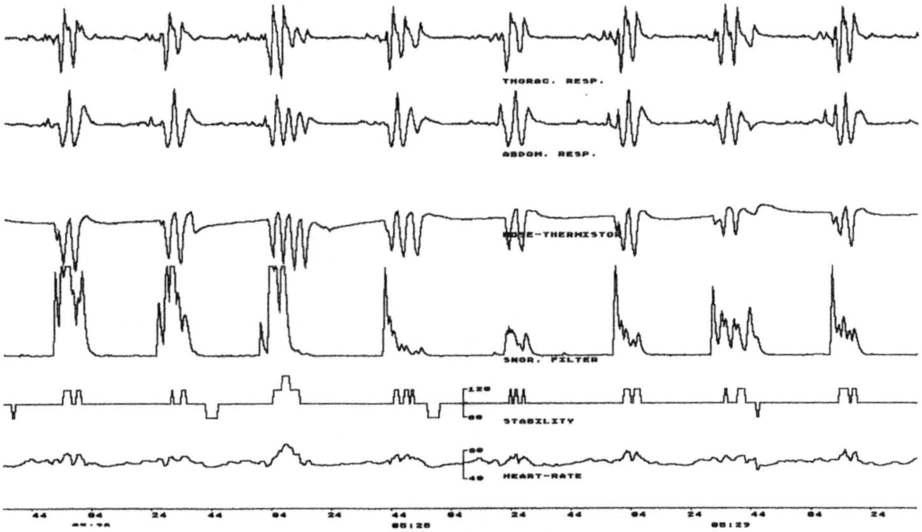

Fig. 3. Recording from the sleep laboratory, including the signal from the filter bank (*snor.* filter) and the calculation of heart rate stability. The moving average of heart rate is added. Both the indications of snoring and of deviations > 20% from constant heart rate correspond to the indications of apnea found in the recordings of the respiratory parameters

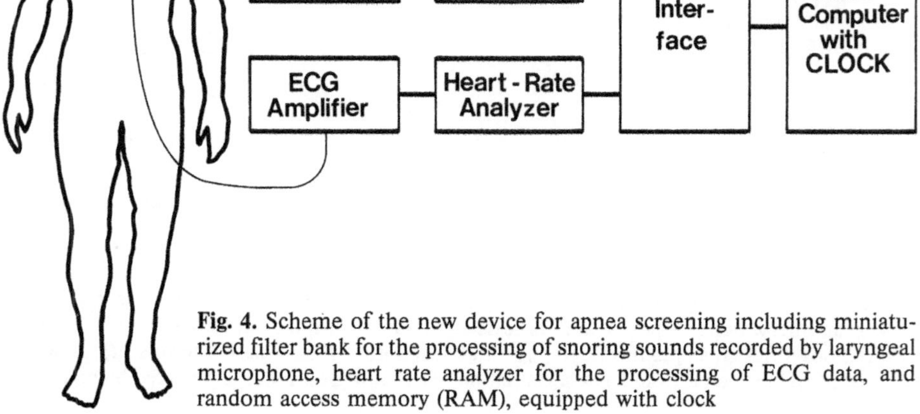

Fig. 4. Scheme of the new device for apnea screening including miniaturized filter bank for the processing of snoring sounds recorded by laryngeal microphone, heart rate analyzer for the processing of ECG data, and random access memory (RAM), equipped with clock

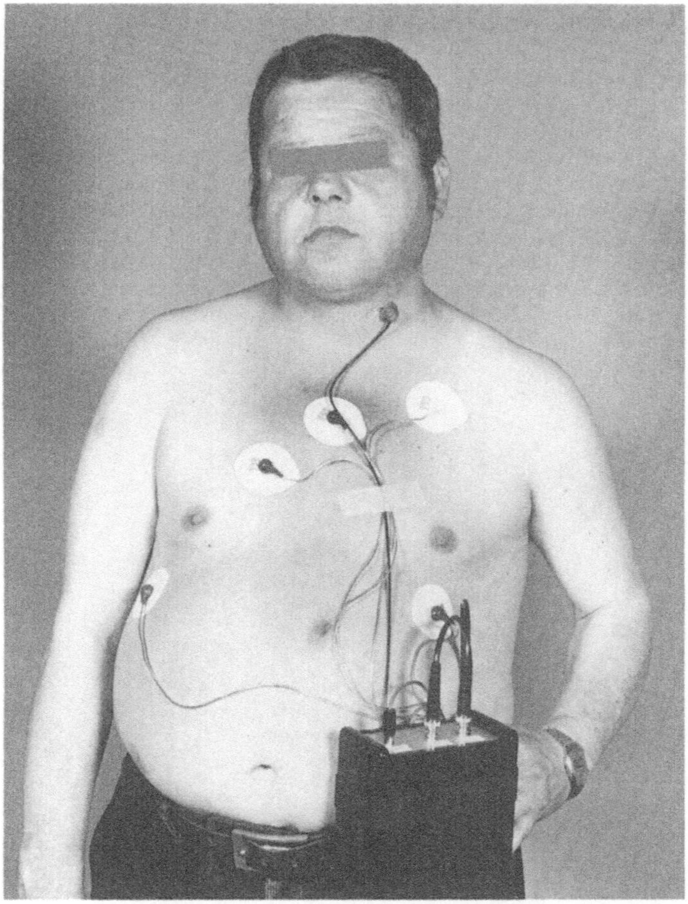

Fig. 5. Prototype of the new recorder in use

phone for sound recordings which then pass through the miniaturized filter bank, and with heart rate analyzer and random access memory. The evaluation of the data thus obtained is accomplished by means of a commercial personal computer. A standardized anamnestic procedure with apnea-specific questions is also stored there. It can be operated interactively by the attending physician.

Figure 5 shows a prototype of the recorder in use. At present, both the filter bank routines and the algorithm for the calculation of heart rate stability are being optimized in a series of studies. This work is about to be completed. The system will be available for purchase in the middle of 1987. (Ing. P. Griebel ME, D-7600 Freiburg, Tullastr. 72).

References

1. Peter JH (1985) Holter monitoring technique in a comprehensive approach: ambulatory monitoring of sleep apnea. In: Hombach V, Hilger HH (eds) Holter monitoring technique. Schattauer, Stuttgart, pp 127–149
2. Tilkian AG, Motta J, Guilleminault C (1978) Cardiac arrhythmias in sleep apnea. In: Guilleminault C, Dement WC (eds) Sleep apnea syndromes. Liss, New York, pp 197–210
3. Guilleminault C, Connolly S, Winkle R, Melvin K, Tilkian A (1984) Cyclical variation of the heart rate in sleep apnoea syndrome. Lancet i:126–131
4. Peter JH, Becker E, Fuchs E, Meinzer K, von Wichert P (1982) Ambulante transkutane Langzeitregistrierung von arterieller Sauerstoffspannung und Herzrhythmusstörungen bei Patienten mit Schlafapnoesyndrom. Verh Dtsch Ges Inn Med 88:390–394

Vigilance and Performance in Sleep Apnea Under Single-Dose Theophylline Therapy

K. WEBER, B. EHRIG, E. FUCHS, T. PENZEL, and J. H. PETER

Introduction

Excessive daytime sleepiness (EDS) is one of the diagnostically most important symptoms of the sleep apnea syndrome (SAS). According to Dement at al. [6] and Guilleminault [11], 37% of patients with EDS suffer from obstructive sleep apnea (SA). Vice versa, EDS was observed as the major psychophysiological symptom in almost 80% of all patients with obstructive SA. Watson and his coworkers have reported a variety of neuropsychological deficiencies which are characteristic of patients with obstructive SA as compared with control groups [31]. Attention, sustained concentration, psychomotor efficiency, and visual motor coordination are affected. EDS and neuropsychological deficiencies are to a large extent responsible for the deterioration in vital capacities and general quality of living which patients with SAS frequently experience.

EDS is considered to be the consequence of sleep fragmentation. Obstructive apnea episodes, in particular, are terminated by EEG arousals which are related to respiration [19, 25, 29, 30]. Stepanski et al. found a significant positive correlation between the number of arousals per night and the degree of daytime sleepiness [28]. Other investigators stress the importance of oxygen desaturation as the main cause of EDS [23, 27]. A pronounced reduction in δ-sleep (deep sleep) as well as REM sleep in patients with severe SA has also been reported [13].

It must be expected that an improvement in the patients' sleep quality will result in diminished daytime sleepiness. However, the medical therapy of SA is still a matter of debate. While theophylline, aminophylline, and caffeine have been successfully used to treat premature infants with idiopathic SA [2, 5, 10, 21], the evidence is contradictory where adult patients are concerned. Guilleminault and Hayes [12] have reported that while theophylline increases diaphragmatic activity during REM sleep-related mixed apnea, it has no effect upon obstructive (upper airway) apnea. Mayer and colleagues, on the other hand, found that theophylline therapy resulted in a distinct improvement of SA in a long-term theophylline therapy study.

A considerable proportion of our patients have reported subjective improvement in their general condition, and particularly their EDS symptoms, after they had been treated with theophylline. We therefore sought to objectify these subjective improvements reported in questionnaire inquiries by using an EEG-assisted vigilance test during the day. In this respect, the present study design, which consists of a single-blind crossover theophylline trial supplemented by a performance and vigilance assessment during the day, has a pilot function for further comprehensive studies in the therapy of SA and its pertinent symptoms.

Methods

Subjects

Ten male patients between 35 and 62 years of age (mean: 49.8 years) were included in the study. They all had clinically relevant sleep apnea, i.e., more than 10 apnea episodes of at least 10-s duration each per h sleep, according to the criterion by Lavie [16]. SA was found to be of the mixed type, i.e., central and obstructive apnea, with a dominant proportion of obstructive apnea. Without therapy, all patients felt severely handicapped by EDS. The problems they reported included falling asleep at work, with the consequence of involuntary changes of job; falling asleep while driving long distances, in some cases resulting in car accidents; and massive psychosocial problems.

Patients with the following diagnoses were not considered for the study: acute cardiac infarction, hyperthyreosis, epilepsy, manifest cardiac insufficiency, pulmonary edema, chronic cor pulmonale, liver function disorders, and renal insufficiency. Those in need of medication which influenced the effect of theophylline, such as allopurinol, xanthines, furosemide, etc., were also excluded. All drugs which could possibly alter the patients' level of vigilance were discontinued. As the patients could not always be supervised, especially in the periods between the individual vigilance tests during the day, it can not be safely asserted that all patients refrained from smoking. A diagnostic account of the study population is given in Table 1.

Table 1. Clinical findings and apnea results in ten patients

	1	2	3	4	5	6	7	8	9	10
Age	35	55	51	47	60	62	50	39	52	47
Obesity		+	+		+	+		+	+	+
Hyperlipoproteinemia	+					+		+	+	
Hypertension			+	+		+	+		+	
Pulmonary hypertension at rest										+
during exercise				+					+	
Coronary heart disease					+		+			
Apnea index	64	64	50	18.7	17.3	18.2	13.2	22.5	17.2	71

Study Design

In a single-blind crossover trial, the drug was tested against placebo. Sustained release theophylline was administered orally at a single dose of 400 mg before sleep on 3 consecutive nights. On the morning of the 4th day, theophylline serum levels were determined by means of a nephelometric inhibition immunoassay (lower detection limit 2.5 mg/liter, and daytime vigilance tests were conducted. After the tests, the patients were given 4 days of rest, allowing the serum levels to normalize, then the series was repeated under crossover conditions.

Daytime vigilance was tested in a 2-h reaction-time test supplemented by EEG, EOG, and EMG recordings plus eye-blink monitoring using a newly developed device. Another series of reaction-time tests, which lasted for 20 min each and were repeated every 2 h over a period of 10 h, included a continuous recording of eye-blink duration and frequency over the entire day. The eye-blink monitor developed by Fuchs [9] is a spectacle-shaped device equipped with infrared emitters and sensors, permitting an indirect monitoring of vigilance via the recording of lid closure time and changes in blink frequency. The EEG was registered according to the international 10/20 system, using the leads F_z–T_4 and C_z–O_2. For the reaction-time test, the subjects were seated one by one in a comfortable position in a quiet room with dimmed lights, to watch a monitor displaying four square geometrical forms. A randomizer causes each of the forms to disappear independently at irregular intervals averaging 25 s. The subjects are asked to call the form back on the screen by pushing the appropriate button on a small task response box. We distinguished three possible reactions: correct response (test status 1), incorrect response (test status 2), and no response (test status 0). In the case of the subject's failure to respond, the missing form is automatically reestablished on the screen after 10 s while an alarm is sounded. All responses and their respective statuses are automatically recorded. A scheme of the design is shown in Fig. 1.

Evaluation

Performance was evaluated by counting correct, incorrect, and missing responses and by assessing reaction time. The EEG records were evaluated using the classification scheme by Loomis [17], modified according to Fruhstorfer and Bergström [8]. Lack of vigilance indicated by missing responses in the test or by instances of lid closure recorded by the eye-blink monitor were verified by visual analysis of the EEG (see Fig. 2 for the classification of vigilance levels). In order to assess and monitor the patients' subjective condition, we used a questionnaire including questions on the degree of EDS and sleep quality.

Results

On the initial measurement before onset of the main investigation, the ten patients (average age 49.8 years) exhibited 35.6 apnea episodes/h on average

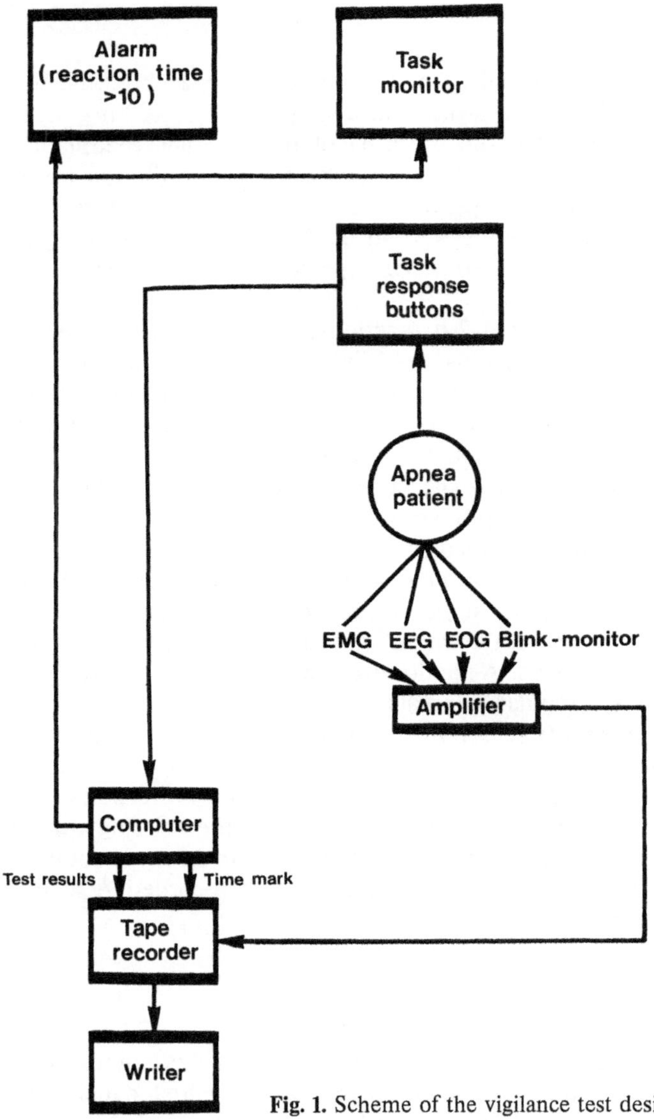

Fig. 1. Scheme of the vigilance test design

(range 13.2–71 apneas/h). After 3 days of 400 mg single-dose theophylline, serum levels averaged 5.23 mg/liter (SD ± 2.05).

In the questionnaire inquiry after therapy, eight of the patients reported a marked reduction of EDS symptoms and/or a distinct improvement in sleep quality. Two patients reported unchanged conditions, and one of those who felt improved complained of initial stomach troubles after theophylline.

In the vigilance test, we found neither a significant deterioration under verum nor a significant improvement under placebo. In agreement with the questionnaire results, there was a significant improvement in reaction times as well as a

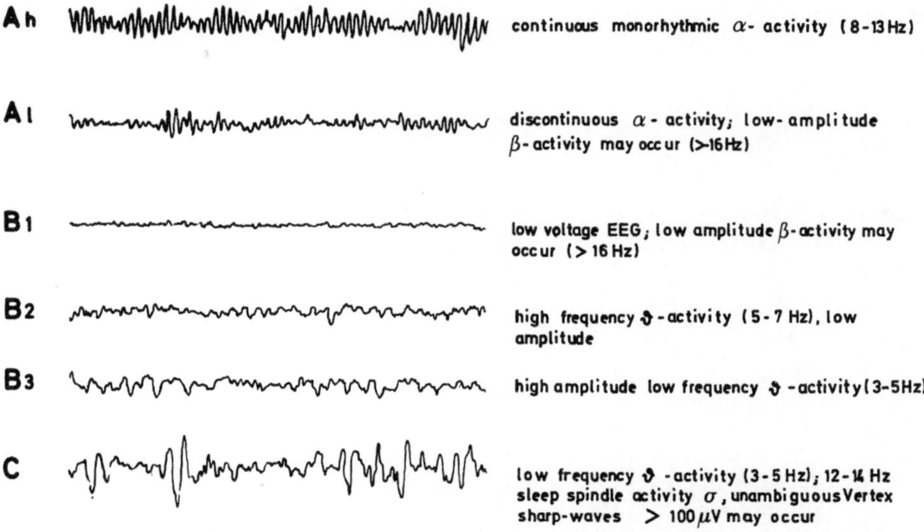

Fig. 2. EEG classification of vigilance. *A*, awake; *B*, intermediary subvigil stages; *C*, light sleep. *Ah* and *Al* include characteristic α-activity. *Bl* is characterized by low voltage EEG. Θ-activity occurs in stage B as well as in stage C, which also includes sleep spindles or vertex sharp waves

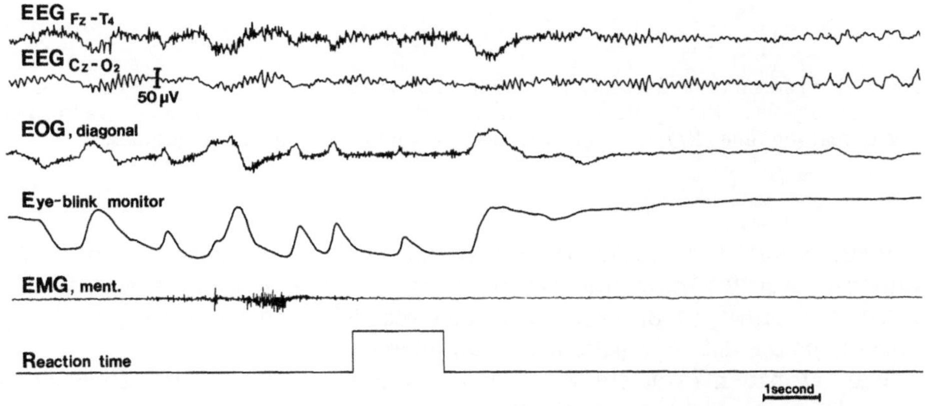

Fig. 3. Example of a vigilance test recording showing a task response with a 1.6-s reaction lag and a subsequent failing of vigilance as indicated by closed eyes (eye-blink monitor) and vigilance B_3 in the EEG

significant decrease in the time spent with eyelids closed in four patients. EEG-defined failings of vigilance were also less frequent among these patients.

Figure 3 shows an example of a test recording, while Fig. 4 documents a particularly impressive improvement in reaction time during the test.

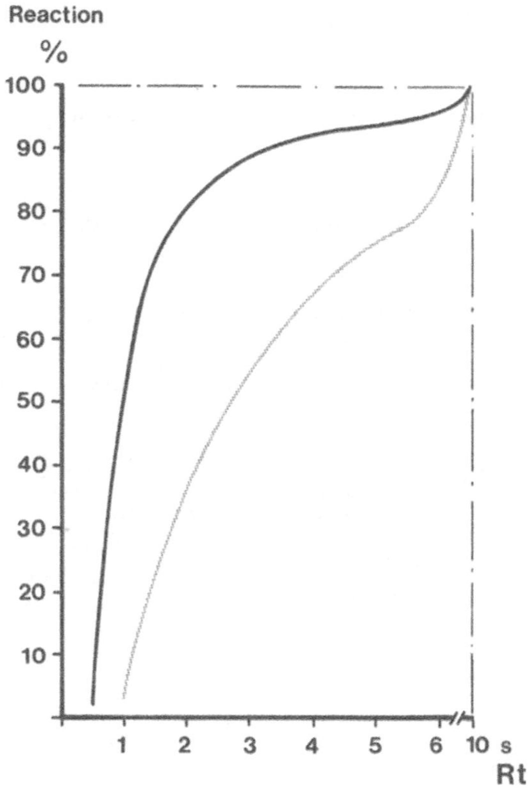

Fig. 4. Comparison of performance in the 2-h vigilance test under drug (———) and placebo (......) for a patient with a particularly pronounced improvement. Cumulative relative frequencies of reaction time *(RT)* in 0.5-s classes (100% ≙ total number of correct responses)

Figure 5 and 6 show the distribution of the reaction time intervals in the six 20-min tests over 10 h during the day. While Fig. 5 shows an improvement, as indicated by a larger proportion of very quick reactions under theophylline, Fig. 6 documents the data of a patient with an unchanged condition.

The four patients who showed a marked improvement under objective conditions also responded better to the theophylline treatment. They were in comparatively good physical condition, although they had reported no less extensive problems with EDS than the others. Two of them had systemic hypertension, and one also suffered from pulmonary hypertension which appeared during exercise. Mean age in this subgroup was lower (47 years, range 35–55 years), and SAA was severe (mean apnea index 49.2, range 18.7–64 apneas/h). In comparison with the other patients, they managed the reaction-time test relatively successfully even without therapy. Table 2 shows that whereas there was a decrease in AI of up to 50% under a single dose of theophylline in this subgroup, a complete therapeutical reversal of apnea did not take place, and the mean duration of the longest apnea episodes was not reduced in two patients.

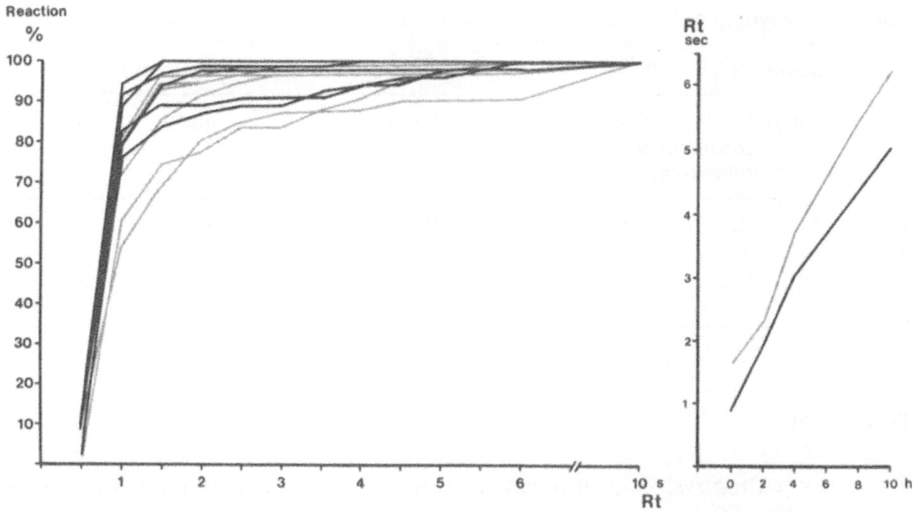

Fig. 5. Cumulative relative frequencies of reaction time (in s) of a patient who improved under theophylline. Results of six 20-min tests over 10 h. Drug (———); placebo (......)

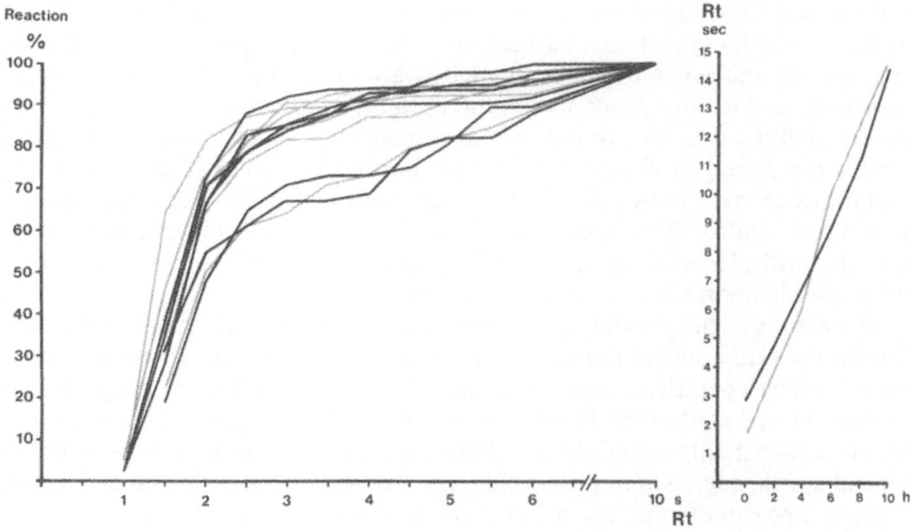

Fig. 6. Same as Fig. 5, giving results for a patient with an unchanged condition

In the present study population of only 10 patients, a statistically significant correlation between the morning theophylline levels and the degree of improvement during the day could not be established.

Table 2. A subgroup of four patients whose performance improved under theophylline

	Apnea index without theophylline (phases/h)	Apnea index under theophylline (phases/h)	Mean duration of 30 longest apnea (s) without theophylline	Mean duration of 30 longest apnea (s) under theophylline
1	64	31.8	33	36
2	64	32.8	64	33.4
3	50	33.3	31.5	38
4	18.7	9.3	26.9	17.1

Discussion

The basic pathophysiological mechanism involved in sleep apnea is assumed to be a disorder of the central nervous system with subsequent instability of respiratory control [4, 15, 18, 22]. Drugs which lower the level of vigilance and have a depressant impact on respiratory control and muscle tone such as sedatives, hypnotics, and alcohol are generally regarded as contraindicated [3, 7, 14]. Although the mechanisms underlying the action of theophylline on respiration are not yet fully understood, the drug presumably has an effect on the CNS; Davi et al. found that theophylline treatment of premature infants with idiopathic apnea reduced the incidence of apnea, increased alveolar ventilation, increased CO_2-sensitivity and led to a pronounced shift of the CO_2-response curve to the left [5]. Aminophylline is known to increase diaphragmatic contractility [1] and hypoxic ventilatory drive [26]. We suggest that the onset of sleep in patients with SAS is accompanied by a critical fall in vigilance, which leads to a destabilization of respiratory control (Fig. 7, compare [24]). Theophylline could possibly antagonize this critical loss of vigilance and thus lead to a stabilization of the neuromuscular coordination which is vital for respiration.

The results of the present pilot study show that a beneficial effect of theophylline on the symptoms of EDS can be observed and verified under 400 mg single-dose therapy conditions with sustained-release theophylline, although further trials will be needed to clarify whether or not specific dosages of theophylline are required by patients with different characteristic conditions such as severity and type of apnea, degree of multimorbidity, or the type of coexisting illnesses. Also, there is a possibility that the daytime improvement which we observed may be due to the generally stimulating effect of theophylline; on the other hand, there was no significant relationship between morning levels of theophylline and performance during the day. For a more discriminating analysis both the study design and the selection of subjects will have to be further refined.

More studies should investigate the effect of theophylline on patients with SAS and its pertinent daytime symptoms. These will involve homogeneous groups of patients, distinguishing according to age and the severity of SAS and concomitant illnesses. In order to assess the possible mechanism underlying the mode of action of this drug, it will also be necessary to analyze in detail the

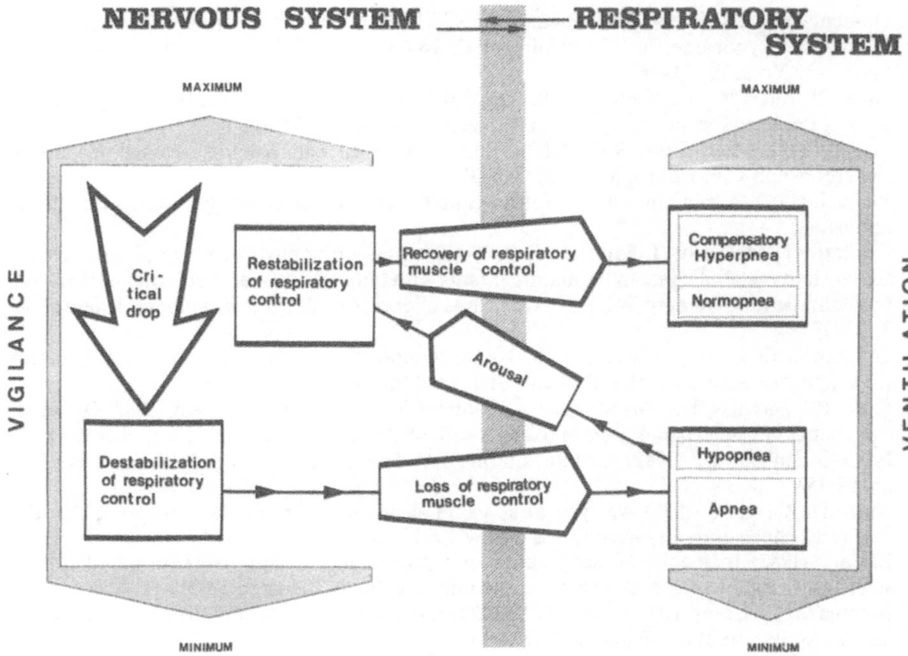

Fig. 7. Scheme of the presumed mechanism of interaction between the nervous system and respiratory system in sleep apnea from [24]

patients' sleep EEGs under theophylline medication and to compare the results with a time-related discrimination of mixed, obstructive, and central apnea as well as the number and duration of the apnea episodes. As a prerequisite to these studies, we are currently working on a computerized evaluation of EEG-defined vigilance in a comprehensive approach including other parameters.

Finally, the verification of vigilance levels during the day by means of the reaction-time test here described should be conducted under conditions of sensory deprivation in order to rule out external distractions and the possibility of false-positive interpretations of performance.

References

1. Aubier M, De Troyer A, Sampson M, Roussos C (1981) Aminophylline improves diaphragmatic contractility. N Engl J Med 305:249–252
2. Autret E, Bretau M, Laugier J, Gold F, Gautier C, Majzoub S (1985) Comparaison de deux doses d'entretien differentes de caffèine dans le traitment des apnées du prématuré. Therapie 40:235–239
3. Bradley D, Phillipson EA (1983) The treatment of sleep apnea. Am Rev Respir Dis 128:585
4. Chokroverty S, Sharp JT (1981) Primary sleep apnea syndrome. J Neurol Neurosurg Psychiatry 44:970
5. Davi MJ, Koravangattu S, Simons KJ, Seshia MM, Rigatto H, Simons ER (1978) Physiologic changes induced by theophylline in the treatment of apnea in preterm infants. Pediatr 92:91–95

6. Dement WC, Carskadon MA, Richardson G (1978) Excessive daytime sleepiness in the sleep apnea syndrome. In: Guilleminault C, Dement WC (eds) Sleep apnea syndromes. Liss, New York, pp 23–46
7. Dilly FR, Block RJ (1982) Effect of flurazepam on sleep disordered breathing and nocturnal oxygen desaturation in asymptomatic subjects. Am J Med 73:239
8. Fruhstofer H, Bergström RM (1969) Human vigilance and auditory evoked responses. Electroenceph Clin Neurophysiol 27:346–355
9. Fuchs E (1987) A miniature device for no-contact eye-blink monitoring. Biomed Eng (to be published)
10. Gerhardt T, McCarthy J, Bancalari E (1979) Effect of aminophylline on respiratory center activity and metabolic rate in premature infants with idiopathic apnea. Pediatrics 63:537–542
11. Guilleminault C, Dement WC (1977) 235 cases of excessive daytime sleepiness. J Neurol Sci 31:13–27
12. Guilleminault C, Hayes B (1983) Naloxone, theophylline, bromocriptine and obstructive sleep apnea: negative results. Bull Eur Physiopathol Respir 19:632–634
13. Hesla PE, Nay KN, Kiel M, Mendez A, Coolidge T, Norman S, Cohn MA (1985) Quantitative changes in sleep parameters in patients with obstructive sleep apnea. Sleep Res 14:164
14. Issa FG, Sullivan CE (1982) Alcohol, snoring and sleep apnea. J Neurol Neurosurg Psychiatry 45:353
15. Kurtz D, Krieger J (1978) Analysis of apnea in sleep apnea. In: Guilleminault C, Dement WC (eds) Sleep apnea sydromes. Liss, New York, pp 145–160
16. Lavie P (1983) Incidence of sleep apnea in a presumably healthy working population: a significant relationship with excessive daytime sleepiness. Sleep 6:312–318
17. Loomis AC, Harvey EN, Hobart GA (1937) Cerebral states during sleep, as studied by human brain potentials. Psychol 21:127–144
18. Lugaresi E, Coccagna G, Mantovani M (1978) Hypersomnia with periodic apneas. In: Weitzman ED (ed) Advances in sleep research (vol. 4). Spectrum, New York London
19. Martin RJ, Pennock BE, Orr WC, Sanders MH, Rogers RM (1980) Respiratory mechanics and timing during sleep in occlusive sleep apnea. J Appl Physiol 48:432–437
20. Mayer J, Fuchs E, Hügens M, Penzel T, Peter JH, Podszus T, von Wichert P (1984) Long term theophylline therapy of sleep apnea syndrome. Am Rev Respir Dis 129 [Suppl. II] : A252
21. Milsap RL, Krauss AN, Auld PAM (1980) Oxygen consumption in apneic premature infants after low dose theophylline. Clin Pharmacol Ther 28 (4):536–540
22. Önal E, Lopata M, O'Connor TD (1982) Pathogenesis of apneas in hypersomnia – sleep apnea syndrome. Am Rev Respir Dis 125:167–174
23. Orr WC, Martin RJ, Imes NK, Rogers RM, Stahl ML (1979) Hypersomnolent and nonhypersomnolent patients with upper airway obstruction during sleep. Chest 75:418–422
24. Peter JH (1985) Holter monitoring technique in a comprehensive approach: ambulatory monitoring of sleep apnea. In: Hombach V, Hilger HH (eds) Holter monitoring technique. Technical aspects and clinical applications. Schattauer, Stuttgart, pp 127–149
25. Remmers JE, De Groot WJ, Sauerland EK, Anch AM (1978) Pathogenesis of airway occlusion during sleep. J Appl Physiol 44:931–938
26. Sanders JS, Berman TM, Bartlett MM, Kronenberg RS (1980) Increased hypoxic ventilatory drive due to administration of aminophylline in normal men. Chest 78:279–282
27. Sink J, Bliwise DL, Dement WC (1986) Self-reported excessive daytime somnolence and related psychological symptoms in patients with impaired respiration in sleep. Chest 90:177–180
28. Stepanski E, Lamphere J, Badia P, Zorik F, Roth T (1984) Sleep fragmentation and daytime sleepiness. Sleep 7 (1):18–26
29. Sullivan CE, Issa FG (1980) Pathophysiological mechanisms in obstructive sleep apnea. Sleep 3:235–246
30. Walsh RE, Michaelson ED, Harkleroad LE, Zighelboim A, Sackner MA (1972) Upper airway obstruction in obese patients with sleep disturbance and somnolence. Ann Intern Med 76:185–192
31. Watson R, Greenberg G, Deptula D (1985) Neuropsychological deficits in sleep apnea. Sleep Res 14:136

Computerization of Respiratory Parameters During Sleep

D. Rose, P. Aubry, T. Veleine, and Z. Rida

Introduction

During the past few years, numerous studies have been devoted to the effect of sleep on breathing. Many breathing disorders have been reported to present nocturnal worsening. Some of these events have a clear relationship to a particular EEG sleep stage; for example appreciable oxygen desaturation occurs almost exclusively in rapid eye movement (REM) sleep in chronic obstructive pulmonary disease. Many patients who were complaining primarily of excessive daytime somnolence have presented with a sleep apnea syndrome. Thus, many centers have systematically monitored patients with breathing disorders during sleep to investigate the relationship between sleep state and respiratory patterns, and polygraphic recording has become an accepted procedure for the evaluation of respiratory abnormalities during sleep. Nevertheless, the interpretation of these recordings is highly time-consuming, due to all the data that must simultaneously be analyzed during the whole night, which corresponds to 6 or 7 h of recording. Thus, the use of a microcomputer system seemed an invaluable and cheap tool for settling this problem. This paper presents a low-cost software solution for measurements based on the popular Apple IIe microcomputer, which is available in many laboratories. Computer assistance enables a reduction in time taken to collect and analyze raw data and gives the investigator an immediacy of access to a wide spectrum of powerful mathematical and graphical techniques. A polygraphic recording of sleep includes:

a) the monitoring of respiratory parameters such as oxygen saturation, carbon dioxide tension, thoracic and abdominal movements, and oral or nasal air flow, and
b) the study of standard sleep variables (electroencephalogram, electrooculogram, and submental electromyogram).

We have selectively computerized the respiratory data. Indeed, the study of sleep variables by means of a microcomputer system is much more difficult and requires a high capacity memory system. We hoped to obtain a reliable analysis of respiratory events, to gain time for our interpretation, and to have a clear and suitable presentation of the final results.

Equipment

The measuring system included:
- Hewlett-Packard 47201A ear oximeter
- Skin sensor for the transcutaneous PCO_2 ($TcPCO_2$) (Model TCM20 Electrode Radiometer)
- Respitrace system using Respibands placed around the rib cage and abdomen for thoracic and abdominal respiratory movement recordings
- Nasal or buccal thermistor for the detection of the best air flow signal

These were connected both to an Apple IIe microcomputer using commercial standard peripheral equipment throughout with an interface between the recorders and computer and a Time II clock card, and to an ink-writing recorder (6 channels, paper speed of 6 cm per min). A computer-generated signal was recorded both on the EEG and on the ink-writing recorder traces every minute.

Data Input Program Description

All the equipment was calibrated before each record, with the subject lying in bed, quiet, and awake confirmed by EEG. We recorded baseline ventilation, i.e., thoracic and abdominal respiratory movements, SaO_2 and $TcPCO_2$. All the signals have to be strictly well-defined and stable before the onset of recording, since their quality determines the reliability of the study.

Determination of the Individual Basic SaO_2 Value

During the first 30-min epoch, with the subject lying in bed, quiet, and awake, SaO_2 signals (frequency 2 Hz) were recorded, and the mean value was chosen as the baseline awake SaO_2.

Calculation of Derived Parameters. SaO_2 signals were recorded during the whole night, except when the ear oximeter was "off ear". The mean value of SaO_2 during the whole night was thereafter computed. Mean SaO_2 was also analyzed by 5-min epochs. Thirdly, throughout the night, the total duration (seconds) of arterial oxygen desaturation (4% below the baseline awake SaO_2) episodes was calculated. The number of desaturation episodes longer than 10 s was recorded, and the time of occurrence, duration, and lowest SaO_2 for each episode noted. The total duration of desaturation episodes below a determined SaO_2 was measured in 2.5% steps.

Determination of the Individual Basic $TcPCO_2$ Value

During the first 30-min epoch, with the subject lying in bed, quiet, and awake, $TcPCO_2$ signals (frequency 2 Hz) were recorded and the mean value was chosen as the baseline awake $TcPCO_2$.

Calculation of Derived Parameters. $TcPCO_2$ was recorded during the whole night. The mean value of $TcPCO_2$ during the whole night was thereafter determined. Mean $TcPCO_2$ was also measured by 5-min epochs. Thirdly, throughout the night, the duration (seconds) of episodes of hypercapnia (8 mmHg over the baseline awake $TcPCO_2$) was calculated. We chose this controlled value of 8 mmHg because a mean increase of 5 mmHg during sleep is quite physiologically normal.

For each episode the time of occurrence, the duration and the highest $TcPCO_2$ were stored. The total number and duration of episodes of hypercapnia were also recorded. The total duration of episodes over a determined $TcPCO_2$ was measured in 2 mmHg steps.

Detection of Apneas

Apneic episodes were defined by the absence of nasal or oral air flow for at least 10 s and were classified by type: central, mixed, or obstructive. Central apnea refers to cessation of nasal or oral air flow with cessation of respiratory effort; obstructive apnea is defined as absence of nasal or oral air flow despite continuing respiratory effort; and mixed apnea is one with both central and obstructive components, the obstructive part usually following the central.

For each apnea, the time, duration (seconds), and type were recorded. The total number and duration of apneic episodes were calculated. The computer then analyzed the thoracoabdominal movement signals and computed the delay between the end of the nasal or oral air flow signal and the first variation of the next thoracoabdominal movement signal: no variation indicated central apnea; variations marked an obstructive apnea. If the computed delay was longer than the mean duration of the five respiratory cycles preceding the detected apnea, this apnea was marked as a mixed apnea.

The Program in Use

First the type of recording must be chosen: SaO_2 alone, SaO_2 and $TcPCO_2$, or SaO_2 and $TcPCO_2$ and apnea measurement. All equipment must be calibrated and captors installed.

Throughout the night of recording, it is important to keep a continuous watch on the screen of some parameters such as the time, how long it has been since the start of the record (in 5-min epochs), the visual alarm for the ear oximeter ("off ear"), both the visual and oral alarm for apneas that are longer than 60 s and the printout of three keywords (desaturation, apnea, hypercapnia) when the computer detects the corresponding event.

All the data are stored during the whole night. At the end of the recording in the morning, the computer edits the results, producing the following details:

Identification of the patient (name, date of birth, weight, height)
Motive of the study
Date of the record

Parameters studied
Clinical remarks
Baseline awake SaO_2 and $TcPCO_2$
Summary of main results
Graphical reconstruction of the evolution of SaO_2 throughout the night
Graphical reconstruction of the evolution of the $TcPCO_2$ throughout the night
Tabulation of all data stored during the whole night
Time of onset and end of the "off ear" alarm
Time of onset, duration (seconds), minimum value of SaO_2, and time of this minimum for each period of the arterial oxygen desaturation ($>$ 10 s)
Time of onset, duration (seconds), maximum value of $TcPCO_2$, and time of this maximum for each period of hypercapnia
Time of onset, duration (seconds), and mean duration of the five respiratory cycles preceding each detected apnea, number of thoracic movements detected during the apnea, computed delay (seconds) between the onset of the apnea and the first thoracic movement, type of apnea
Outline of the SaO_2 and $TcPCO_2$ curves throughout the night (scale: 1 h = 13 cm)

Conclusion

The reliability of this program is still under study but the first results are very convincing, particularly for the detection and analysis of the SaO_2 and $TcPCO_2$ signals. Concerning apneas, the reliability of the analysis strictly depends on the quality of the thoracoabdominal movement signals (calibration, amplitude). We have used the program for nearly a year and are quite satisfied. We think that it can greatly improve continuous monitorings of respiratory parameters during sleep and allow easier analysis of polygraphic records.

EEG-Analysis Among Patients with Sleep Apnea by Means of a Microcomputer

H.-G. Daun

Introduction

The idea for this project arose from observations made during the analysis of EEG sleep recordings from patients with sleep apnea. It appeared that during periods of apnea, the transition from one sleep stage to another happened very quickly, with stages sometimes lasting only a few seconds. Manually classifying the sleep stages from these recordings proved to be a cumbersome task, especially when the data were later to be analyzed by computer. It meant handling large rolls of registration paper, keeping track of the time in the recording, and writing the beginning of each sleep stage as well as the stage classification on a notepad. The same had to be done for recordings from the abdominal and thoracic belts. Then all the data had to be typed into the computer before we could correlate the EEG changes with breathing parameters, such as the beginning or termination of an apnea period. On the other hand we did not want to use automatic classification techniques at this stage, because the resolution of automated analysis becomes increasingly more difficult for very short durations of sleep stages and because we felt that manual classification was necessary as a basis for the future evaluation of different algorithms and strategies. So we decided to use the computer for the time-consuming work and to develop a system simplifying the manual analysis.

System Hardware

The system is based on an Apple Macintosh computer, which is widely available, relatively portable, and features a graphically oriented user interface and a mouse device for controlling the computer's actions. There is a disk drive for 3.5-in. (8.75 cm) magnetic disks built into the computers while a second disk drive can be added as an external unit. Each drive holds about 800 kilobytes information, and the internal memory has a capacity of 1 megabyte.

The particular computer model was chosen because it was available, not because it was considered best suited for the task. Still, its graphic abilities and the mouse, which makes control of the computer almost as easy as pointing a finger, are excellent advantages in a system designed to simplify something. The only problem with the computer was the (then) unavailibility of an analogue-to-digital converter required to digitize the polygraphic recordings in order to make them "readable" for the computer. Our solution was to use the Intertechnique computer at the Marburg sleep laboratory for the conversion and then employ both computers' serial ports to move the data from the Intertechnique to the Macintosh. Finally, the Imagewriter II printer for the Macintosh was used for printing out data from the analysis.

System Software

For programming the system, the MacMeth development system from the Eidgenössische Technische Hochschule Zürich (ETHZ) was used. MacMeth is a very fast system for programming in the Modula-2 language also developed at ETHZ by Prof. N. Wirth. This language supports modular programming at a relatively high level of abstraction. The program realizing the analysis system itself leans heavily on routines of the Macintosh computer's operating system called the Macintosh Toolbox. These routines provide easy access to the computer's graphic abilities and its user interface, which helps make the program simple to use and understand. The operating system also offers ways of exchanging data between programs, so that data prepared by the analysis program can be transferred to other programs, such as ones for creating graphics or the drawing program that was used to create the poster presented at the symposium.

Key Features of the Program

The program can process up to eight tracks of a polygraphic recording. In the current version these tracks are being digitized on the Intertechnique computer and then transferred to the Macintosh's magnetic disks. From there the data is read into the computer's memory. The length of the recording stored on one disk is dependent on the number of tracks and their sampling rates, i.e., the number of times per s that the signal is measured. In this project we have used sampling rates of 128 Hz for the EEG and 16 Hz for the other three channels, so that each second of the recording requires 176 words or 352 byte of storage. A single magnetic disk with a capacity of 800 kbyte can thus store 2300 s or about 38 min of a sleep recording. For longer recordings several disks are required. This can be avoided by using one of the hard disks offered for the Macintosh, thus extending the recording length to 16 h (for 20 megabyte) or more.

There are three modes of operation: scroll through, classification, and analysis modes. In the first two the tracks are displayed on the screen. The user may choose the time base, the amplitude scaling factor, and other parameters for each track as desired (Fig. 1).

The horizontal lines between the tracks can be dragged up and down with the mouse to assign more or less space to a track. In the middle of the screen a time reference marker is displayed. In scroll through mode, the amplitude of each track at the time marked by the reference bar and the time passed since the start of the recording are displayed on the upper part of the screen. It is possible to set

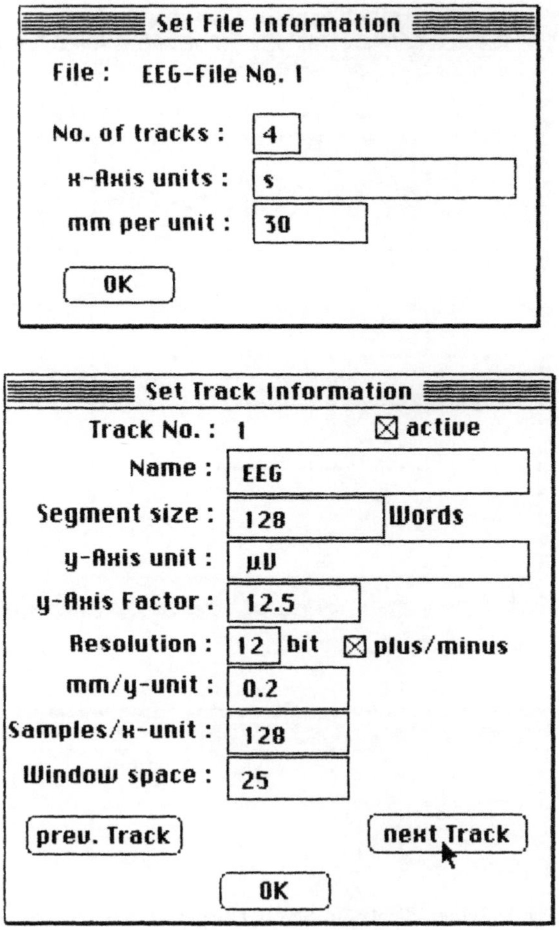

Fig. 1. Dialogue boxes for setting the parameters for the whole recording file *(above)* and for each of the tracks *(below)*

time markers at any point of the recording, the time interval between the reference bar and these markers also being displayed. A horizontal scroll bar at the bottom of the screen can be used to scroll backwards and forwards through the recording. Double-clicking the mouse button on one of the arrows on either side of the screen selects continous scrolling, which is especially useful in classification mode.

Classification mode is similar to scroll through mode. In the upper part of the screen, however, the user may install "buttons" referring to the classification stages (Fig. 2). Each button is assigned to a particular track, so that classification of multiple tracks in one run is possible. When one of these buttons is pressed by clicking the mouse button on it, the time and the stage are recorded in a classification file. If a recording has been classified already, the buttons show the classification stages previously chosen for that point in the recording.

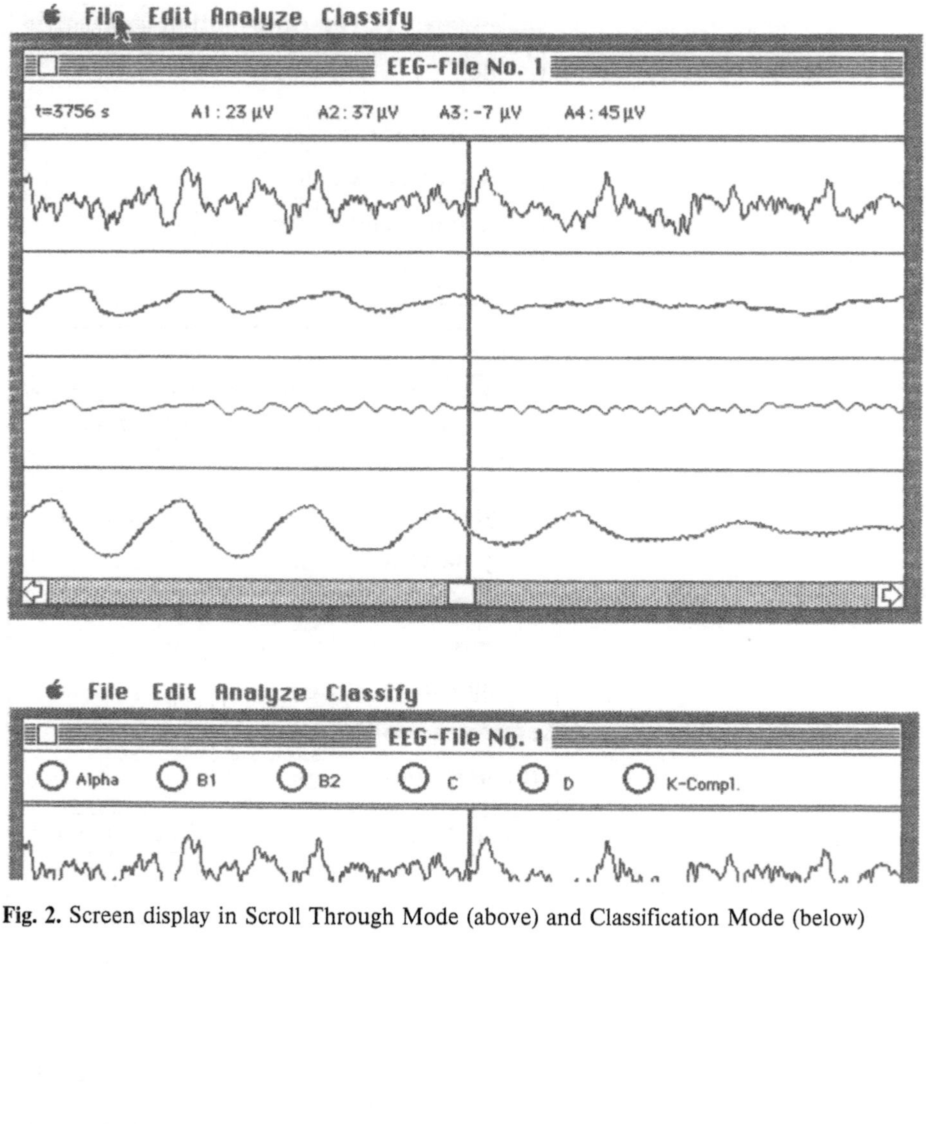

Fig. 2. Screen display in Scroll Through Mode (above) and Classification Mode (below)

In analysis mode both the recording data and the data in the classification files can be analyzed in different ways. So far we have implemented histograms showing the distribution of sleep stages and amplitude classes, and have developed a technique for displaying the event-correlated distribution of sleep stages, which is illustrated in Fig. 3. It shows the distribution of sleep stages at the point of apnea termination in a patient with sleep apnea. As can be seen from the graph, the termination of apnea is marked by the occurrence of K-complexes followed by spindle activity. After a few seconds this activity is followed by stage C, in most cases with a short transition through stage B2. The part of the program realizing the analysis mode has been designed to allow easy expansion, so that new ideas for analyzing the data can be implemented in a very short time.

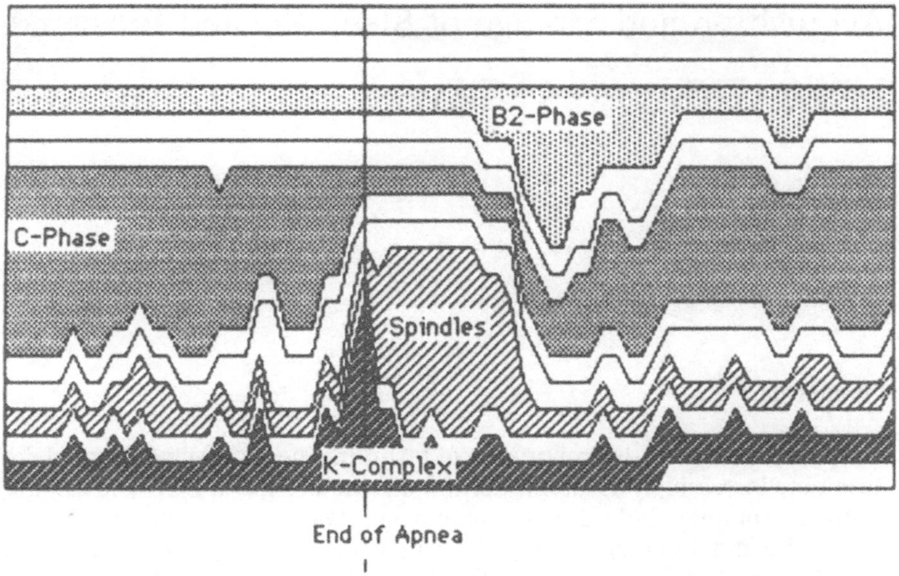

Fig. 3. Example of graphic output: sleep stage distribution before and after apnea termination (–30 to + 40 s)

Conclusion

The system described above was designed to simplify manual classification of sleep stages in polygraphic sleep recordings and may be used as well for analyzing other biosignals. It eliminates most of the time-consuming steps involved in manual classification and offers several techniques for further analysis of the data. The graphically oriented user interface makes the compact system easy to use and helps in creating graphs from the data. Thus the system assists with various steps of analysis, such as classifying sleep stages, analyzing the sleep stage pattern, and preparing a graphical output. All the "bookkeeping" is done by the computer, so the user can concentrate on the evaluation of the data.

Acknowledgements. I would like to thank colleagues at the Sleep Laboratory in the Department of Internal Medicine here in Marburg for their help and encouragement, especially Thomas Penzel, Katja Weber, and, of course, Hermann Peter. Comments or questions regarding this article are welcome.

Acquisition and Storage of Sleep-Related Biosignals

T. PENZEL, K. MEINZER, and J. H. PETER

Introduction

In internal medicine, the importance of recording measured physiological data is becoming increasingly apparent. Continuous monitoring of ECG and respiration is already common, indeed indispensable, in intensive care units. For an investigation of pathophysiology during sleep, however, it is necessary to record many more biosignals. Since it is also desirable to analyze their complex interrelations off-line in the computer [3], it is important to be able to make reproducible recordings which contain all the relevant information. Within the framework of our project Time Series Analysis and Sleep Apnea, we have developed ways of producing both analogue and digital recordings (Fig. 1).

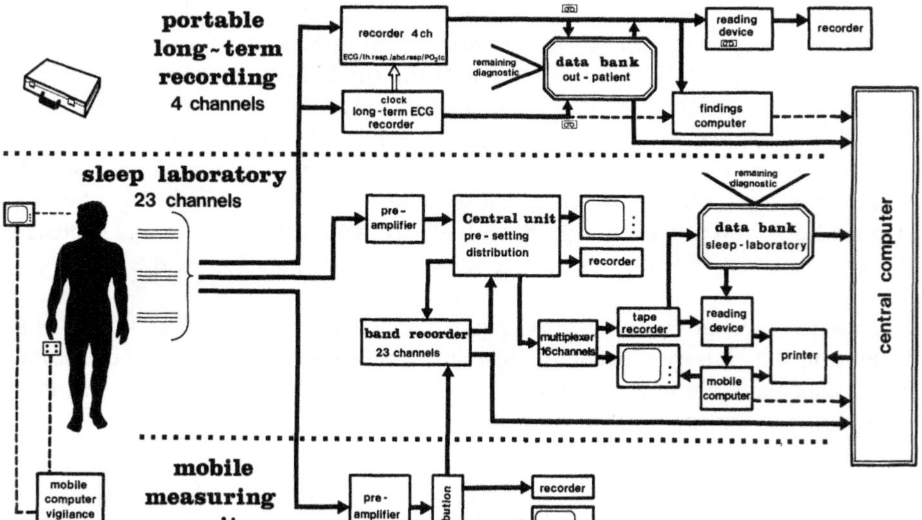

Fig. 1. The data flow plan illustrates the interaction between analogue and digital recordings with data storage and data evaluation as employed in the Time Series Analysis and Sleep Apnea project

Analogue Acquisition

Analogue recording modes are used both for stationary investigations in the sleep laboratory and for ambulatory monitoring. In the sleep laboratory, 23 physiological parameters can be continuously recorded in analogue form by means of a tape recorder. Such an elaborate approach is necessary if one seeks to be able to determine how the various pathophysiological functions are interconnected. We use a microcomputer to generate date and time codes which are incorporated in the recording as a square-wave signal. This is required to define the actual time at which the various events occur. For ambulatory monitoring, an Oxford Medilog Mark IV recorder has proved effective. The system we use records ECG, thoracic and abdominal respiratory activity, and partial arterial oxygen tension [5, 6]. Every 10 min the time indication is inserted into the pO_2 recording in the form of calibration marks. The disadvantages of this method are well-known, e.g., tape-speed variation [2] and a limited number of parameters.

Digital Acquisition

Digital acquisition permits real-time processing of incoming data. This means that the data can be selectively reduced by recording all relevant information whilst discarding any redundant information. Here it would be desirable to condense time by a factor of 20–60.

Audiocassettes used in start-stop operation have been found to be an ideal low-cost means of recording data. Since 1971, we have been using this method with a data recording density of 50 bit/mm (or 2400 bit/s). With more advanced techniques we have since 1982 been able to record at twice this density (100 bit/mm or 4800 bit/s; Fig. 2). This enables us to store about 8 megabytes of data on one C-120 audiocassette.

Data Compression

In recording digitized data, we can draw on the knowledge gained from space technology. We have combined start-stop recording on cassettes with blocked format recording [1]. Even in off-line processing, blocked format recording

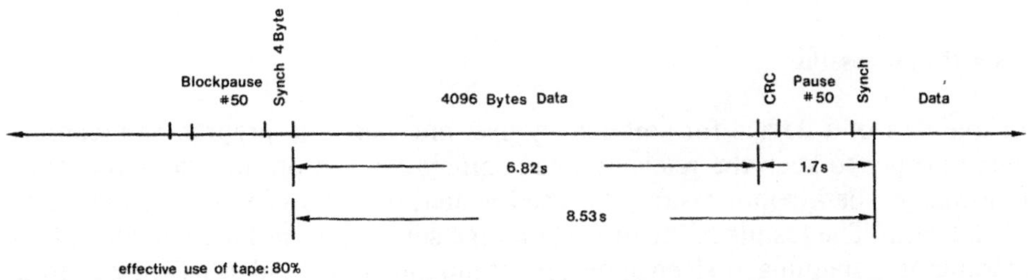

Fig. 2. Audiocassette tape exploitation with block structure of data recording at 4800 bit/s

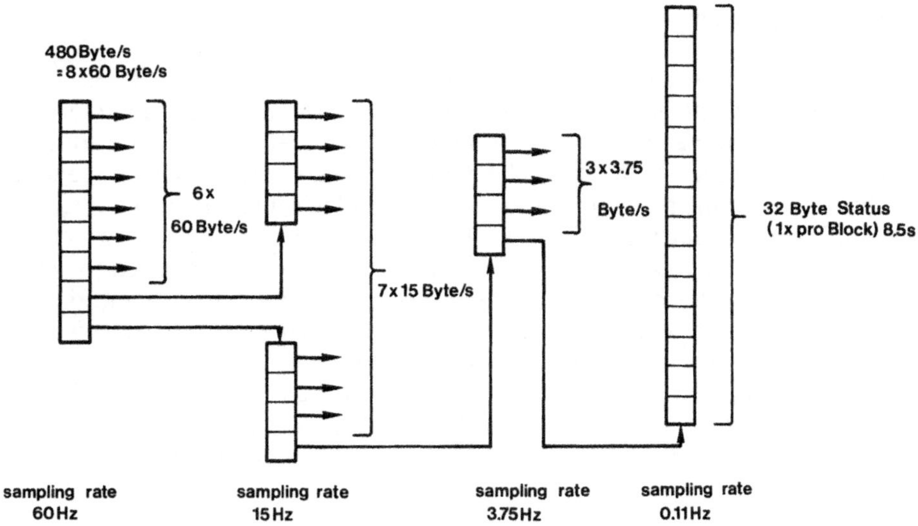

Fig. 3. Supercommutation of medical parameters for adaptation to physiological variables changing at varying speeds (1 byte resolution of analogue-digital converter)

through the use of cyclic buffers permits continuous computation of correlations and other evaluations with moving windows [4]. Since physiological parameters change at greatly varying speeds (EEG, respiration, body temperature), it is necessary to use a suitably adapted mode of recording. For this purpose we use data supercommutation (Fig. 3).

With this technique it is possible to record 16 different physiological signals. Six rapidly variable parameters such as ECG, EEG, and arterial blood pressure are read at 60 samples/s, seven less rapidly variable parameters such as respiration and integrated EMG activity are read at 15 samples/s, and three slowly variable parameters such as oxygen tension and carbon dioxide tension are read at 3.75 samples/s. Furthermore, a "status" part records coded data for time, date, patient name, and date of birth (time, 4 bytes; date, 2 bytes; patient name, 22 bytes; date of birth and serial number, 4 bytes).

A module which meets these requirements has been built for an Apple computer and has proved effective in more than 100 recordings.

Data Preprocessing

In the case of a device for ambulatory use, one needs to preprocess incoming data in order to keep the relevant data compressed. For on-line data processing followed by data compression, we used a method consisting of analogue and digital parts. The results of the project on time series analysis have shown that for ambulatory screening of sleep apnea, recording heart rate and processing snoring and breathing sounds provides sufficient indication of sleep apnea. We have

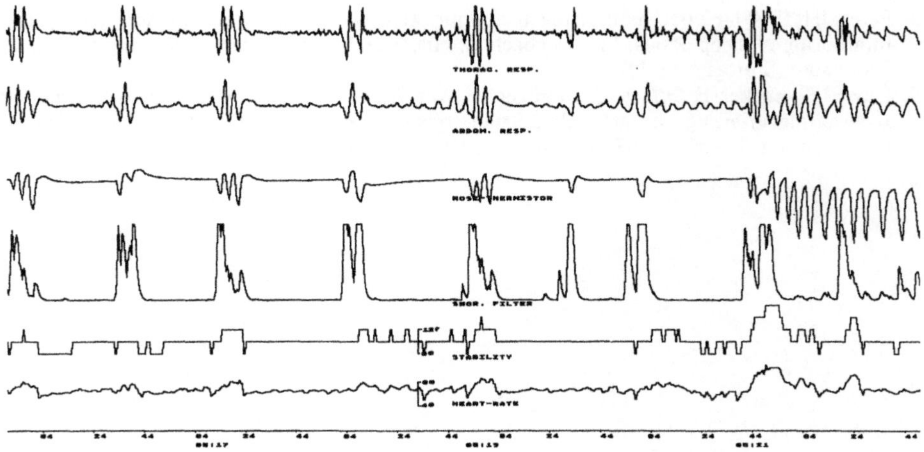

Fig. 4. Sample recording of a patient with sleep apnea including preprocessing of the snoring and breathing sounds

therefore combined a filter for detecting snoring and a program for computing the duration of phases of constant heart rate. For further information compare Peter et al. (this volume, pp 140–146). The results are recorded with high data density and permit clear interpretation (Fig. 4.).

Conclusion

The use of digital data acquisition and recording methods permits an effective on-line reduction of data. The methods are suitable for both stationary and ambulatory use. They permit rapid data evaluation with the assistance of set programs, as well as comprehensive documentation of data on a low-cost, space-saving medium. The principle of data reduction is the retention of all relevant information and the rejection of all redundant information on the basis of selecting programs.

References

1. Meinzer K (1978) IPS – eine neue Programmiertechnik für Mikrocomputer. Elektronik 15:35–42
2. Mitchell RH, Ruff S, Jenkins JG (1980) The correction of timing errors due to tape speed variation in the tape recording of physiological data. Med Biol Eng Comput 18:353–357
3. Oppenheim AV, Schafer RW (1975) Digital signal processing. Prentice-Hall, Englewood Cliffs
4. Penzel T, Fuchs E, Mayer J, Peter JH (1984) Pattern recognition of sleep apnea. In: Kimmich HP, Klewe HJ (eds) Biotelemetry VIII. Kimmich, H.-J. Klewe (eds) Proceedings of the Eighth International Symposium on Biotelemetry, Dubrovnik. Döring-Druck, Braunschweig, pp 435–438

5. Peter JH (1985) Holter monitoring technique in a comprehensive approach: ambulatory monitoring of sleep apnea. In: Hombach V, Hilger HH (eds) Holter monitoring technique. Schattauer, Stuttgart, pp 127–149
6. Peter JH, Becker E, Fuchs E, Meinzer K, von Wichert P (1982) Ambulante transkutane Langzeitregistrierung von arterieller Sauerstoffspannung und Herzrhythmusstörungen bei Patienten mit Schlafapnoe-Syndrom. Verh Dtsch Ges Inn Med 88:390–393

Part 3: Epidemiology I

Sleep Disturbances and Cardiovascular Risk: A Biopsychosocial Approach

J. SIEGRIST

It is common to analyze the relation between sleep disturbances and cardiovascular risk in a unidirectional way: advanced cardiovascular pathology is seen as a relevant cause of disordered sleep. It is well-known that pain associated with nocturnal unstable angina provokes awakenings, and similar experiences happen in patients with severe peripheral artery occlusion. Poor sleep is often reported in patients with congestive heart failure and may be present in other cardiovascular syndromes. In this presentation, however, a less common approach is outlined, taking sleep disturbances as a starting point and cardiovascular pathology as a possible outcome.

During the past few years increasing evidence on this type of relationship has been found at three levels. First, longitudinal epidemiological studies have reported an association between sleep characteristics and subsequent cardiovascular excess morbidity and mortality. Second, clinical medicine and epidemiology have been able to advance our understanding of adverse cardiovascular effects of disturbed sleep associated with sleep apnea. Finally, sleep disturbances have been analyzed in the framework of central neuronal control of the cardiovascular system and especially of impaired regulation due to experiences of severe socioemotional distress.

In the main part of this chapter, recent evidence along these three lines will be presented, including findings from our own research. Finally, some suggestions for further research are briefly outlined.

Epidemiology

Several, large-scale, longitudinal studies have reported an association between sleep disturbances and subsequent cardiovascular excess morbidity or mortality. A 6-year follow-up of a very large sample of adults conducted by the American Cancer Society revealed a relative risk of 2.8 in men sleeping 4 h or less as compared to those sleeping 7–8 h per night. This excess mortality was found for ischemic heart disease, stroke, suicide, and cancer and was established by multiple discriminant analysis after controlling for a large set of possibly confounding variables [9]. The study also found cardiovascular excess mortality of 1.8 in those sleeping more than 10 h. The same trend was evident in the Alameda county study in which approximately 7000 adults were followed over 9 years. The mortality rate for ischemic heart disease was 1.7 in those sleeping less than 7 h or more than 9 h at entry as compared to those with 7–8 h regular sleeping time. There was still a significant excess mortality of poor or long sleepers after controlling for 12 moderating variables [24].

Sleep disturbances to some extent were predictive of future cases of myocardial infarction in the Kaiser Permanente epidemiological study [3]. A further study investigated the effect of "tiredness" in different occupations on the incidence of hospitalization during a 1-year follow-up in Sweden. For women aged 20–64, occupations with a high percentage of members who were markedly tired "during the last 2 weeks" showed a significantly elevated incidence of hospitalization for myocardial infarction and ischemic heart disease, among others [21]. The Finnish twin cohort study included information on sleep habits in about 5400 male twin pairs. It should be mentioned that the study was not prospective but established a significant effect of quality of sleep on the history of pain of possible myocardial infarction by means of multiple logistic regression analysis [14].

Very recently, the same group has presented findings from a 6-year follow-up study of 10 778 persons aged 35–59 years where poor quality of sleep was associated with life dissatisfaction, stress of daily activities, unemployment, and neuroticism. Age-adjusted risk ratios for bad sleep quality as compared to good quality were calculated for men and women using death certificates and hospital records as criteria. Among other findings, the study could demonstrate a significantly increased risk ratio of 2.04 (men) and of 2.23 (women) for ischemic heart disease (death or hospitalization; [8]).

Taken together this information shows that poor sleep is associated with a moderately increased risk of future cardiovascular morbidity or mortality. In addition it shows that somatic as well as psychosocial conditions are involved in the association between poor sleep and cardiovascular morbidity. Yet as few if any prospective epidemiological studies have included polysomnographic registration or clinical screening so far, we are left with considerable uncertainty about the nature of possible links between both phenomena. In the next sections, two approaches towards analyzing those links in more detail are outlined.

Sleep Apnea

Depending on definition criteria as well as on the risk factors included, the prevalence of sleep syndrome apnea (SAS) in the middle-aged male population has been observed to range from 1% to 15%. The group of P. Lavie was the first one to investigate the prevalence of SAS in a large sample of otherwise healthy male workers. Between 1, 2, and 5.9% of men were suggested as having SAS [11]. As the population under study was nonobese and probably nonhypertensive, the prevalence of SAS may have been slightly underestimated. Our group has recently published data from a prospective study on 416 middle-aged, male, blue-collar workers who, although free from overt ischemic heart disease at entry, exhibited coronary risk factors to a considerable degree. A representative sample of those 78 workers who reported frequent sleep disturbances during the past 4 weeks underwent ambulant polysomnographic registration for at least 1 night. When applying a rigid definition of SAS (10 or more apneic episodes lasting more than 10 s each per h sleeping time, or a total of more than 100 apneic episodes per night), 15% of registered men had to be defined as suffering from SAS [16].

Table 1 compares mean age, weight, and blood pressure between workers with and without sleep disturbances (A vs B) as well as between the group with increased sleep apnea activity and the group without signs of SAS (B_1 vs B_2). Interestingly, workers with increased sleep apnea activity did not exhibit significantly increased coronary risk factors as compared to workers without SAS but with sleep disturbances. Given the prevalence of sleep disturbances, mild hypertension, and overweight in middle-aged male populations, one may expect an impressive number of people with undetected SAS in these groups.

SAS has been related to the development of systemic hypertension and pulmonary hypertension [15, 17], to left ventricular hypertrophy [2] and to cardiac arrhythmias with increased risk of nocturnal sudden cardiac death [1, 13, 22].

Table 1. Characteristics of the study population (354 male blue-collar workers) and its subsamples (mean and standard deviation) [16]

	Age (years)	Overweight (Broca) (kg)	Blood pressure (systolic/ diastolic) (mm Hg)	Mean frequency of apneic episodes (lasting at least 10 s each) (N)	Mean apnea index[a]
A Workers without frequently disrupted sleep ($n = 276$)	41.8 ± 9.7	113.6 ± 14.1	135.2 ± 1.2 88.1 ± 10.6	-	-
B Workers with frequently disrupted sleep ($n = 78$) Subgroups with polysomnographic registration:	45.7 ± 8.5	114.9 ± 14.7	135.5 ± 16.1 88.3 ± 10.2	-	-
B1: Workers without increased sleep apnea[b] ($n = 12$)	49.7 ± 4.6	119.5 ± 12.9	141.6 ± 19.1 89.6 ± 12.3	27.1 ± 19.9	3.5 ± 2.3
B2: Workers with increased sleep apnea[b] ($n = 8$)	48.8 ± 5.1	121.3 ± 13.3	138.0 ± 12.8 90.8 ± 7.5	97.6 ± 42.7	13.3 ± 6.2
T-test	4.36 $p < 0.001$ (A vs B)	ns (A vs B)	ns (A vs B)	5.0 $p < 0.0001$ (B1 vs B2)	7.2 $p < 0.0001$ (B1 vs B2)

[a] Number of apneic episodes/h sleeping time
[b] ≧ 50 apneic episodes pernight lasting at least 10 s each.

These somatic consequences of SAS might well be an important link between sleep disorders and cardiovascular disease. Therefore, it is important to monitor groups at high risk by means of polysomnographic registration in order to detect and prevent premature cardiovascular pathology.

Other contributions in this volume illustrate the clinical importance of SAS in a much more sophisticated way. Nevertheless, it should be emphasized again how intimately SA and cardiovascular risk are intertwined. In the blue-collar study mentioned above, workers with increased sleep apnea activity underwent echocardiography. Despite normal to borderline levels of blood pressure these men exhibited an enlarged end-diastolic diameter of the left ventricle (64.0 ± 9.5 mm), an enlarged diameter of the septum (10.8 ± 0.5 mm), and greater posterior wall thickness (10.2 ± 1.2 mm) [16]. This suggests that hypoxemia and recurrent adrenergic activity could be associated with SAS [2] as promotors of left ventricular hypertrophy even under conditions of moderate volume load. In this context it should be remembered that left ventricular hypertrophy is an important risk factor of cardiac death even after correcting for the level of blood pressure. This has been clearly demonstrated in the Framingham study by Kannel et al. [6].

Distress-Induced Sleep Disturbances

Cardiovascular consequences of recurrent sleep apneas probably form the most important link bridging the observed association between sleep disturbances and cardiovascular morbidity. Do they constitute the only possible link? Today we are not in a position to give definitive answers. However, as the title of this contribution alludes, another and fairly new argument, a biopsychosocial approach, is presented here.

It is known that sleep and cardiovascular function to some extent are regulated by common morphological structures such as the brain reticular formation [10]. It is also known that serotonin in the nerve endings of nucleus tractus solitarii is involved in the control of circulation as well as in the control of NREM sleep. β-blockers at the same time reduce sympathetic cardiovascular tone and disturb serotenergically triggered sleep stages [7].

Other examples of interactions in central nervous system functions can be found. They suggest that aggravated sleep disturbances might be interpreted as a sign of impaired neuronal regulation within these common centers and that such dysregulation has an impact on cardiovascular function as well. What causes impaired neuronal regulation? One possible explanation is that chronic adverse environmental stimuli, and especially sustained experiences of socioemotional distress, activate a fronto-cortical-brainstem pathway, resulting finally in the triggering of dysregulation [20]. Is there evidence for a relationship between sustained neocortical stimulation, disrupted sleep, and altered cardiovascular function?

In this context we propose to introduce the term "distress-induced sleep disturbances" (DISD), which is defined both in terms of subjective and objective indicators.

Subjectively, DISD is present if specific, stressful, socioemotional conditions in the individual prevail (see below), if sleep disturbances have been aggravated in the recent past, and if trivial causes such as noise, pain, shift work etc. have been ruled out.

Objectively, DISD is assessed

a) by exclusion of SAS and
b) by indicators of altered heart rate on the Holter ECG such as increased cyclical variation of heart rate during the night or a decreased shift in the pattern of heart rate between daytime (waking) and nighttime (sleep, bed rest, see below).

Subjectively assessed indicators of DISD include chronic or subacute severe socioemotional distress due to adverse working conditions or interpersonal difficulties as well as cognitions and emotions associated with impaired individual coping ability. Table 2 presents results from our prospective study on blue-collar workers in which several indicators of work-related distress are connected with severity of sleep disturbances in the recent past. High demand at work (e.g., time urgency, increase of workload), tensions at work, and low control over occupational career are associated with poor sleep.

In addition, as can be seen from Table 2, sustained feelings of hopelessness over the last 12 months are linked very strongly with poor sleep. Of those reporting frequent sleep disturbances 41% have definite feelings of hopelessness, but only 14.6% of those who report minor or no sleep disturbances have such feelings.

We have shown elsewhere that a distinct pattern of cognitions and emotions associated with impaired coping ability in occupational life is often present in patients with premature ischemic heart disease as compared to healthy controls [18]. This pattern, called "immersion," reflects a state of exhaustive struggling

Table 2. Associations between indicators of severe socioemotional distress and aggravated sleep disturbances ($n = 310$ male blue-collar workers)

	Difficulties during past 4 weeks								
	Falling asleep			Maintaining sleep					
				During night			Early in morning		
	χ^2	df	p	χ^2	df	p	χ^2	df	p
Inability to improve occupational status	5.8	2	0.05	17.1	2	0.001	7.6	2	0.05
Perceived time urgency at workplace	10.9	4	0.05	10.5	4	0.05	15.2	4	0.005
Tensions at workplace		ns		14.2	4	0.01		ns	
Increase of workload during last year	6.5	2	0.05		ns			ns	
Sustained feelings of hopelessness/helplessness	17.6	4	0.001	16.6	4	0.01	18.2	4	0.001

Table 3. Analysis of variance: mean score of "immersion" in male workers with severe sleep disturbances (SSD) vs undisturbed sleep, correcting for age

	Score "immersion" mean sd	F	2.tailed p	T separate estimate	2-tailed p
Workers with SSD ($n = 57$)	4.86 ± 2.22				
		1.29	0.208	-5.26	0.0001
Workers without SSD ($n = 211$)	3.15 ± 1.96				

Covariant age: F = 16.0 $p < 0.0001$
Main effect SSD F = 23.8 $p < 0.0001$
Grand mean, 3.52; adjusted: group with SSD +1.18 group without SSD -0.32 multiple R = 0.36

with occupational demands. One of the six scales of the construct "need for control," whose measurement by a standardized questionnaire has been developed in our group, is able to represent the latent factor "immersion" quite adequately [12]. It consists of nine items on a unidimensional scale. In Table 3 the mean score of this scale is demonstrated in a group with severe recent sleep disturbances as compared to a group with minor or no sleep disturbances. Severe recent sleep disturbances is defined as waking up during night and/or waking up early in morning without falling asleep again at least eight times during the past 4 weeks.

As can be seen from Table 3, the group with disrupted sleep exhibits significantly higher scores on the scale "immersion." This holds true after correcting for age which, as is well-known, influences sleep very markedly, and for possible bias due to two sleep-related items on the scale.

As far as objective measures are concerned, only preliminary findings can be reported here. Heart rate monitored by Holter ECG (system Oxford 4000) indicates a typical shift in the condensed diurnal pattern between daytime (waking) and nighttime (sleep or bedtime) in normal subjects without recurrent sleep disturbances. However subjects with symptoms of DISD exhibit a decreased or even vanished shift in the diurnal pattern of heart rate. This observation is illustrated in Fig. 1 where mean heart rate on a 24-h ECG in a normal subject (upper part) is compared with mean heart rate (16-h ECG) in a worker with severe subjective symptoms of DISD (lower part). Altered heart rate as a consequence of severe socioemotional stress experienced during the day has been reported in experimental animal studies in tree shrews [23] where a single defeat during the day impairs nocturnal heart rate for several weeks. Of course, more detailed studies are needed to explore this association.

Cyclical variation of heart rate has been postulated as characteristic of SAS [4]. However, when monitoring our blue-collar workers with reported sleep disturbances, we observed an even greater amount of nocturnal cyclical variation of heart rate in those without SAS but with signs of DISD as compared to those

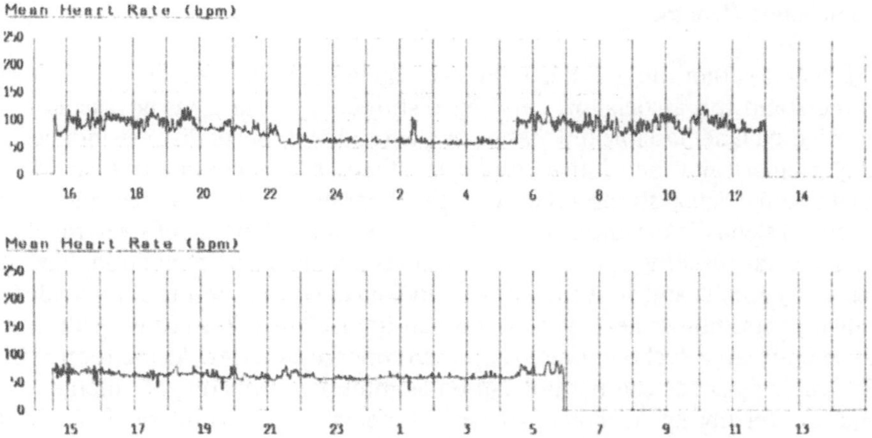

Fig. 1. Mean heart rate (Holter ECG; Oxford 4000) in a subject without sleep disturbances (male blue-collar worker; *upper part*) and in a subject with sleep disturbances in the recent past as well as with severe socioemotional distress (severe life events, sustained feelings of hopeleness and anger; *lower part*)

with SAS but without signs of DISD. A comparison of the central tendency in the extent of heart rate variation between the DISD-positive group and a control group without DISD and without SAS, based on ECG data from a reprensentative "window", showed a significantly higher median in the DISD-positive group (T = 3.33, $p < 0.01$; Z = -2.84; $p < 0.01$).

Very recently we have shown that workers with severe socioemotional distress (including severe sleep disturbances) react to a standardized psychomental stress test at the end of a working day with a reduced maximal heart rate and a reduced increase of blood pressure. Analysis of variance with age as the covariant showed significant main effects of indicators such as "sutained feelings of hopelessness" and "high degree of quantitative overload at work" on reduced maximal difference from baseline in heart rate and blood pressure.

The main effects of indicators of recent sleep disturbances were in the same direction but slightly beyond the defined level of statistical significance [19].

Nocturnal alteration in heart rate associated with DISD may have no meaning in a healthy cardiovascular system. In an organism with advanced atherosclerosis, thrombotic developments, and silent or manifest ischemia, however, impaired central neuronal control of sleep and of cardiovascular function might trigger overt disease. Again, preliminary findings from the prospective blue-collar study show that subjects who during their last interview reported severe sleep disturbances were at a higher risk of developing their first lethal or nonlethal myocardial infarction within the 2 subsequent years as compared to those with normal sleep. The relative risk was 3.8 in those reporting frequent early wakings in the morning without falling asleep again and 2.6 in those reporting frequent difficulties staying asleep during night. These findings are based on small numbers of subjects, and it will be important to extend such studies to larger sample groups and longer observation periods.

Concluding Remarks

As stated earlier, links other than sleep apnea have to be explored in order to understand the association between disturbed sleep and cardiovascular excess morbidity. One possible link has been analyzed in terms of distress-induced sleep disturbances and their impact on heart rate. As a final comment, I would like to make some suggestions relating both phenomena, sleep apnea and distress-induced sleep disturbances, to a more general understanding of sleep regulation.

Two, far-reaching, general assumptions about sleep regulation have been made by Koella and Jouvet [7, 5] who looked at sleep in terms of a broader, vigilance-controlling system and interpreted undisturbed sleep as a result of a balance between catecholaminergic and serotonergic systems. As mentioned in Fig. 2. apneic episodes can be understood as multiple intrusions of emergency vigilance, interrupting sleep at all stages. Immediate and secondary effects of these intrusions are listed in Fig. 2.

On the other hand, distress-induced sleep disturbances can be assumed to be the result of vigilance-enhancing mechanisms due to excessive adrenergic stimulation during the day. Adrenergic activation associated with experiences of socioemotional distress may override sleep-inducing and sleep-maintaining serotonergic (and peptidergic) influences. According to these ideas, DISD-related nocturnal awakenings are expected to occur more often during NREM sleep than during REM sleep. In comparison with SAS, secondary effects of DISD are much more attenuated. As a consequence, the potential of DISD to trigger cardiovascular pathology is probably much smaller than the potential of SAS.

- Sleep as vigilance-controlling system (Koella)
- Balance between catecholaminergic and serotonergic system (Jouvet)

Apneic episodes:

- intrusion of emergency (vigilance) into sleep (multiple, all sleep stages)

→ immediate effects: altered heart rate, risk of severe arrhythmia
blood pressure ↑
hormonal release ↑

→ secondary effects: fatigue due to sleep fragmentation (EDS), psychophysiologic alteration during day

Distress-induced sleep disturbances:

- vigilance-enhancing mechanisms override serotonergic sleep-inducing mechanisms (difficulties falling asleep; waking up during NREM sleep)

→ immediate effects: altered heart rate
hormonal release (?)

→ secondary effects: decrease in cardiovascular reactivity to challenges during day (?) mild fatigue due to sleep fragmentation.

Fig. 2. Conceptual approach to sleep disturbances

Nevertheless, DISD may be regarded as an important precipitating factor in an already compromised cardiovascular system.

These concluding remarks demonstrate how many questions still have to be answered. In the near future EEG, ECG, and hormonal assessment should be taken in populations at cardiovascular risk. At the same time, psychosocial conditions have to be integrated into a comprehensive approach in order to gain new insights into the fascinating phenomenon of human sleep regulation and its impact on premature cardiovascular disorder.

References

1. Bolm-Audorff U, Köhler U, Becker E, Fuchs E, Meinzer K, Peter JH, von Wichert P (1984) Nächtliche Herzrhythmusstörungen bei Patienten mit Schlafapnoe-Syndrom. Dtsch Med Wochenschr 109:853–856
2. Bondoulas H, Schmidt HS, Clark RW, Geleris P, Schaal SF, Lewis RP (1983) Anthropometric characteristics, cardiac abnormalities and adrenergic activity in patients with primary disorders of sleep. J Med 14:223–238
3. Friedman GD, Ury HK, Klatsky AL (1974) A psychological questionnaire predictive of myocardial infarction: results from the Kaiser permanente epidemiologic study of myocardial infarction. Psychosom Med 36:327–343
4. Guilleminault C, Connolly S, Winkle R, Melvin K, Tilkian A (1984) Cyclical variation of heart rate in sleep apnea syndrome; mechanisms and usefulness of 24h ECG as a screening technique. Lancet i:126–131
5. Jouvet M (1969) Biogenic amines and the states of sleep. Science 163:32–41
6. Kannel WS, Sorlie P (1981) Left ventricular hypertrophy in hypertension: prognostic and pathogenetic implication (the Framingham study). In: Strauer BE (ed) The heart in hypertension. Springer, Berlin Heidelberg New York, pp 223–241
7. Koella WP (1984) The organization and regulation of sleep. Experientia 40:309–338
8. Koskenvuo M, Kaprio J, Partinen M, Langinvainio H, Sarna S, Rita H, Heikkilä K (1987) Poor sleep quality, emotional stress and morbidity. (to be published)
9. Kripke DF, Simons RN, Garfinkel L, Hammond EC (1979) Short and long sleep and sleeping pills. Is increased morbidity associated? Arch Gen Psychiatry 36:103–116
10. Langhorst P, Schulz G, Lambertz M, Krienke B (1980) Funktionelle Organisation eines gemeinsamen Hirnstammsystems für Kreislauf, Atmung und allgemeine Aktivitätsmessung. In: Schiffer R (ed) Zentralvegetative Regulationen und Syndrome. Springer, Berlin Heidelberg New York, pp 39–55
11. Lavie P (1983) Sleep apnea in industrial workers. In: Guilleminault C, Lugaresi E (eds) Sleep-wake disorders: natural history, epidemiology and longterm evolution. Raven, New York, pp 127–135
12. Matschinger H, Siegrist J, Siegrist K, Dittmann KH (1986) Type A as a coping career. In: Schmidt TH, Dembroski TM, Blümchen G (eds) Biological and psychological factors in cardiovascular disease. Springer, Berlin Heidelberg New York Tokyo, pp 104–126
13. Miller WP (1982) Cardiac arrhythmias and conduction disturbances in the sleep apnea syndrome. Am J Med 73:307–321
14. Partinen M, Putkonen PTS, Kaprio J, Koskenvuo M, Hilakivi I (1982) Sleep disorders in relation to coronary heart disease. Acta Med Scand [Suppl] 660:69–83
15. Peter JH, Bolm-Audorff U, Becker E, Eble R, Fuchs E, Meinzer K, Penzel T, von Wichert P (1983) Schlafapnoe und essentielle Hypertonie. Verh Dtsch Gesch Inn Med 89:1132–1135
16. Peter JH, Siegrist J, Podszus T, Mayer J, Selzer K, von Wichert P (1985) Prevalence in sleep apnea in healthy industrial workers. Klin Wochenschr 63:807–811
17. Schroeder JS, Motta J, Guilleminault C (1978) Hemodynamic studies in sleep apnea. In: Guilleminault C, Dement WC (eds) Sleep apnea syndromes. AR Liss, New York, pp 177–196

18. Siegrist J (1987) Impaired quality of life as a risk factor in cardiovascular disease. J Chronic Dis (to be published)
19. Siegrist J (1987) Disturbed sleep in blue-collar workers suffering from "occupational stress". (to be published)
20. Skinner JE (1985) Psychosocial stress and sudden cardiac death: brain mechanisms. In: Beamish RE, Singal PK, Dhalla NS (eds) Stress and the heart. Nijhoff, Boston, pp 44–59
21. Theorell T, Akerstedt T, Alfredsson L, Spetz CL (1987) Tired occupations and hospitalization (to be published)
22. Tilkian AG, Motta J, Guilleminault C (1978) Cardiac arrhythmias in sleep apnea. In: Guilleminault C, Dement WC (eds) Sleep apnea syndromes. New York AR Liss, pp 197–210
23. von Holst D (1986) Psychosocial stress and its pathophysiological effects in tree shrews *(Tupaia belangeri)*. In: Schmidt TH, Dembroski TM, Blümchen Cr (eds) Biological and psychological factors in cardiovascular disease. Springer, Berlin Heidelberg New York, pp 476–490
24. Wingard DL, Berkman LF (1983) Mortality risk associated with sleeping pattern among adults. Sleep 6:102–107

Sleep and Stress

T. ÅKERSTEDT

In previous chapters it has been shown that disturbed sleep constitutes a major medical problem both in itself and as a component in the development of other diseases, and thus probably also in mortality. Obviously then, it is of particular importance to understand the causes of disturbed sleep, not only in clinical populations but also in the population at large. Many causative factors may be involved, although one of the most widely recognized ones is psychosocial stress. It is the purpose of the present paper to review and discuss the arguments for a connection between stress and sleep.

Clinical Observations and Survey Studies

Most of the arguments of a connection between stress and disturbed sleep derive from clinical observations. It is a frequent observation, for example, that patients with insomnia exhibit problems at work, with their families or in life in general [8, 21, 50]. Such conditions may lead to increased tension and difficulties initiating or maintaining sleep. Patients with insomnia have also been shown (in retrospective studies) to have a pronounced increase of life change scores immediately before the outbreak of insomnia [30]. Furthermore on personality inventories their scores often indicate psychopathology and the tendency to internalize stress which, presumably, leads to physiological activation interfering with sleep [34].

In survey studies of nonclinical populations it has been observed that those individuals who complain of disturbed sleep often have more worries in life [44]. Such individuals may also report that they need help for tension, depression, and loneliness [13]. Retrospective studies of nonclinical groups also indicate that psychosocial stress often precedes periods of less satisfactory sleep [16].

The role of psychosocial stress is also reflected in the classification of sleep disorders [7]. The major stress-related categories are transient situational insomnia and chronic psychophysiological insomnia. The latter is presumed to develop from the former after long-term or repeated exposure to stress, together with a negative conditioning to the sleep situation [28]. In addition, psychosocial stress may also be involved in insomnia related to psychiatric disturbances and drug abuse.

It should be emphasized that these observations may suffer from certain biases since they derive from self-reports and are obtained retrospectively. Thus, it is possible that a deteriorated state of health at the time of reporting may have influenced the interpretation of the psychosocial circumstances contributing to that state of health. However, Bixler et al. [13] also used less easily distorted variables, such as occupation and education, and found that disturbed sleep was more common in lower educational and occupational strata. Partinen et al. [45] in a survey study also found that difficulties of sleep maintenance were greater in occupations with physically heavy work, whereas increased sleep latency and early morning awakenings were common in occupations with mental strain.

In a somewhat similar approach to that of Partinen et al. [45] we used aggregated data to study the covariation between sleep and work characteristics. We first obtained data on 271 occupations ($n = 14\,500$) with respect to work characteristics and well-being [6]. We then computed gamma correlation coefficients *across occupations* (manuscript in preparation). Table 1 shows that, for males, occupations leading to disturbed sleep are characterized by higher proportions of individuals having a more instrumental attitude towards work, experiencing more monotony, feeling unable to plan ahead, feeling unable to learn new skills, etc. Correlations for females show similar patterns. Among work characteristics not showing significant correlations are, for example, accident risk, sweating, feeling rushed, and full-time/part-time work. Among occupations with the highest proportion of workers complaining of poor sleep were waiters, kitchen personnel, cleaning personnel, and textile workers. The lowest proportion was found in occupations like forest foreman, physician, music and art teacher, and dental nurse. The results clearly suggest an association between disturbed sleep and negative work characteristics.

The only way to obtain conclusive data on cause and effect is through prospective studies. Such studies of sleep and stress are extremely rare, however. That reported by Dr Siegrist (this volume) is one of the few, and it demonstrates

Table 1. Significant gamma correlations between reports of disturbed sleep and various work characteristics. The correlations are computed across occupations ($n = 271$)

Gamma	Variable
Males 20–64 years	
0.31***	Instrumental attitude
0.31***	Monotonous work
0.29**	Inability to plan ahead
0.24**	No opportunities to learn new skills
0.23*	Noisy work environment
0.23*	Heavy work
0.23*	Hot work environment
Females 20–64 years	
0.39**	Not being able to talk during work
0.38**	Draughty environment
0.30*	Monotonous work
0.30*	Instrumental attitude
0.29*	Piece wage work
0.28*	Bad lighting

* $p < 0.05$; ** $p < 0.001$; *** $p < 0.001$

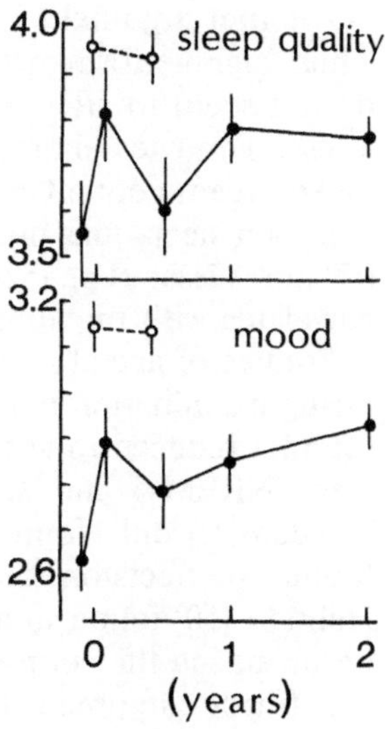

Fig. 1. Ratings of sleeps quality *(above)* and mood *(below)* before and after becoming unemployed (*filled circles*, $n = 60$) as well as corresponding measurements for a control group (*open circles*, $n = 50$) with stable employment. Unemployment starts at 0

that negative conditions, particularly in working life, precipitate disturbed sleep and, eventually perhaps, cardiovascular disease. Interestingly, this research group sees disturbed sleep and feelings of hopelessness as indicators of breakdown of the coping mechanisms of the individual.

In another prospective study we followed the reactions of a group of workers who faced imminent unemployment due to a factory closure [15]. An extended analysis of the data (manuscript in preparation) is presented in Fig. 1 and shows that during the month preceding the closure mood and sleep quality were low.

Immediately after closure both variables indicated improvement. This was interpreted as relief at the final certainty - perhaps in combination with the realization that unemployment might have some advantages as long as unemployment benefits could be collected and the free time made useful. This state remained for half a year, when suddenly pessimism and disturbed sleep reappeared, presumably because a new job had not appeared, and uncertainty about the future had started to grow. The data clearly demonstrate a covariation between the psychological reactions to unemployment and reports of disturbed sleep.

EEG Studies

Clinical and epidemiological studies suggest a connection between psychosocial stress and disturbed sleep. Support for this connection from polysomnographic/physiological studies has, however, seldom been sought, and most of the evidence is circumstantial. One type of support is based on the observation that poor sleepers are characterized by higher physiological arousal (heart rate, 17-hydroxycorticosteroids, etc.) than good sleepers [26, 33, 43]. Johns et al. [33] also claimed that sleep may be the most sensitive indicator of stress.

Another argument is based on experimental induction of stress or tension. Thus, high performance demands shortly prior to bedtime delay sleep onset but do not seem to affect sleep length or sleep architecture [27, 29]. Furthermore, stressful movies shortly before bedtime seem to intensify REM sleep and to make dream content more unpleasant [9, 19, 25, 41]. The ability to initiate and maintain sleep does not, however, seem to be affected. Still, Cluydts and Visser [17] and Visser et al. [52] have found that the (self-rated) anger induced by a film correlates with the amount of waking during the subsequent sleep.

Studies of actual real-life stress have, to a large extent, focussed on students facing examination periods. Holdstock and Veerschor [31] and Lester et al. [40] found a reduced total sleep time (TST). The latter authors also found reduced stage NREM-4 and an increased number of awakenings. Becker-Carus and Heyden [11] only found a small increase in REM time. Beaumaster et al. [10] found no effects on sleep in inexperienced sky divers before a dive. Schneider-Helmert [50] found in a few subjects that major life events, which happened to occur during the course of a laboratory study, reduced sleep efficiency.

A further argument for stress effects on sleep may be the transient insomnia that is often seen during the first sleep episode in a sleep laboratory, i.e., the so-called first night effect [3]. Admittedly, this disturbance could often be regarded as an effect of psychosocial stress. Still, it may equally well result from the lack of experience at coping with the physical aspects of wearing electrodes and cables.

To us, the results cited above seem rather inconclusive. The effects are weak and very variable and hardly indicate any close connection between stress and sleep. One reason for this could be that sleep, simply, is insensitive to stress. In most studies cited, however, the amount of stress induced seems to have been rather low, and it is unclear how the laboratory setting has affected the amount of perceived stress. Another problem is that the necessity of having a subject report to a sleep laboratory will interfere with the possibilities of recording sleep under severe life stress. In addition, the traditional sleep scoring method [47] fails to account for more than a fraction of the variance of the EEG [14] - most of the variability takes place *within* sleep stages.

In a small study of our own we recorded the sleep of ship's engineers (on transatlantic routes) who spend every 2nd or 3rd night "on call." That is, they sleep in their own quarters but are awakened by one or two alarms per night. This is perceived as unpleasant and disturbing. It is also associated with reports of apprehension and disturbed sleep quality.

We recorded the sleep of the engineers through portable tape recorders (Medilog) and found that TST and the amounts of all major sleep stages were reduced during nights on call [51] (Fig. 2). We also subjected the recordings to spectral analysis (Fast Fourier Transformation FFT) and found very strong reductions in accumulated power in the δ- and ϑ-bands (0.5–7.9 Hz). This reduction may have been a trivial consequence of spending a given amount of time ($\approx$ 1 h) out of bed attending to alarms, were it not for the fact that mean power/min was also reduced. Furthermore, the first sleep cycle which, by chance, was never interrupted by alarms, showed a very strong reduction of spectral power density (Fig. 2). This was accompanied by an increased heart rate and presleep feelings of uneasiness.

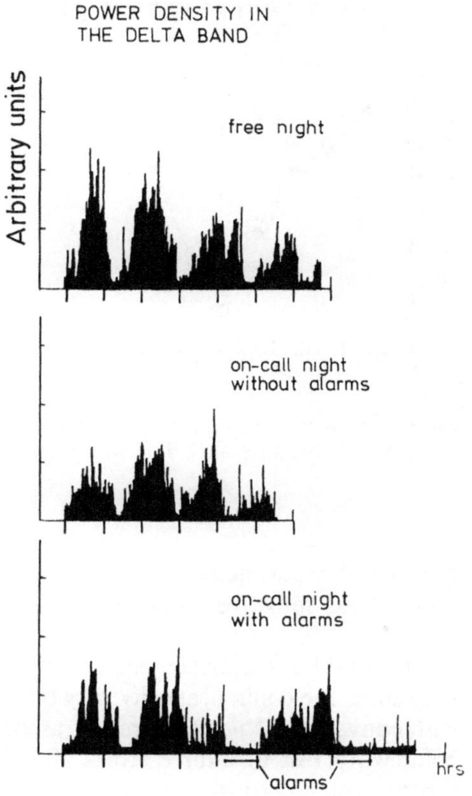

Fig. 2. Results from spectral analysis of one subject during a free night *(top)*, an undisturbed night on call *(middle)*, as well as an on-call night with two alarms *(below)*. The spectral power density (in the δ-band) units on the y-axis are arbitrary

The results suggest that even the rather moderate stress of expecting an alarm causes some type of apprehension that suppresses the normal augmentation of EEG spectral power during the first sleep cycle and, possibly, also during later cycles. Presumably, many types of day-to-day life stress might cause much larger effects. They and their long-term results remain to be demonstrated, however.

Sleep Loss as a Stressor

Another aspect of the link between stress and sleep is the reverse of that discussed above, that is, does sleep loss not only result from stress, but cause it as well? We are all aware of the fact that complaints of reduced sleep often seem to covary with irritation and other putative consequences of stress. This may be particularly evident in small children. As was discussed above, however, there has been no successful attempt to substantiate such assumptions. In our own studies we have found that 2 or 3 days of continuous wakefulness do not cause any change in traditional stress indicators such as adrenaline or noradrenaline excretion or stress ratings [4, 22–24]. Figure 3 illustrates the pattern of adrenaline excretion found in these studies. There is no change in adrenaline excretion as sleep loss increases, and the circadian rhythmicity remains imperturbed. A large

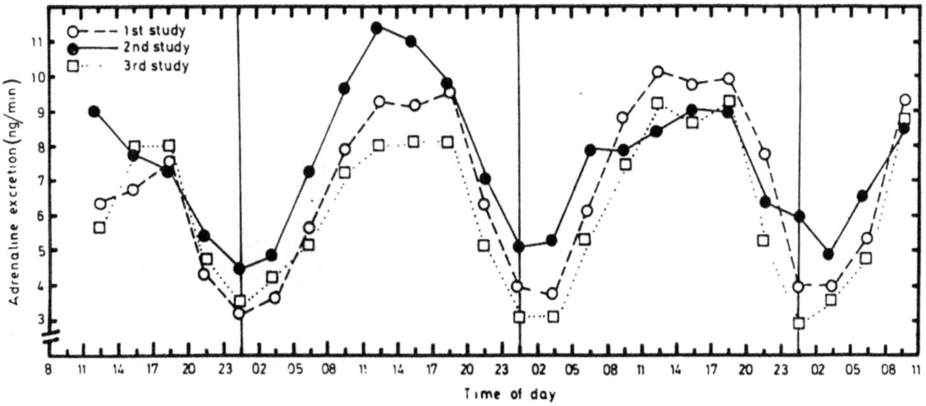

Fig. 3. Adrenaline excretion (3-h intervals) from three studies of 75 h of continuous wakefulness. *1st study* [23], *2nd study* [24]; *3rd study* [4, 22] ($n = 91$, ≈ 30 each)

number of experiments have been conducted to study the effects of sleep loss on other stress-sensitive parameters, but no conclusive pattern has been observed [32].

One could also expect sleep loss to potentiate the effects of a stressor, particularly since the coping capacity may be reduced. This does not seem to be the case with conventional performance stressors. We have, for example, used the Stroop color word test to induce stress after 28, 40, and 53 h of wakefulness [5]. The Stroop test did cause significant responses of adrenaline excretion, but none differed from control group levels. Similar results have been obtained by Bergström et al. [12] who exposed subjects to electric shocks after 80 h of sleep loss: only the normal heart rate response was found. Also, Kollar et al. [35] administered ACTH to their subjects during sleep deprivation but found only the normal cortisol response.

In hindsight, it may seem logical that fairly trivial, nonego-threatening stressors fail to interact with sleep loss. It may still be suspected that the effects of more stressful events in everyday life will be potentiated by sleep loss. This remains to be demonstrated, however. Clearly, there is a great need for more field studies, preferably longitudinal ones.

Sleep as Recuperation from Stress

Even if sleep loss may not be a stressor in itself, sleep may still serve a vital function in the recuperation from stress. Rest and sleep are the usual recommendation to patients recovering from physical illness or psychological trauma. Surprisingly little systematic knowledge is available, however.

Adam and Oswald [2] have argued that sleep provides an anabolic state supporting, for example, tissue restoration. There are several arguments in favor of this anabolic role. For example, there is a pronounced secretion of human growth hormone related to sleep, particularly slow-wave sleep [46, 49]. Stress-related changes in growth hormone, prolactin, and testosterone secretion are reversed through short sleep episodes [1]. The immune system seems activated by sleep, and particularly by slow-wave sleep [42]. Furthermore, sleep deprivation in laboratory rats leads to their death [48], often through bleeding ulcers, myocardial infarctions, etc. The latter study may be compared with that of Kripke et al. [39] demonstrating an increased mortality ratio in humans sleeping less than 4 h (or more than 10 h) per 24 h.

Another argument supporting a restorative role is that sleep may have a mood-regulating function [37] especially through dreams [36]. It was observed earlier that Cohen [19] found increased amounts of REM sleep after pre-bedtime threatening experiences. It was also found that those who exhibited the largest REM response were those who had the lowest neuroticism indices - and thus presumably were more adept at coping with stress. Furthermore, those who incorporated stressful events in their dreams felt better in the morning [20]. This correlates with psychodynamic concepts that dreaming is a part of a problem-solving process.

Taken al together, the results above tend to support the common sense notion of sleep as recuperation from stress. Hard, conclusive evidence is still lacking, however.

Conclusions

The literature reviewed indicates that the relationship between stress and sleep has not been conclusively established. It would seem that there is a great need for

a) prospective studies that evaluate the effects of spontaneously or predictably occurring life stress;
b) interdisciplinary studies merging polysomnography with endocrinology, immunology, and other specialties, including psychology;
c) studies in the normal environment of individuals; and
d) more sensitive methods of EEG analysis.

The approach suggested demands sizeable resources, but the growing interest in sleep and internal medicine may make such studies feasible.

References

1. Aakvaag A, Sand T, Opstad PR, Fonnum F (1978) Hormonal changes in serum in young men during prolonged physical strain. Eur J Appl Physiol 39:283–291
2. Adam K, Oswald I (1977) Sleep is for tissue restoration. J Coll Phys 11:376–388
3. Agnew HW, Webb WB, Williams RL (1966) The first night effect: an EEG study of sleep. Psychophysiology 2:263–266
4. Åkerstedt T, Fröberg JE (1977) Psychophysiological circadian rhythms in women during 72 h of sleep deprivation. Waking Sleep 1:387–394

5. Åkerstedt T, Fröberg JE (1979) Sleep, stress and sleep deprivation in relation to circadian rhythms in catecholamine excretion. Biol Psychol 8:69–80
6. Alfredsson L, Spetz G-L, Theorell T (1985) Type of occupation and near-future hospitalization for myocardial infarction and some other diagnoses. Int J Epidemiol 14:378–388
7. ASDC-Association of Sleep Disorders Centers (1979) Diagnostic classification of sleep and arousal disorders. Sleep 2:1–137
8. Baastians J (1981) The psychosomatic approach of sleep disturbances. In: Koella WP (ed) Sleep 1980. Karber, Basel, p 86
9. Baekeland F, Koulack D, Lasky R (1968) Effects of a stressful presleep experience on electroencephalograph-recorded sleep. Psychophysiology 4:436–443
10. Beaumaster EJ, Knowles JB, MacLean AW (1978) The sleep of sky divers: a study of stress. Psychophysiology 15:209–213
11. Becker-Carus C, Heyden T (1979) Stress-Wirkungen in Labor- und Realsituation in Abhängigkeit von REM-Schlaf und psychophysiologischer Aktivation. Z Exp Angew Psychol 1:37–52
12. Bergström B, Gillberg M, Arnberg P (1973) Effects of sleep loss and stress upon radar watching. J Appl Psychol 58:158–162
13. Bixler EO, Kales A, Soldatos CR, Kales JD, Healey S (1979) Prevalence of sleep disorders in the Los Angeles metropolitan area. Am J Psychiatry 136:1257–1262
14. Borbély AA, Baumann F, Brandeis D, Strauch I, Lehmann D (1981) Sleep deprivation: effect on sleep stages and EEG power density in man. Electroencephalogr Clin Neurophysiol 51:483–493
15. Brenner S-O, Arnetz B, Levi L (1983) Effekter av otrygghet i arbetet, förlust av arbetet och arbetslöshet: de tre första mätningarna på gruppen arbetslösa som deltar i ett åtgärdspaket. (Effects of insecurity at work, loss of work, and unemployment) Stressforskningsrapporter 120:1–58
16. Cernovsky ZZ (1984) Life stress measures and reported frequency of sleep disorders. Perceptual and Motor Skills 58:39–49
17. Cluydts R, Visser P (1980) Mood and sleep I: effects of the menstrual cycle. II. Effects of aversive pre-sleep stimulation. Waking Sleep 4:193–203
18. Cluydts RJG, Visser P (1981) Emotional stress, mood state and sleep. In: Koella WP (ed) Sleep 1980. Karger, Basel, p 102
19. Cohen DB (1975) Eye movements during REM sleep: the influence of personality and presleep conditions. J Pers Soc Psychol 32:1090–1093
20. Cohen D, Cox C (1975) Neuroticism in the sleep laboratory: implications for representational and adaptive properties of dreaming. J Abnorm Psychol 84:191–198
21. Dement WC (1983) Rational basis for the use of sleeping pills. Pharmacology [Suppl] 2:3–38
22. Fröberg J (1977) Twenty-four-hour patterns in human performance, subjective and physiological variables and differences between morning and evening active subjects. Biol Psychol 5:119–134
23. Fröberg J, Karlsson C-G, Levi L, Lidberg L (1975a) Circadian variations of catecholamine excretion, shooting range performance and self-ratings of fatigue during sleep deprivation. Biol Psychol 2:175–188
24. Fröberg J, Karlsson C-G, Levi L, Lidberg L (1975b) Psychobiological circadian rhythms during a 72 hour vigil. Försvarsmedicin 11:192–201
25. Goodenough DR, Witkin HA, Koulack D, Cohen H (1975) The effects of stress films on dream affect and on respiration and eye-movement activity during rapid-eye-movement sleep. Psychophysiology 12:313–320
26. Goodyear MDE (1973) Stress, adrenocortical activity and sleep habits. Ergonomics 16:679–681
27. Hauri P (1968) Effects of evening activity on early night sleep. Psychophysiology 3:267–277
28. Hauri P, Fischer J (1986) Persistent psychophysiologic (learned) insomnia. Sleep 9:38–53
29. Haynes SN, Fitzgerald SG, Shute G, O'Meary M (1985) Responses of psychophysiologic and subjective insomniacs to auditory stimuli during sleep: a replication and extension. J Abnorm Psychol 94:338–345
30. Healey ES, Kales A, Monroe LJ, Bixler EO, Chamberlain K, Soldatos CR (1981) Onset of insomnia: role of life stress events. Psychosom Med 43:439–451

31. Holdstock TL, Verschoor GJ (1974) Student sleep patterns before, during and after an examination period. SA J Psychol 4:16–24
32. Horne JA (1978) A review of the biological effects of total sleep deprivation in man. Biol Psychol 7:55–102
33. Johns MW, Gay TJA, Masterton JP, Bruce DW (1971) Relationship between sleep habits, adrenocortical activity and personality. Psychosom Med 33:499–508
34. Kales A, Caldwell AB, Soldatos CR, Bixler EO, Kales JD (1983) Biopsychobehavioral correlates of insomnia. II: pattern specificity and consistency with the Minnesota multiphasic personality inventory. Psychosom Med 45:341–355
35. Kollar EJ, Slater GR, Palmer JO, Docter RF, Mandell AJ (1966) Stress in subjects undergoing sleep deprivation. Psychosom Med 28:101–113
36. De Koninck J (1981) Dreaming and mood regulation in stressful situations. In: Koella WP (ed) Sleep 1980. Karger, Basel, p 91
37. Kramer M, Roehrs T, Roth T (1976) Mood change and the physiology of sleep. Compr Psychiatry 17:161–165
39. Kripke DF, Simons RN, Garfinkel L, Cuyler-Hammond E (1979) Short and long sleep and sleeping pills. Is increased mortality associated? Arch Gen Psychiatry 36:103–116
40. Lester BK, Burch NR, Dossett RC (1967) Nocturnal EEG-GSR profiles: the influence of presleep states. Psychophysiology 3:238–248
41. McGrath MJ, Cohen D (1980) REM drive and function: a study of the interactive effects of personality and presleep condition. J Abnorm Psychol 89:737–743
42. Moldofsky H, Lue FA, Eisen J, Keystone E, Gorczynski RM (1986) The relationship of interleukin-1 and immune functions to sleep in humans. Psychosom Med 48:309–318
43. Monroe LJ (1967) Psychological and physiological differences between good and poor sleepers. J Abnorm Psychol 72:225–264
44. Palmer CD, Harrison GA (1983) Sleep latency and life style in Oxfordshire villages. Ann Hum Biol 10:417–428
45. Partinen M, Eskelinen L, Tuomi K (1984) Complaints of insomnia in different occupations. Scand J Work Environ Health 10:467–469
46. Quabbe HJ, Schilling E, Helge H (1976) Pattern of growth hormone secretion during a 24 hour fast in normal adults. J Clin Endocrinol Metab 26:1173–1177
47. Rechtschaffen A, Kales A (eds) (1968) A manual of standardized terminology, techniques and scoring system for sleep stages of human subjects. UCLA brain information service Brain Research Institute, Los Angeles
48. Rechtschaffen A, Gilliland MA, Bergmann BM, Winter JB (1983) Physiological correlates of prolonged sleep deprivation in rats. Science 221:182–184
49. Sassin JF, Parker DC, Mace JW, Gotlin RW, Johnson LC, Rossman LG (1969) Human growth hormone release: relation to slow wave sleep and sleep-waking cycles. Science 165:513–515
50. Schneider-Helmert D (1981) Clinical and conceptual aspects of sleep and emotional stress. In: Koella WP (ed) Sleep 1980. Karger, Basel, p 107
51. Torsvall L, Åkerstedt T, Fröberg J (1986) On-call duty, sleep and wakefulness. An EEG-study of engineers on ships in the Swedish merchant marine. In: Koella WP (ed) Sleep 1986. Gustav Fischer, Stuttgart
52. Visser P, Hofman WF, Kumar A, Cluydts R, de Diana IPF, Marchant P, Bakker HJ, van Diest R, Poelstra PAM (1979) Sleep and mood: measuring the sleep quality. In: Priest RG, Pletscher A, Ward J (eds) Sleep research. MTP Press, Lancaster, p 135

Prevalence of Sleep Complaints Among Swedish Men - An Epidemiological Study

T. Gislason

Introduction

Several surveys based on questionnaires have revealed a high prevalence of insomnia and of excessive daytime sleepiness in the population [1–5]. Some somatic diseases [6–8] and also some medications [9] have been known to cause sleep disturbances. Sleep-induced respiratory disorders such as the sleep apnoea syndrome (SAS) have a well-known relationship to sleep complaints, of which the main ones are heavy snoring and daytime sleepiness [10]. Recently some authors have reported a high frequency of SAS among patients with systemic hypertension and also among those with various other manifestations of cardiovascular disturbances [11–13]. Even snoring alone has been discussed as a risk factor for hypertension and angina pectoris [14, 15].

As shown in Table 1, previous investigations into the prevalences of SAS have been based on: presumably healthy and selected populations [16, 17]; in-patient populations [18, 19]; a healthy, working male population [20]; or apparently healthy, elderly individuals [21]. Both the designs and results of these studies have varied considerably. None of the investigated groups constitute a cross section of the general population. On the contrary, they consist of special categories of subjects, who happened to be available for investigation at the time. In only two studies [19, 20] were defined procedures for subject selection employed, i.e. the subjects were from specified background populations. Lavie's report [20] is the only one in which statistical considerations are presented.

Aim of the Study

The basic strategy of this study was to recruit from a Swedish population a cohort of men with symptoms that are known to be associated with SAS, using a mailed questionnaire. It was planned that from among these a group of 60 subjects should be studied for a whole night in a sleep laboratory to estimate the prevalence of SAS. Apart from information on symptoms possibly indicating this syndrome, the questionnaires also provided basic data for calculating the prevalence of insomnia and daytime sleepiness and the association of these conditions with systemic hypertension, diabetes mellitus, rheumatic diseases and obstructive pulmonary diseases. The relationship between snoring, age, body weight and hypertension was also to be investigated.

Table 1. Construction and results of previous studies on the prevalence of sleep apnoea syndrome (SAS)

Reference	Population	Sample size *(n)* and criteria	Sex	Mean Age (Range) (years)	No. of such subjects with SAS
Bixler et al. [16]	Volunteers, students, technical staff and friends	$n = 100$, without complaints of sleep disorders	41 M 59 F	39 (18–74) 41 (18–74)	0[a]
Block et al. [17]	Medical and nursing staff and patients	$n = 49$, no breathing complaints	30 M 19 F	38 (24–62) 29 (20–31)	?
Kreis et al. [18]	Patients from a general medical service	$n = 26$, not medicallv unstable, not demented or not expected to be discharged withing 3 days	26 M	62 (38–88)	7[b]
Franceschi et al. [19]	All patients ($n = 2518$) admitted to S. Raffaele Hospital during 1 year	$n = 87$, selected on the basis of questionnaires and clinical data			SAS:8 M, 18 F
Lavie [20]	Industrial workers	$n = 78$, males, selected on the basis of questionnaires	78 M	43 (median 35)	SAS:17 M
Carskadon et al. [21]	Elderly volunteers from nonmedical sources	$n = 40$, without serious medical disorders not complaining spontaneously of sleep problems	18 M 22 F	73 (63–86) 74 (62–82)	SAS:8 M, 7 F

[a] Six males and six females had 3–29 apnoeas.
[b] Another three men had 24–27 apnoeas.

Material and Methods

Population. The survey was carried out in the municipality of Uppsala, Sweden, during the winter of 1984–1985. The total population of the municipality at the time of the study was 150 579 (77 444 women and 73 135 men). Among the men, 35 779 were between 30 and 69 years of age. Systematic (random) sampling of approximately every ninth man was performed, comprising 4064 men or 11.4% of all men aged 30–69 years.

Questionnaire. The questionnaire consisted of eight specific questions, to be answered by yes or no, concerning high blood pressure, heart diseases, psychiatric disorders, diabetes mellitus, bronchitis and asthma. There were three general questions concerning regular medical examinations, medication, and previous hospital care. Weight and height were reported and the body mass index (BMI) was calculated as Quetelet's index (weight in kg)/(height in m^2). Thirteen questions of the multiple choice type dealt with sleep disturbances and daytime symptoms, mainly those that could be expec ted to occur concomitantly with SAS. The subjects were asked to state the severity of their sleep complaints and snoring by means of a 5-point scale.

Procedure. The 4064 questionnaires were mailed at the beginning of December, 1984, and to those who did not reply, two reminding letters were mailed at intervals of 5 weeks. Some advertisement was published in a local newspaper.

Results

A total of 3201 acceptably answered questionnaires were analysed, giving a net response rate of 79.6%. The age distribution of the responders was almost the same as for the target population in the municipality. All the following questions were answered by at least 98.0% of the 3201 responders.

Insomnia

Difficulty in Initiating Sleep (DIS). Of all subjects 6.9% complained of great difficulty in falling asleep at night and 14.3% had moderate problems of the same kind (Table 2).

Difficulty in Maintaining Sleep (DMS). Great problems with frequent awakening were reported by as many as 7.5% of the men and moderate problems of this kind by 14.9% (Table 2).

Excessive Daytime Sleepiness (EDS). Complaints of moderate daytime sleepiness were made by 16.7% and 5.8% reported that this was a major problem (Table 2).

Table 2. Percentage of men with different sleep complaints concomitant with somatic diseases. *DIS*, difficulty in initiating sleep; *DMS*, difficulty in maintaining sleep; *EDS*, excessive daytime sleepiness.

	DIS		DMS		EDS	
	moderate	major	moderate	major	moderate	major
All men ($n = 3201$)	14.3	6.9	14.9	7.5	16.7	5.8
Men attending regular medical checkups ($n = 879$)	18.8	12.6***	23.5	14.5***	17.9	10.2**
Systemic hypertension ($n = 299$)	18.9	8.4***	26.1	13.5***	18.2	8.8*
Bronchitis/bronchial asthma ($n = 113$)	15.2	11.6	23.2	18.8***	22.1	12.4**
Diabetes mellitus ($n = 74$)	19.7	21.1***	20.5	21.9***	29.7	12.2***
Joint complaints/low back pain ($n = 176$)	17.9	13.3***	19.4	15.9***	20.2	10.4

* $p < 0.05$; ** $p < 0.01$; *** $p < 0.001$

Somatic Diseases and Sleep Complaints

Of the 3201 men, 879 (27.5%) were attending regular medical examinations. The prevalence of major complaints of insomnia (both DIS and DMS) and of EDS was almost twice as high among them (Table 2). A further analysis of the most common somatic diseases in relation to sleep complaints is presented in Table 2.

Snoring

Habitual snoring was reported by 487 subjects (15.5%) and occasional snoring by 928 (29.6%). There was an age-related increase in snoring up to 60 years, but subsequently there was some decline (Fig. 1). The frequency of snoring also rose with increased body weight.

Systemic Hypertension and Snoring

Altogether 299 subjects (9.3%) reported hypertension, and this was more common in the older age groups. Among them 21.5% were habitual snorers and 32.6% snored occasionally. Statistically there was a higher frequency of habitual snorers among hypertensives than among non-hypertensives ($\chi^2 = 12.18$, $p < 0.01$). This difference was greatest in the age group 40–49 years.

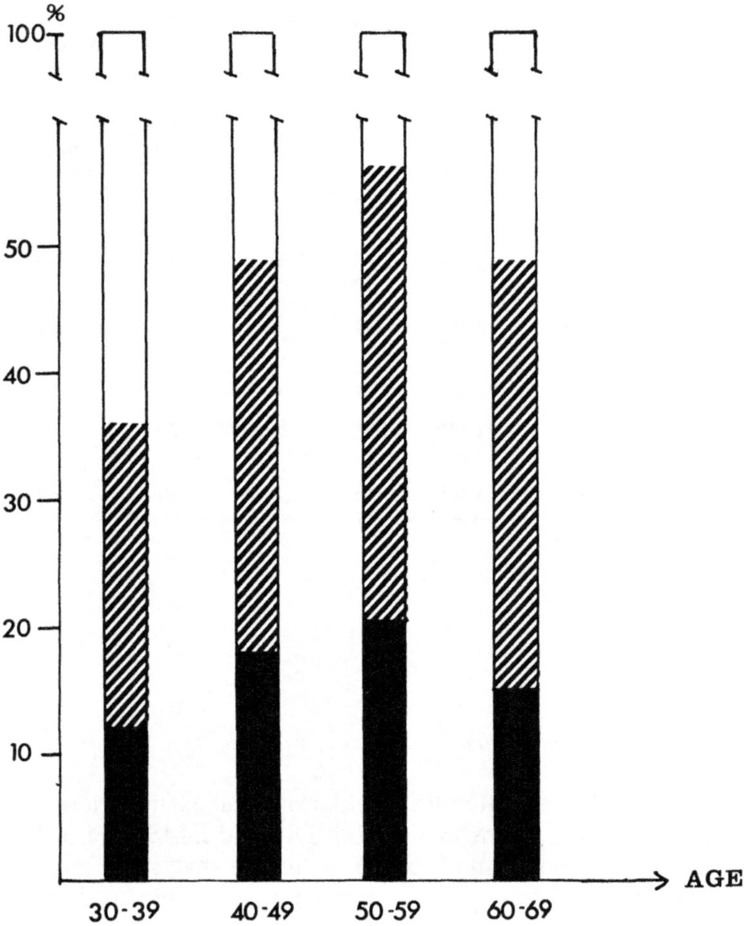

Fig. 1. Prevalence of snoring in each age group (years): habitual *(black bars)*, occasional *(hatched)* and non-snorers *(open)*

Prevalence of SAS

The complaints of snoring and daytime sleepiness were used for identification of the high-risk group. Those with the greatest complaints of both were highly suspected of suffering from SAS. Thus a group of 166 men was so identified, and eventually 61 of them submitted to a whole-night polysomnographic study with simultaneous recording of sleep stages, respiratory effort, air flow and oxygen saturation. According to preliminary results 15 men had more than 30 respiratory events (both apnoeas and hypopnoeas). If we assume that the 61 investigated are representative of all the 166 men highly suspected of having SAS, the lower prevalence of SAS will be 16/61 × 166/3201, or 1.3% with a standard error of 0.3%.

Discussion

With an almost 80% response rate and with the same age distribution among the responders as among the population at large, the results should be representative of the prevalence of sleep complaints among all those 30–69 years old. The reliability of the diagnoses reported by the participants themselves in the questionnaire cannot be assessed, but the prevalence of hypertension and obstructive pulmonary disease found in this study is close to figures from other counties in Sweden.

Insomnia. Our findings that 6.9% complained of major difficulty in falling asleep and that 14.3% had moderate problems of this kind are not readily comparable with reports from other studies, as the sampling techniques and questions differ [1–5]. From a study in Florida [2], it was reported that 13.4% complained of having difficulty in sleeping "often" or "always", and in another study 14.7% of Italian males over the age of 20 years were found to suffer from subjective insomnia [4].

Sleep complaints were almost twice as common among men who were attending regular medical checkups for somatic disease (Table 2). There is a logical explanation for these complaints among men suffering from pain, such as those with rheumatic diseases [8]. Among subjects with obstructive pulmonary disorders, breathing problems [6] or the pharmacological treatment [9] might be the underlying cause. The question whether the sleep complaints are an expression of higher activity of the basic somatic disease or a complication of the treatment, cannot be answered on the basis of this study. The results presented give reason to ask how often complaints of insomnia might be caused by an undiagnosed underlying somatic disease.

Snoring. The age-related increase in the frequency of snoring up to the age of 60 years, followed by a decline, has been described previously [14], as has the relationship between snoring and cardiovascular diseases [11–14]. In the present study, however, it was only in the 40–49-year age group that a statistically significant increase in the frequency of hypertension was found. It is noteworthy that in another investigation the relative risk of angina pectoris among habitual snorers was also highest in men aged 40–49 years, and fell with age [15]. The decrease in risk with age could be explained by the well-known fact that a single factor can lose its effect with increasing age at the same time as the relative effects of other factors become greater.

Prevalence of SAS. The 1.3% prevalence of SAS is similar to that found by Lavie in an investigation of healthy male industrial workers [20] but much lower than the figures reported in other studies. Objective comparison is difficult, however, as indicated in Table 1. If we apply these preliminary results to the whole male population of Sweden, we estimate that there are some 20 000 cases of SAS among men aged 30–69 years, with the majority in the age group 50–59 years.

References

1. McGhie A, Russell SM (1962) The subjective assessment of normal sleep patterns. J Ment Sci 108:642–654
2. Karacan I, Thornby JI, Anch M, Holzer CE, Warheit GJ, Schwabb JJ, Williams RL (1976) Prevalence of sleep disturbance in a primarily urban Florida county. Soc Sci Med 10:239–244
3. Bixler EO, Kales A, Soldatos CR, Kales JO, Healey S (1979) Prevalence of sleep disorders in the Los Angeles metropolitan area. Am J Psychol 136:1257–1262
4. Lugaresi E, Cirignotta F, Zucconi M, Mondini S, Lenzi P, Coccagna G (1983) Good and poor sleepers: an epidemiological survey of the San Marino population. In: Guilleminault C, Lugaresi E (eds) Sleep/wake disorders: natural history, epidemiology and long-term evolution. Raven, New York, pp 73–85
5. Partinen M, Kaprio J, Koskenvuo M, Langinvainio H (1983) Sleeping habits, sleep quality, and use of sleeping pills: a population study of 31140 adults in Finland. In: Guilleminault C, Lugaresi E (eds) Sleep/wake disorders: natural history, epidemiology and long-term evolution. Raven, New York, pp 29–35
6. Branscomb BV (1984) The difficult asthmatic. Clin Chest Med 5:695–713
7. Johns MWW, Egan P, Gay TJ, Mastenon JP (1970) Sleep habits and symptoms in male medical and surgical patients. Br Med J 2:509–512
8. Cohen L (1978) A controlled study of Trancopal in sleep˙disturbances due to rheumatic disease. J Int Med Res 6:111–114
9. Hendeles L, Bighley L, Richardson RH, Hepler CD, Carmichael J (1977) Frequent toxicity from IV aminophylline infusions in critically ill patients. Drug Intell Clin Pharm 11:12–18
10. Guilleminault C, Cummisky J, Dement WC (1980) Sleep apnea syndromes: recent advances. Adv Intern Med 26:347–374
11. Lavie P, Ben-Yosef R, Rubi AE (1984) Prevalence of sleep apnea syndrome among patients with essential hypertension. Am Heart J 108:373–376
12. Kales A, Bixler E, Cadieux R, Schneck DN, Shaw LC, Locke TW, Vela-Bueno A, Soldatos CR (1984) Sleep apnea in a hypertensive population. Lancet II:1005–1008
13. Williams AJ, Houston P, Finberg S, Lam C, Kinney JL, Santiago S (1985) Sleep apnea syndrome and essential hypertension. Am J Cardiol 55:1019–1022
14. Lugaresi E, Cirignotta F, Coccagna G, Piana C (1980) Some epidemiological data on snoring and cardiocirculatory disturbances. Sleep 3:221–224
15. Koskenvuo M, Kaprio J, Partinen M, Langinvainio H, Sarna S, Heikkilà K (1985) Snoring as a risk factor for hypertension and angina pectoris. Lancet II:893–895
16. Bixler EO, Kales A, Soldatos CR, Bueno AV (1982) Sleep apneic activity in a normal population. Res Commun Chem Pathol Pharmacol 36(1):141–152
17. Block AJ, Boysen PG, Wynne JW, Hunt LA (1979) Sleep apnea, hypopnea and oxygen desaturation in normal subjects – a strong male dominance. N Engl J Med 300:513–517
18. Kreis P, Kripke DF, Ancoli-Israel S (1983) Sleep apnea: a prospective study. West J Med 139:171–173
19. Franceschi M, Zamproni P, Crippa D, Smirne S (1982) Excessive daytime sleepiness: A 1-year study in an unselected inpatient population. Sleep 5:239–247
20. Lavie P (1983) Incidence of sleep apnea in a presumably healthy working population. Sleep 6:312–318
21. Carskadon M, Dement WC (1981) Respiration during sleep in the aged human. J Gerontol 36:420–423

Part 4: Epidemiology II – Snoring

Clinical Approach to Heavy Snorers' Disease and Other Sleep-Related Respiratory Disorders

E. Lugaresi, F. Cirignotta, and P. Montagna

The advent of polysomnographic techniques has vastly improved our understanding of respiratory disorders arising during sleep. Our studies in this field have already been discussed in previous reviews [1–3]. We will now attempt to delineate briefly the clinical features of the main nosological categories of sleep-related respiratory disorders, from snoring and the obstructive sleep apnea syndromes (OSAS) to central apneas and the idiopathic central alveolar hypoventilation (ICAH) syndromes.

Snoring

In the 1960s, when we began our studies on patients affected by OSAS, we were impressed by the fact that these patients had been heavy snorers for years or even decades. We wondered then whether snoring and OSAS were conditions related to each other. Polygraphic studies of snoring confirmed our hypothesis.

Snoring is an inspiratory noise due to stenosis of the upper airways during sleep. This is demonstrated by the increased activity of inspiratory intercostal muscles and by the abnormal increase in negative endothoracic pressure. Heavy snorers undergo obstructive apneas especially during sleep stages 1–2 and REM sleep. Apneas are favored by a phasic weakening of central ventilation. Series of obstructive apneas may occur in heavy snorers and, in this situation, snoring becomes intermittent. In heavy snorers, values of systemic arterial and pulmonary pressures, and PaO_2 and $PaCO_2$ during sleep are intermediate between normal controls and patients with OSAS. As far as systemic arterial pressure (AP) is concerned, nonsnoring normal subjects show a 10%–15% decrease during sleep, with lowest values during stages 3–4. Snorers instead show a slight but significant increase in AP, with the highest values during REM sleep.

On the basis of these findings, we wondered whether chronic snoring, even when it does not progress into manifest disease, could in itself represent a risk factor for the heart and circulation. Therefore we conducted an epidemiological survey on snoring on a sample of about 6000 people in the small Republic of San Marino [4]. We found that habitual snoring is quite common: 19% of all people snore habitually, 24% of males and 14% of females. Snorers increase with age, and about 50% of all males over 40 years snore habitually. Snoring is significantly related to weight; 16% of thin against 45% of obese people snore habitually in the

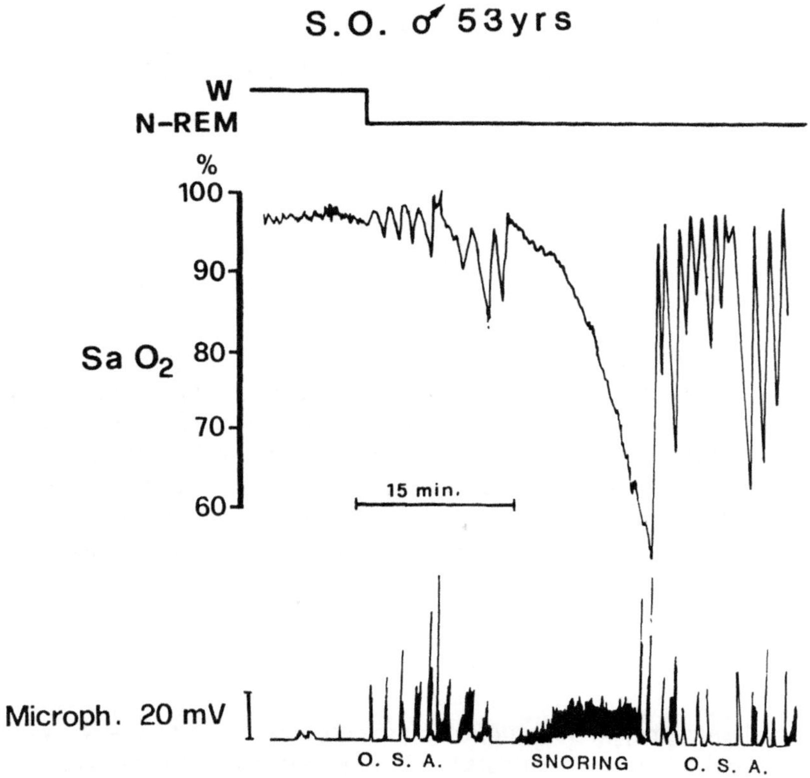

Fig. 1. Patient with OSAS. Snoring was associated with decrease of SaO_2 to levels lower than during apneas

age range 30–59 years. An even more interesting finding of our survey was that habitual snorers, whether thin, moderately overweight, or markedly obese all had pressure values higher than nonsnorers. Our epidemiological findings have been duplicated by other surveys, which have all confirmed our hypothesis that snoring can exert negative effects on the cardiocirculatory system.

Finally, it should be noted that even when snoring does not represent the principal complaint, its presence may aggravate pre-existing disorders. Thus profound detrimental changes in blood gas exchanges may be caused by snoring in pathological conditions characterized by respiratory impairment. This may be the case, for instance, in patients affected with OSAS (Fig. 1) or with ICAH syndromes (Fig. 2).

Heavy Snorers' Disease (OSAS)

Having shown that snoring and obstructive apneas represent variants of the same mechanism, i.e., incomplete or complete stenosis of the upper airways, we tried to define the evolutive stages through which trivial snoring may progress into

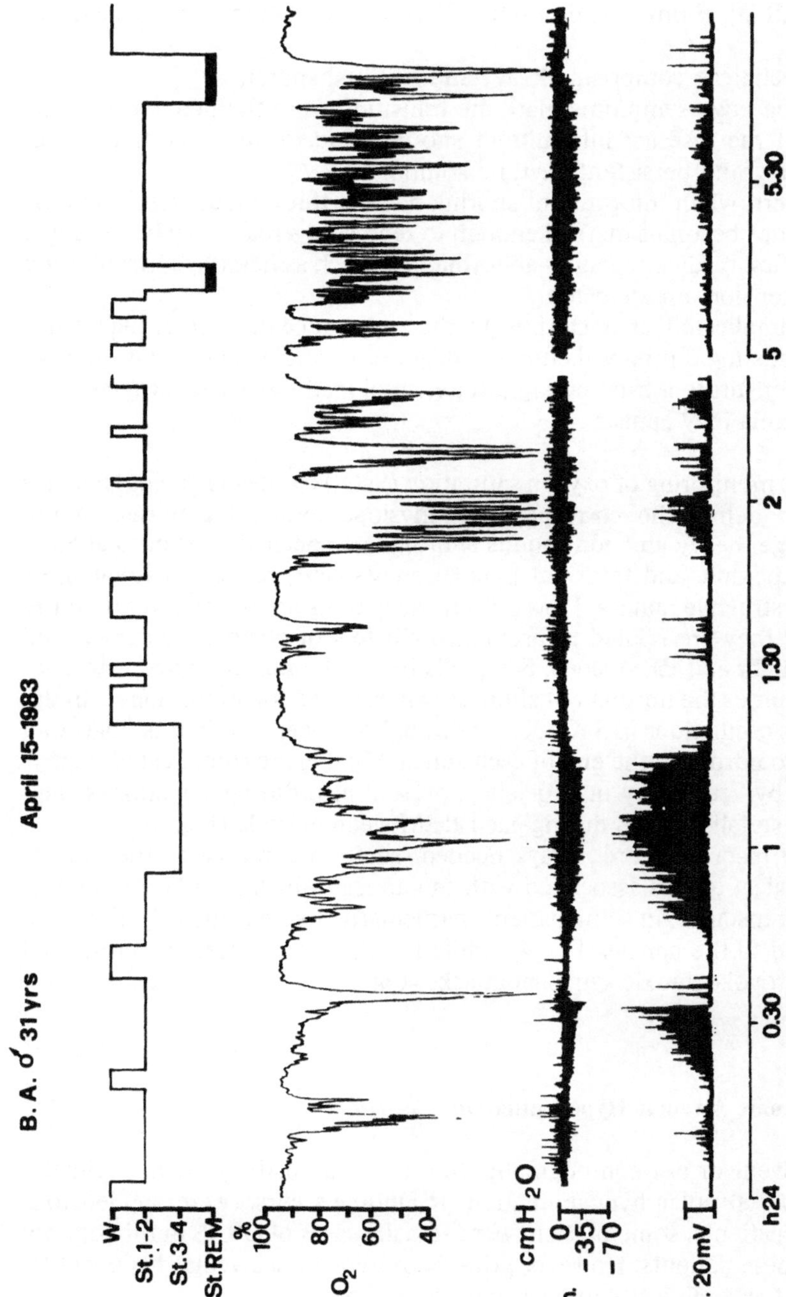

Fig. 2. Patient with ICAH. Peaks of severe O_2 desaturation are seen during snoring (*microph.*)

manifest OSAS [5]. From a clinical point of view, this process can be staged in four phases:

Stage 0 or preclinical; comprising heavy and habitual snorers

Stage I or initial; two symptoms mark the transition from the preclinical to the initial stage of the disease: intermittent snoring, due to rather protracted obstructive apneas, and persistent daytime somnolence

Stage II or overt; when intermittent snoring persists throughout sleep and daytime somnolence becomes marked enough to represent a real social handicap; at this stage the first cardiocirculatory abnormalities, such as heart hypertrophy and arterial hypertension, are detected

Stage III or complicated; characterized by the appearance of alveolar hypoventilation also persisting during wakefulness; daytime somnolence now becomes so severe as to constitute a true lethargic state; cardiopathy worsens progressively and polycythemia may appear

Continuous monitoring of oxygen saturation (SaO_2) by means of ear oxymetry allowed us to define the corresponding physiopathological patterns. In the preclinical stage, heavy and continuous snoring is associated with normal SaO_2 values; only sporadic and transient hypoxia may occur, related to isolated, or clusters of, obstructive apneas. Phasic SaO_2 oscillations are instead found in the initial stage I; they are related to prolonged clusters of obstructive apneas and occur during light and REM sleep. SaO_2 falls below the normal range with each apnea, but resumes the normal wakefulness values at the end of the apnea. In the overt stage the oscillations in SaO_2 persist throughout sleep, but in this stage, too, SaO_2 returns to normal at the end of each apnea. Finally, the complicated stage is characterized by ventilatory insufficiency, present also during wakefulness and by a progressive fall in SaO_2 during each REM sleep episode (Fig. 3).

Polygraphic recordings are always needed, since in some cases they reveal other pathological events associated with the apneas which may be relevant to treatment. For instance, in some patients particularly severe cardiac dysrhythmia may be related to the apneas (Fig. 4), while in others the extremely protracted apneas may provoke anoxic syncopal attacks (Fig. 5).

Idiopathic Chronic Alveolar Hypoventilation

Before the advent of polysomnography, the terms idiopathic, central, primary, and neurogenic alveolar hypoventilation or Ondine's curse were applied to a wide range of patients; some of them were actually cases of OSAS in thin or only moderately obese patients. However primary or idiopathic alveolar hypoventilation does exist as a clinical entity separate from OSAS.

The clinical history of patients with ICAH is characterized by episodes of ventilatory failure arising during sleep. In mild cases, symptoms are limited to a stuporous state associated with headache on awakening in the morning. Severe cases show lethargy or coma with onset during sleep. These episodes of breathing insufficiency during sleep are often favored by even trivial acute respiratory

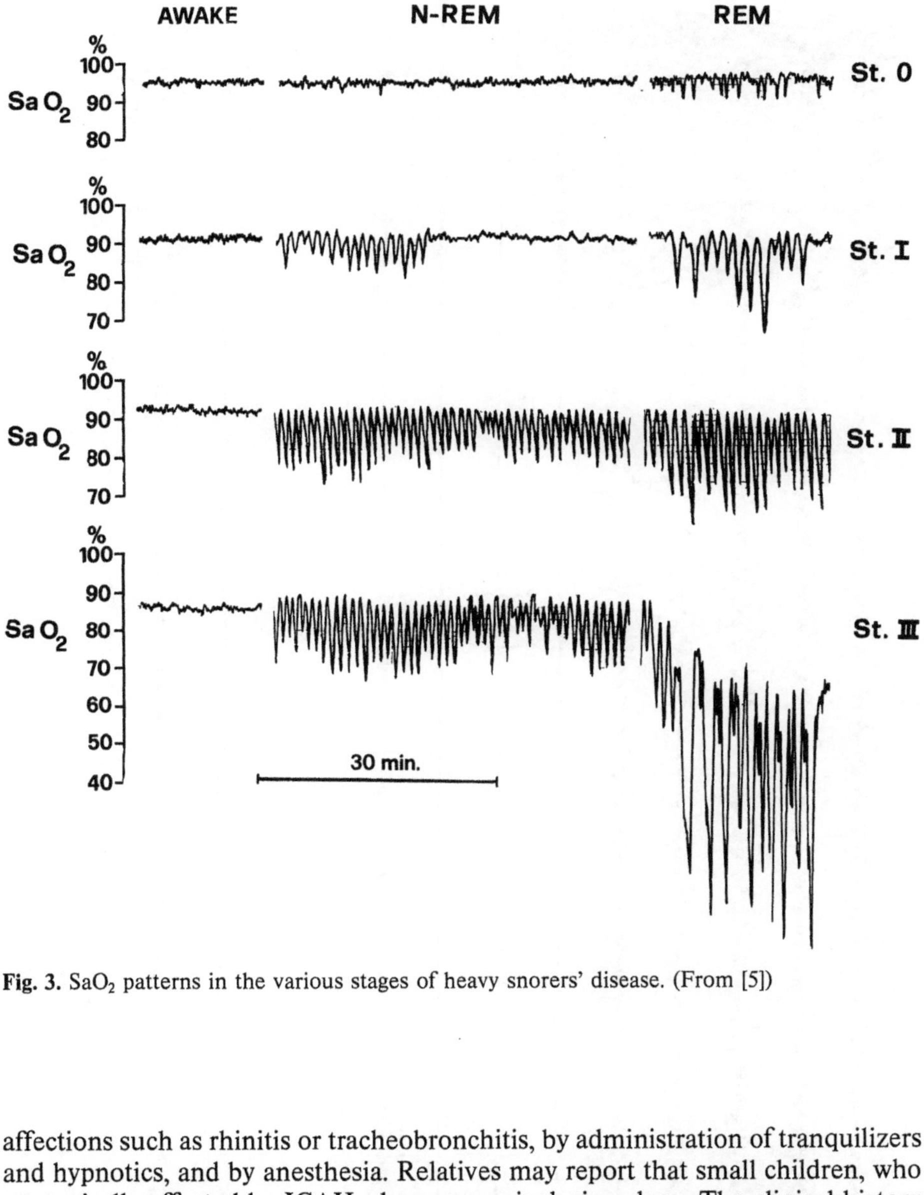

Fig. 3. SaO_2 patterns in the various stages of heavy snorers' disease. (From [5])

affections such as rhinitis or tracheobronchitis, by administration of tranquilizers and hypnotics, and by anesthesia. Relatives may report that small children, who are typically affected by ICAH, show cyanosis during sleep. The clinical history of these patients is often characterized by repeated admissions to intensive care units.

Compared to OSAS, the patterns of breathing and ventilation are quite different in ICAH. In fact, SaO_2 decreases quickly and progressively with sleep onset, reaching very low values without any phasic oscillations related to apneas, which in these patients never occur in prolonged series. The lowest values of SaO_2 are seen during REM sleep in adult patients, or during NREM sleep in small children (Fig. 6).

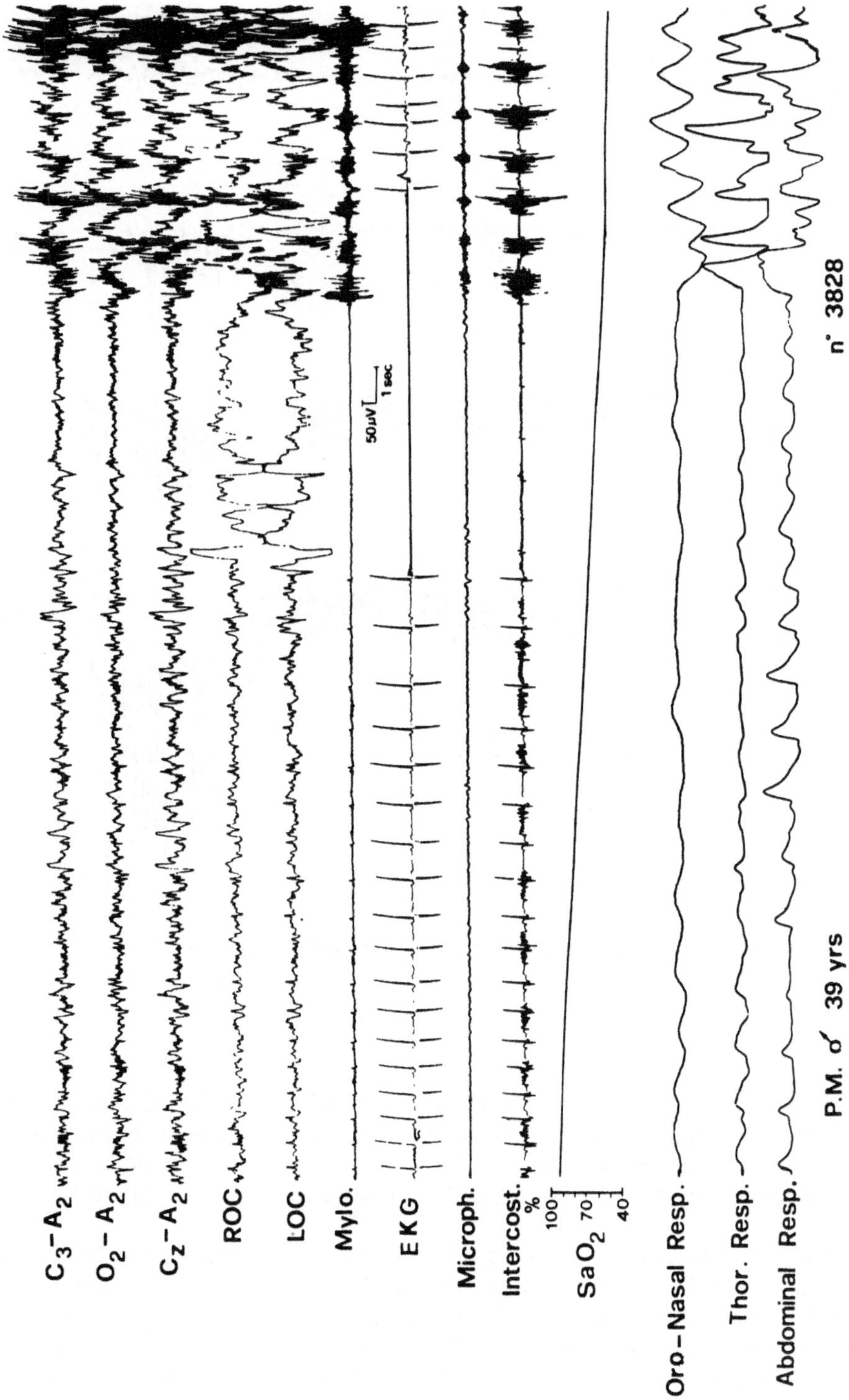

Fig. 4. Heart block lasting 11 s during an obstructive apnea

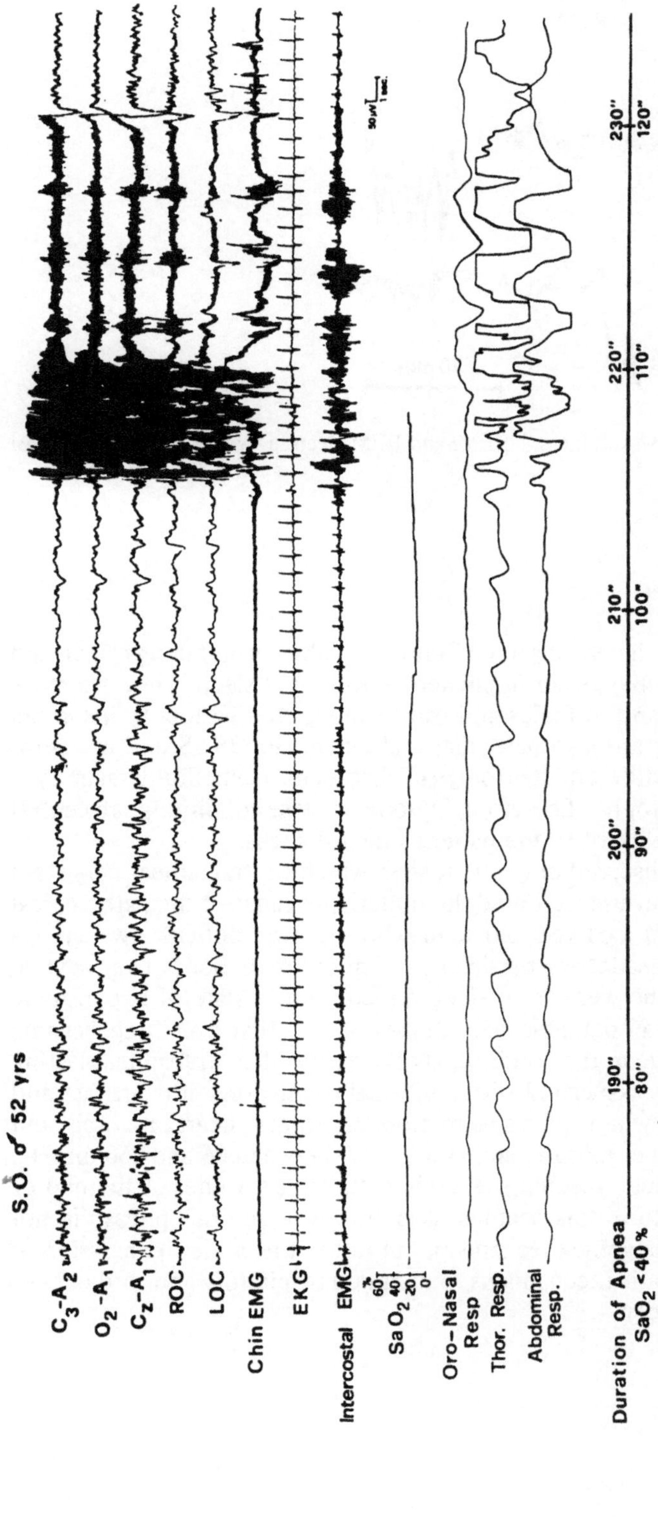

Fig. 5. Syncopal anoxic attack induced by a long-lasting obstructive apnea

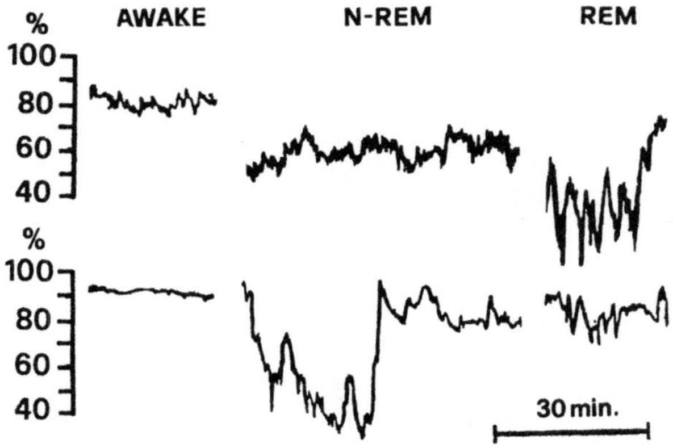

Fig. 6. SaO_2 patterns during wakefulness, NREM, and REM sleep in two cases of ICAH *(upper and lower tracings)*

Central Apnea Syndromes

Central apneas are sporadically observed in normal subjects on falling asleep and during REM sleep, and may occur in clusters during light sleep. They are more frequent in the elderly and in males and can be associated with both insomnia and hypersomnia. They are also particularly abundant in OSAS and are commonly seen in widely different neurological disorders, from Shy-Drager syndrome to myotonic dystrophy. Therefore, in none of these conditions can central apneas be considered relevant to the patient's disturbances.

In 20 years we have observed only one case in which central apneas persistent throughout sleep may have represented the underlying cause of the pathological condition. This involved a 51-year-old man who reported difficult awakenings with somnolence and headaches persistent for minutes or hours over several years. In one instance, he went from sleep directly into a state of hypercapnic coma. Repeated polysomnographic recordings showed that breathing became periodic during sleep, due to the continuous occurrence of central apneas lasting 20–40 s. Each apnea was associated with abnormal oscillations of heart rate and AP. During REM sleep, when apneas were more prolonged, heart rate oscillated between 56 an 96 beats per minute, and systolic AP between 66 and 250 mmHg. SaO_2 also oscillated widely, reaching severely pathological values at the end of each apnea (Fig. 7). Even in this peculiar case, however, central apneas did not represent the major pathogenic mechanism, but rather the clinical expression of the inability of homeostatic mechanisms to maintain respiratory and cardiocirculatory balance during sleep.

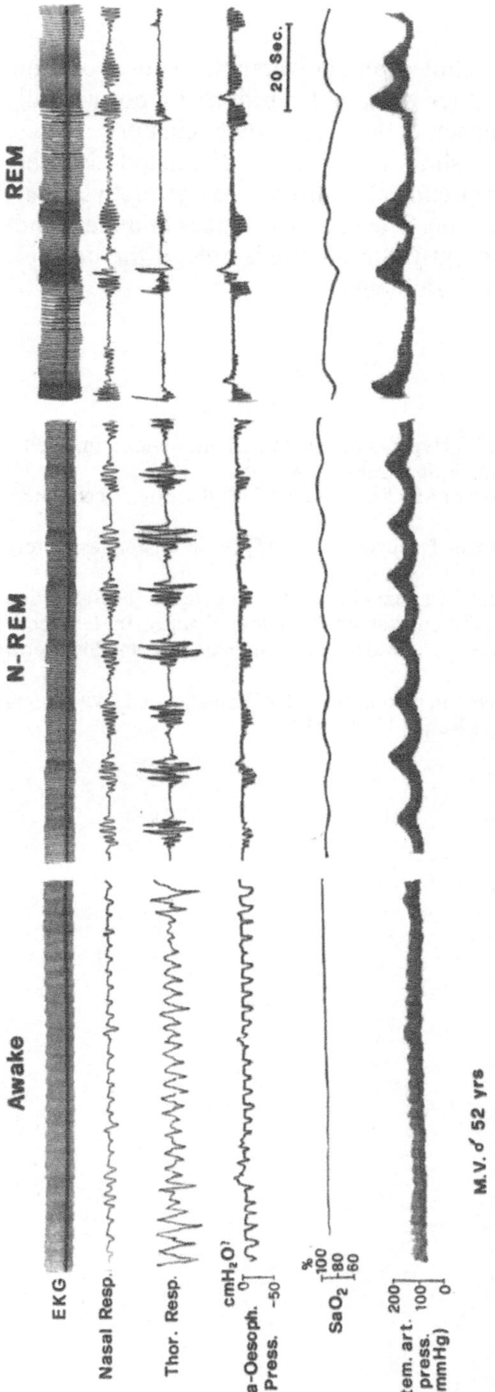

Fig. 7. Severe apnea-associated oscillations of heart rate, SaO_2 and systemic AP in a peculiar case of ICAH

Comment

We have tried to summarize the major clinical and polygraphic features of some sleep-related respiratory disorders. Further work will clarify many not yet fully understood points, especially the impact upon the cardiocirculatory system. Here, by way of conclusion, we only wish to stress that sleep-related disorders border several medical disciplines, from clinical neurology to neurophysiology, ear, nose, and throat, and internal medicine. The recent advances in understanding these pathological conditions represent yet another example of the need for an interdisciplinary approach to medical problems.

References

1. Lugaresi E, Coccagna G, Mantovani M (1978) Hypersomnia with periodic apneas. In: Weitzman E (ed) Advances in sleep research, vol 4. Spectrum, New York
2. Lugaresi E, Coccagna G, Farneti P, Mantovani M, Cirignotta F (1975) Snoring. Electroencephal Clin Neurophysiol 39:59–64
3. Lugaresi E, Cirignotta F, Mondini S, Montagna P, Zucconi M (1985) Sleep-related respiratory disorders. Ital J Neurol Sci 6:389–399
4. Mondini S, Zucconi M, Cirignotta F, Aguglia U, Lenzi PL, Zauli C, Lugaresi E (1983) Snoring as a risk factor for cardiac and circulatory problems: an epidemiological study. In: Guilleminault C, Lugaresi E (eds) Sleep/wake disorders. Natural history, epidemiology, and long-term evolution. Raven, New York, pp 99–105
5. Lugaresi E, Mondini S, Zucconi M, Montagna P, Cirignotta F (1983) Staging of heavy snorers disease. A proposal. Bull Eur Physiolpathol Respir 19:590–594

Snoring as a Risk Factor for Ischaemic Heart Disease and Stroke in Men*

M. Koskenvuo, J. Kaprio, T. Telakivi, M. Partinen, K. Heikkilä, and S. Sarna

Introduction

Heavy snoring, which is practically always present in obstructive sleep apnoea, seems to correlate with arterial hypertension [1–6]. During sleep, apnoeic patients may develop hypoxaemia and hypercapnia in association with a rise in pulmonary and systemic arterial pressure, and there may be increased susceptibility to cardiac arrhythmias [7–11]. Cardiac index decreases during an apnoeic episode and increases significantly on resumption of ventilation [12]. There is increasing evidence for a correlation of snoring with cardiovascular disease. Cross-sectional surveys have indicated an association with ischaemic heart disease (IHD) [13] and with angina pectoris [6]. A case-control study [14] of stroke patients found a relative risk (RR) of 2.8 for snoring, and 10.8 for habitual snoring. Prospective studies of snoring in relation to cardiovascular disease have not been reported.

We present a 3-year prospective follow-up for ischaemic heart disease and stroke in a population of 4388 men aged 40–69 years.

Methods

The Finnish twin cohort includes adult twin pairs born in Finland before 1958. A postal questionnaire study of these twins was carried out in October–November 1981. The responses of men aged 40–69 years (response rate 75%) were selected for analysis. Among other things, the questionnaire asked whether the subject never snored, sometimes snored, frequently snored, almost always snored, or could not say. Snoring status could not be given by 6.4% of the men. The snoring question was not answered by 0.6% of the men. Thus 4388 responses remained for analysis. Those who reported snoring almost always were considered as "habitual" snorers. Those who reported that they sometimes snored were considered as "occasional snorers". The questionnaire also asked whether a diagnosis of hypertension, angina pectoris or myocardial infarction had been made by a doctor. Current drug treatment for hypertension was also surveyed. History of hypertension was analysed using three categories:

Note by the Editors:
While the present volume was prepared, a revised version of this chapter was submitted to the British Medical Journal and published, not altered in substance, in Vol. 294 on Jan 3, 1987. The editors are grateful to the editor of British Medical Journal for permission to include the paper in the present context.

a) current drug treatment,
b) temporarily increased blood pressure but no drug treatment;
c) no history of hypertension.

Weight and height were recorded and body mass index (BMI) (weight/height × height) was calculated. Smoking was grouped into two categories:
a) non-smokers, occasional smokers and ex-smokers ($n = 2873$);
b) current smokers ($n = 1384$).

Reported amount of alcohol used (amount of beer, wine and spirits separately per month) was converted to grams of absolute alcohol. Records of IHD ($n = 149$) (ICD-8 410–414) and stroke ($n = 42$) (ICD-8 431–438) from computerised nationwide hospital discharge registers were linked for 27 months from October 1st. Records of death ($n = 105$) from computerised nationwide population registers were linked from for 35 months October 1st. Death certificates were collected from the Central Statistical Office.

The reliability of Finnish death certificate and hospital discharge data on IHD and stroke for epidemiological studies is satisfactory [15–17].

The incidence (death or hospital record) of IHD and stroke were analysed by snoring status contrasting:
a) habitual + frequent snorers and non-snorers;
b) habitual + frequent snorers and occasional + non-snorers using logistic models expressed as RR [18].

The effect of age, BMI, history of hypertension, smoking status and alcohol use were adjusted. Analyses were also done separately for IHD-free men (not reporting angina pectoris or myocardial infarction at the beginning of follow-up) and for men with IHD. Possible bias towards the non-snoring category was accounted for by excluding from the analysis single men without a cohabiting partner ($n = 410$).

Table 1. Occurrence of snoring among men by age groups

Age group	Snoring category				
	Habitual and frequent (%)	Occasional (%)	Never (%)	Total (%)	Total n
40–49	27	61	12	100	2202
50–59	32	59	9	100	1548
60–69	31	55	14	100	638
Age-adjusted	29	60	11	100	
Total number	1294	2614	480		4388

Table 2. Incidence of ischaemic heart disease and stroke by age and snoring

Age group	Snoring category			
	Habitual and frequent (%) (*n*)	Occasional (%) (*n*)	Never (%) (*n*)	Total (%) (*n*)
Ischaemic heart disease				
40–49	2.5 (15)	1.4 (19)	0.0 (0)	1.5 (34)
50–59	6.7 (33)	3.7 (34)	6.1 (8)	4.8 (75)
60–69	6.5 (13)	6.6 (23)	4.5 (4)	6.3 (40)
Total	4.6 (61)	3.0 (76)	2.8 (12)	3.4 (149)
Stroke				
40–49	0.8 (5)	0.3 (4)	0.0 (0)	0.4 (9)
50–59	1.4 (7)	1.3 (12)	0.0 (0)	1.2 (19)
60–69	2.0 (4)	2.9 (10)	0.0 (0)	2.2 (14)
Total	1.2 (16)	1.0 (26)	0.0 (0)	0.9 (42)

Results

The distribution of men by age and snoring category is shown in Table 1. During follow-up, IHD was recorded for 149 men (48 deaths and 120 hospital patients), and stroke for 42 men (5 deaths and 42 hospital patients). The total number of men with IHD and stroke was 187 (four men with both IHD and stroke) (Table 2). Mortality (during 35 months) is shown in Table 3. The age-adjusted mortality ratio between habitual + frequent snorers and occasional + non-snorers was 1.58 ($p < 0.05$) for cardiovascular diseases, 0.71 (NS) for other diseases, and

Table 3. Age-adjusted mortality and snoring

	Snoring category		Relative risk	
	Habitual and frequent	Occasional and never	(and 95% confidence limits)	Deaths *n*
	Mortality (%)	(%)		
Cardiovascular	1.88	1.19	1.58 (1.05–2.38)	61
Other diseases	0.52	0.73	0.71 (0.31–1.63)	29
Violent	0.45	0.29	1.55 (0.63–3.81)	15
Total	2.85	2.21	1.29 (0.92–1.81)	105

1.55 (NS) for violent deaths. Forty-eight men died from IHD during follow-up: 19 habitual + frequent snorers, 27 occasional snorers, and two non-snorers. IHD mortality (per 100 000 per year) of the cohort was 155, 509 and 806 for age groups 40–49, 50–59 and 60–69 respectively. The corresponding figures for the Finnish population were 145, 537 and 1305, respectively in 1982. IHD mortality was 503 in habitual + frequent snorers, 354 in occasional snorers, and 143 in non-snorers. RR of IHD mortality was 3.52 ($p < 0.05$) between habitual + frequent and non-snorers, and 1.48 ($p > 0.05$) between habitual + frequent and occasional + non-snorers. RR of stroke mortality was 3.59 ($p > 0.05$) between habitual + frequent and occasional + non-snorers.

Age-adjusted RR between habitual + frequent snorers and non-snorers for IHD incidence (death or hospital episode) was 1.91 ($p < 0.01$) (Table 4). The group of non-snorers did not include any men with stroke (O/E = 0/4.33, $p = 0.013$ according to Poisson distribution).

The age-adjusted RR between habitual + frequent snorers and occasional + non-snorers was 1.61 ($p < 0.01$) for IHD and 1.40 (NS) for stroke.

The adjustment for age, BMI, history of hypertension, smoking and alcohol use did not significantly decrease the correlation of snoring and disease incidence: RR between habitual + frequent snorers and non-snorers for IHD was 1.71 ($p > 0.05$) (Table 4).

Table 4. Snoring and relative risk of IHD in multiple logistic models

Age-adjusted relative risk and 95% confidence limits:	Habitual + frequent versus occasional + never	Habitual + frequent versus never
Snoring (alone)	1.61 (1.15–2.26)	1.91 (1.18–3.09)
Snoring	1.40 (1.15–1.71)	1.71 (0.96–3.05)
Body mass index	1.07 (1.01–1.13)	1.07 (1.01–1.13)
Hypertension	1.86 (1.49–2.32)	1.86 (1.49–2.32)
Smoking	2.16 (1.44–3.25)	2.17 (1.44–3.27)
Alcohol use	0.98 (0.90–1.02)	0.98 (0.93–1.02)

The exclusion of single men from the analysis did not essentially change the results: RR between habitual + frequent snorers and non-snorers for IHD incidence was 1.81 ($p < 0.05$).

At the beginning of the follow-up, 462 men reported angina pectoris or myocardial infarction. IHD was recorded in 80 cases and stroke in ten cases for men with previous IHD. The RR of IHD between habitual + frequent and non-snorers was 1.30 (NS), and between habitual + frequent snorers and occasional + non-snorers 1.03 (NS). In men without previous IHD the corresponding ratios were 2.72 ($p < 0.05$) and 1.89 ($p < 0.05$). The age-adjusted incidence and RR of IHD and stroke for men with and without previous IHD by snoring categories are given in Table 5.

Table 5. Age-adjusted cumulative incidence and relative risk of IHD and stroke by snoring category during follow-up in men without and with previous IHD

	Cumulative incidence		Relative risk [a]	
	Habitual and frequent %	Occasional and never %	Habitual and frequent versus occasional and never	Habitual and frequent versus never
IHD incidence				
IHD-free men	2.6	1.4	1.89 (1.17–3.07)	2.72 (1.24–5.97)
All men	4.6	2.9	1.61 (1.15–2.26)	1.91 (1.18–3.09)
Men with previous IHD	19.0	15.8	1.03 (0.63–1.70)	1.30 (0.63–2.68)
Stroke incidence				
IHD-free men	1.1	0.7	1.66 (0.82–3.38)	NA
All men	1.2	0.9	1.40 (0.82–2.38)	NA
Men with previous IHD	1.9	2.1	0.69 (0.18–2.71)	NA

[a] Relative risk in logistic regression model adjusted for age and 95% confidence limits.
NA, not applicable because no men with stroke among non-snorers.

Discussion

The response rate was 75% for males aged 40–69, while it was 84% for the whole cohort. IHD mortality of the males who responded, however, did not differ much from IHD mortality of Finnish males of the same age in general. The proportion of IHD mortality of the cohort in comparison to the corresponding population figures was 107% in the age group 40–49, 95% in the age group 50–59 and 62% in the age group 60–69. Thus, the selection was only significant in the oldest age group.

In 1986 a sample ($n = 38$: 17 habitual, 10 occasional and 11 non-snorers) of the individuals of this study underwent a single night's sleep recording using the static-charge-sensitive bed method (Bio-Matt) of measuring body and respiratory movements, a microphone to record snoring sound and an oximeter (BIOX III) to measure blood oxygen saturation transcutaneously [19]. The percentage of habitual snorers with an apnoea index exceeding 10 was 35%, indicating sleep apnoea syndrome. Thus, the preliminary estimate of the prevalence of sleep apnoea in males aged 40–69 was 3% (0.35×0.09) ($0.09 =$ the prevalence of habitual snoring). The mean oxygen saturation level during sleep was significantly lower in habitual snorers than in non-snorers. In habitual snorers, 25% of subjects were found to have arterial hypertension requiring medication, while the corresponding figure for non-snorers was 9%. The analysis of snoring spikes per hour of sleep showed that all individuals reporting snoring in the 1981 questionnaire also snored in recordings. Of individuals who had reported never snoring in the questionnaire, however, 36% (4/11) showed snoring during sleep. Thus, self-reported snoring seems to correspond well with sleep-laboratory findings in the case of habitual snorers, but seems not to be equally reliable in the case of non-snorers, in which group one man (1/11) had an apnoea index over 10 with a snoring index over 7. Thus the estimated RR between snorers and non-snorers is probably underestimated.

The validity of self-reported hypertension and previous IHD can be questioned. The predictive value of these risk factors, however, was significant and expected in magnitude. The self-reported use of alcohol (in the Finnish twin cohort) covers 41% of the sales figures, which is higher than reports obtained by interview studies. The non-response rate of the questionnaire study of the Finnish twin cohort showed the following results: 11% for the whole cohort, 27% for those with a period of hospitalisation due to alcoholism during the 3 years prior to the questionnaire study, and 42% correspondingly for alcohol intoxication. It was not possible to estimate the role of heavy alcohol use in this study [20].

Earlier findings on the correlation of snoring with IHD [1, 2, 6, 13] and stroke [14] are cross-sectional. In this first prospective study, snoring correlated with the age-adjusted risk of IHD. RR between snorers and non-snorers was 1.91 ($p <$ 0.01). These results are consistent with earlier cross-sectional findings, which indicated that habitual snorers might be in a high-risk category of having myocardial infarction. The association of snoring with IHD was quite independent of BMI, hypertension, smoking and alcohol use. RR of IHD by snoring category was significant in healthy men (not reporting a history of angina pectoris or myocardial infarction) but not in men with previous IHD. The role of snoring as a risk factor seems to decrease after the first IHD event, i.e. the role of other risk factors increases. The incidence of IHD, however, was high (17%) for men with previous IHD compared to men without previous IHD (2%). It is possible that the self-reporting of snoring is not as valid among men with IHD compared to men without IHD.

Snoring also correlated with the risk of stroke. It was not possible to calculate the RR between habitual + frequent and non-snorers, as there were no stroke cases among the non-snorers ($p = 0.013$).

Present knowledge on the pathophysiology of sleep apnoea suggests that the increased incidence of cardiovascular diseases in snorers is best explained by obstructive sleep apnoea. Some reports on working-aged populations suggest a prevalence of 1%–2% [21, 22]. Obstructive sleep apnoea is characterised by periodic apnoeas and total collapse of the upper airway during sleep. The frequency and duration of apnoeas vary. In the most severe cases there can be more than 300 apnoeic episodes during 1 night with a duration of 10–30 s [3, 4]. In heavy snorers with sleep apnoea, the blood oxygen saturation level during sleep decreases significantly. In severe sleep apnoea, the oxygen saturation level can fall to below 70%, while it is normally over 95% [4]. After an apnoeic episode, the pulmonary and systemic arterial pressure increase temporarily [12] straining the heart, especially the right side, and the susceptibility to cardiac dysrhythmias is increased [7–11].

The results of this study suggest that snoring is possibly a significant determinant of risk for IHD, and that the risk associated with snoring is quite independent of BMI, hypertension and smoking. Snoring also predicted stroke, but the number of cases was too small for detailed analysis.

Summary

The association of snoring with IHD and stroke was studied prospectively in 4388 men aged 40–69 years. Snoring was surveyed using a mailed questionnaire. Hospital records and death certificates were collected for the next 3 years: there were 149 men with IHD and 42 men with stroke.

Snoring was analysed in three groups:

a) habitual and frequent snorers ($n = 1294$);
b) occasional snorers ($n = 2614$), and
c) non-snorers ($n = 480$).

Age-adjusted RR of IHD between habitual + frequent snorers and non-snorers was 1.91 ($p < 0.01$). There were no stroke cases among the non-snorers. The adjustment for age, BMI, history of hypertension, smoking and alcohol use did not significantly decrease the RR, which was 1.71 for IHD ($p > 0.05$).

At the beginning of follow-up in 1981, 462 men reported a history of angina pectoris or myocardial infarction. For them, RR of IHD between habitual + frequent snorers and non-snorers was 1.30 (not significant-NS) and for men without previous IHD 2.72 ($p < 0.05$).

We conclude that snoring is a potential determinant of risk in the manifestation of IHD and stroke.

Acknowledgements. This study was supported by a grant from the Council for Tobacco Research Inc. USA. MP was supported by Te Paavo Nurmi Foundation.

References

1. Lugaresi E, Cirignotta F, Coccagna G, Piana C (1980) Some epidemiological data on snoring and cardiocirculatory disturbances. Sleep 3:221–224
2. Partinen M, Alihanka J, Lang H, Kalliomäki L (1983) Myocardial infarction in relation to sleep apneas. Sleep Res 12:272
3. Lavie P, Ben-Yosef R, Rubin AE (1984) Prevalence of sleep apnea among patients with essential hypertension. Am Heart J 108:373–376
4. Kales A, Bixler E, Cadieux RJ et al (1984) Sleep apnoea in a hypertensive population. Lancet II:1005–1008
5. Fletcher EC, De Behnke RD, Lovoi MS, Gorin AB (1985) Undiagnosed sleep apnea in patients with essential hypertension. Ann Intern Med 103:190–195
6. Koskenvuo M, Kaprio J, Partinen M et al (1985) Snoring as a risk factor for hypertension and angina pectoris. Lancet I:893–896
7. Schroeder JS, Motta J, Guilleminault C (1978) Hemodynamic studies in sleep apnoea. In: Guilleminault C, Dement WC (eds) Sleep apnea syndromes. Liss, New York, pp 177–196
8. Tilkian AG, Motta J, Guilleminault C (1978) Cardiac arrythmias in sleep apnoea. In: Guilleminault C, Dement WC (eds) Sleep apnoea syndromes. Liss, New York, pp 197–210
9. Deedwania PC, Swiryn S, Dhingra RC, Rosen KM (1979) Nocturnal atrioventricular block as a manifestation of sleep apnea syndrome. Chest 76:319–321

10. Motta J, Guilleminault C (1985) Cardiac dysfunction during sleep. Ann Clin Res 17:190–198
11. Ingbar DH, Gee JBL (1985) Pathophysiology and treatment of sleep apnea. Annu Rev Med 36:369–395
12. Guilleminault C, Motta J, Mihm F, Melvin K (1986) Obstructive sleep apnea and cardiac index. Chest 89:331–334
13. Norton PG, Dunn EV (1985) Snoring as a risk factor for disease: an epidemiological survey. Br Med J 291:630–632
14. Partinen M, Palomäki H (1985) Snoring and cerebral infarction. Lancet II:1325–1326
15. Penttilä A (1975) Mortality from arteriosclerotic and other degenerative heart diseases in Finland in 1968. Health services research of the National Board of Health in Finland 12/1974, Helsinki
16. Koskenvuo M, Kaprio J, Kesäniemi A, Sarna S (1980) Differences in mortality from ischaemic heart disease by marital status and social class. J Chronic Dis 33:95–106
17. Heliövaara M, Reunanen A, Aromaa A, et al (1984) Validity of hospital discharge data in a prospective epidemiologic study on stroke and myocardial infarction. Acta Med Scand 216:309–316
18. BMDP statistical software (1981) Dixon WJ, Brown MD, Engelman L et al (eds) University of California Press, Los Angeles
19. Telakivi T, Kajaste S, Salmi T et al (1986) Breathing and blood oxygen satturation during sleep, cardiovascular disease and cognitive function in snorers and non-snorers. 8th European Congress of sleep research, Szeged (Hungary), Sept. 1-5. p 362
20. Koskenvuo M, Kaprio J, Kesäniemi A et al (1986) Alcohol-related diseases associated with ischaemic heart disease: a three-year follow-up of middle-aged male hospital patients. Alcohol Alcoholism 21: (to be published)
21. Lavie P (1983) Sleep apnoea in industrial workers. In: Guilleminault C, Lugaresi E (eds) Sleep/wake disorders: natural history,epidemiology, and long-term evolution. Raven, New York, pp 127–135
22. Peter JH, Siegrist J, Podszus T et al (1985) Prevalence of sleep apnea in healthy industrial workers. Klin Wochenschr 63:807–812

Snoring, Sleep Apnea, and Hypertension in a Field Study

M. ZAHORKA, U. HESS, H. HIMMELMANN, U. KÖHLER, J. MAYER, J. H. PETER, T. PODSZUS, J. SIEGRIST, and E. SOHN

Introduction

The formerly accepted view that snoring is, at worst, an annoying or irritating factor in human sleep can no longer be maintained in the light of recent medical evidence. Snoring has been discovered to be an important pathophysiological and pathogenic factor, particularly in two fields: sleep apnea (SA) syndromes and essential hypertension. For patients with SA, histories of many years or even decades of loud and irregular snoring have been described [1]. Habitual snoring must be evaluated as an early symptom of obstructive SA [2, 3].

The role of snoring as a risk factor in cardiovascular diseases, on the other hand, has also been described by various investigators. Mondini et al. were able to show that essential hypertension was significantly more frequent, independently of body weight and age, in snorers than in nonsnorers [4]. Jennum et al. stress the significance of habitual snoring in the development of essential hypertension [5].

With the high prevalence of SA [6, 7] and of systemic arterial hypertension, and with strong evidence for the high correlation of both pictures with snoring, it must be expected that snoring occupies an important, if largely unexplored, position in the spectrum of general morbidity and mortality.

The present study is an advance report on the coincidence of snoring, SA, and hypertension, taken from a series of investigations in nonpreselected and presumably healthy high-voltage technicians working for a local power distribution company (compare the paper on "Sleep Apnea Activity and General Morbidity in a Field Study" by J. H. Peter et al., in the present volume).

Methods

The population of the present study consisted of 95 unselected male electricians between 20 and 62 years of age, mean age 38. All subjects underwent thorough internal examinations at our outpatients' department. Apnea was measured after a normal working day by means of continuous nocturnal recordings of thoracic and abdominal respiration (inductive plethysmography), partial arterial oxygen tension, and ECG. The apnea measurements were conducted at the subjects' homes by means of our portable recording unit [8]. Snoring was evaluated on the basis of anamnestic scores.

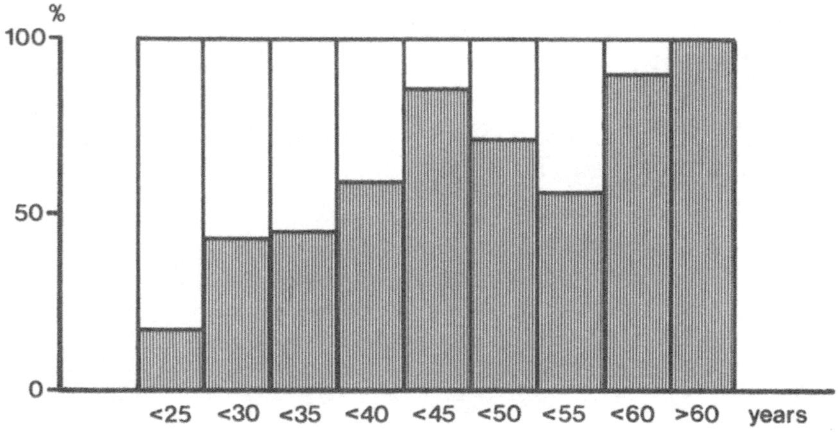

Fig. 1. Snoring in relation to age in 95 unselected subjects. While the prevalence of snoring increases with age, an overproportional increase can be observed in men between 40 and 50, the age group which is also the highest risk group in terms of sleep apnea

Results

Figure 1 shows the distribution of snoring in the study population in terms of age groups. While snoring increases with age, the proportion of snorers does not show a linear increase. There is an intermediary peak between 40 an 50 years of age. A closer analysis of the data shows that the higher proportion of snorers in this age group corresponds to a higher proportion of sleep apnea activity (SAA). In the group as a whole, 55 subjects (58%) reported habitual snoring, while 40 (42%) denied that they ever snored, or only admitted to occasional snoring.

For the apnea results, we distinguished insignificant SAA ($<$ five episodes per hour), moderate SAA [apnea index (Ai) $\geqq 5$, but < 10], and clinically relevant SAA (Ai $\geqq 10$). Moderate SAA was found in all age groups, but clinically relevant SAA (Ai $\geqq 10$) appeared exlusively in the age group 40–60. Significantly more snorers than nonsnorers had elevated apnea values. The figures are 33% and 13%, respectively ($p < 0.01$). Seven snorers, or 13% of this subgroup, had an Ai > 10, as compared to two subjects, or 5%, of the subgroup of nonsnorers. In other words: every third snorer had at least moderate SA (Ai $\geqq 5$), and more than every third subject within this subgroup had a clearly pathological finding of 10 episodes per hour or more. On the whole, the average Ai was 4 in the group of snorers, and 2 in the group of nonsnorers.

According to a systolic blood pressure reading of > 160 mmHg, or a diastolic value of > 95 mmHg, as criteria for the definition of systemic arterial hypertension, 15 subjects, or 15.7%, had hypertension. Of those, 12 subjects, or 80%, were also snorers. Figure 2 shows the proportions of hypertensives in different age groups. The diagram shows that hypertension was chiefly diagnosed in the age groups of 40 and more, and also mainly in snorers.

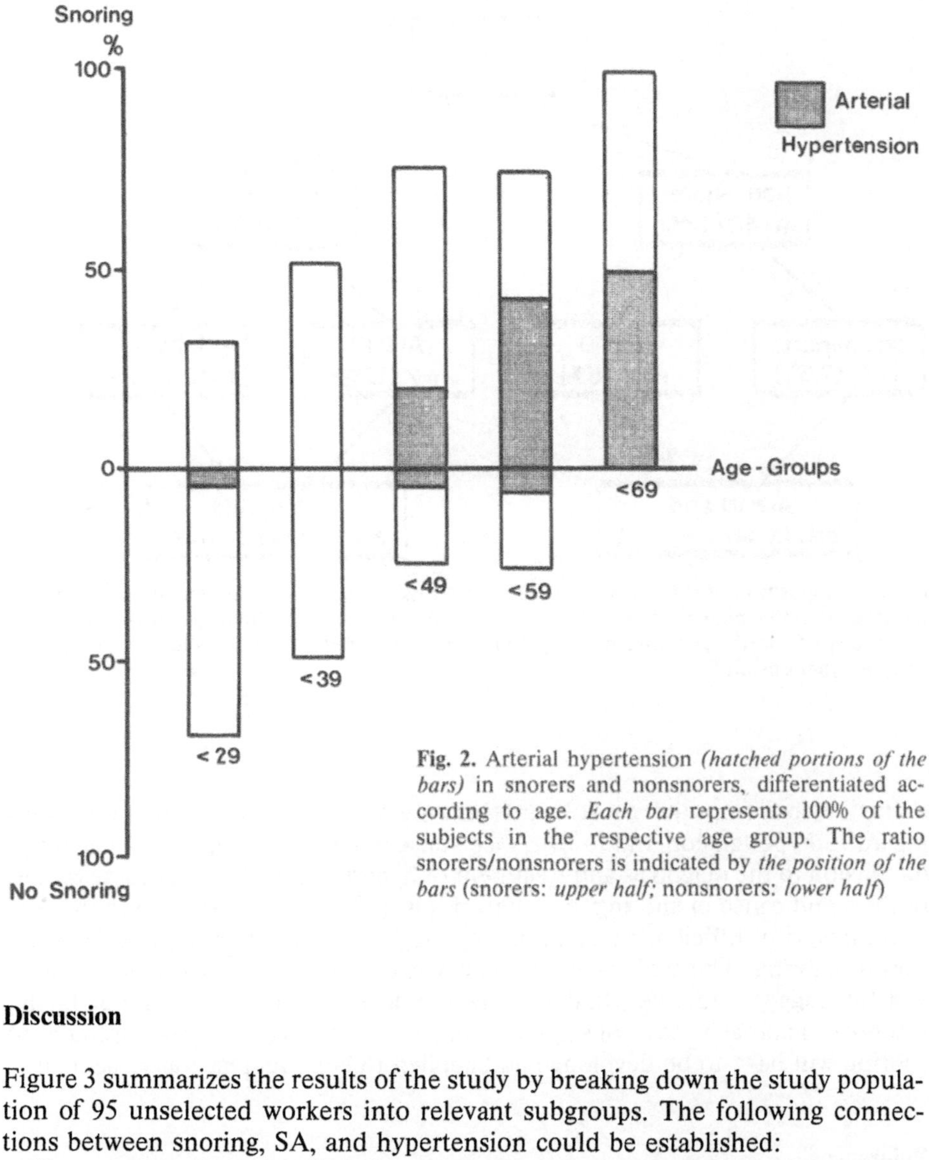

Fig. 2. Arterial hypertension *(hatched portions of the bars)* in snorers and nonsnorers, differentiated according to age. *Each bar* represents 100% of the subjects in the respective age group. The ratio snorers/nonsnorers is indicated by *the position of the bars* (snorers: *upper half;* nonsnorers: *lower half*)

Discussion

Figure 3 summarizes the results of the study by breaking down the study population of 95 unselected workers into relevant subgroups. The following connections between snoring, SA, and hypertension could be established:

- Hypertension was more frequent among snorers than among nonsnorers. The same applies to SA.
- All patients with hypertension had at least moderately increased SAA with an Ai $\geqq$ 5. All patients with pathological SA (Ai $\geqq$ 10) had hypertension. As the absolute number of subjects with both these results is comparatively small, the relationship between hypertension and high SAA will have to be qualified on the basis of larger field samples.
- Excluding the patients with pathologically high SAA, there was still a significantly higher porportion of subjects with hypertension in the subgroup of snorers than among nonsnorers.

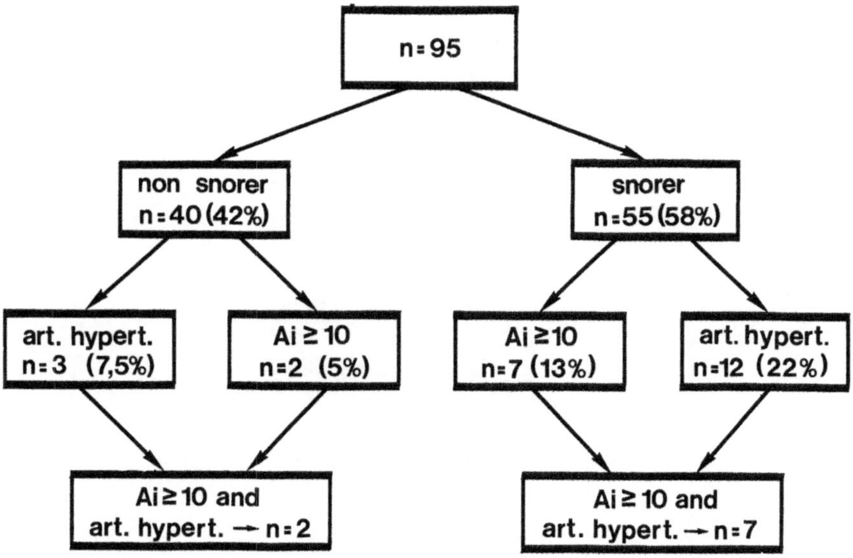

Fig. 3. Composition of the study population in terms of diagnoses, differentiating findings of hypertension and high SAA, as well as the combination of both findings, in the two main subgroups of snorers and nonsnorers. Moderate SAA (Ai ≧ 5) is not included. *Art. hypert.*, arterial hypertension

It is obvious from these results that snoring plays an important part both with regard to hypertension and to SA. Vice versa, SA adds an important diagnostic dimension to the diagnosis and treatment of hypertension. The exact assessment of the significance of snoring in diagnostics is difficult at present due to the lack of studies with sufficiently discriminating methods for the recording and evaluation of snoring. The high rates of coincidence between snoring, hypertension, and SA suggest, however, that snoring should be used as a parameter in the diagnostic approach. As a consequence, precise methods for the measurement of snoring will have to be developed and applied to large representative samples.

References

1. Guilleminault C, van den Hoed J, Mitler MM (1978) Clinical overview of the sleep apnea syndromes. In: Guilleminault C, Dement WC (eds) Sleep apnea syndromes. Liss, New York, pp 1–12
2. Lugaresi E, Coccagna G, Farneti P, Mantovani M, Cirignotta F (1975) Snoring. Electroencephalogr Clin Neurophysiol 39:59–64
3. Lugaresi E, Coccagna G, Cirignotta F (1978) Snoring and its clinical implications. In: Guilleminault C, Dement WC (eds) Sleep apnea syndromes. Liss, New York, pp 221–224
4. Mondini S, Zucconi M, Cirignotta F, Aguglia U, Lenzi PL, Zault C, Lugaresi E (1983) Snoring as a risk factor for cardiac and circulatory problems: an epidemiological study. In: Guilleminault C, Lugaresi E (eds) Sleep/wake disorders. Raven, New York, pp 99–106

5. Jennum P, Schultz-Larsen K, Wildschiødtz G (1985) Snoring as a medical risk factor. I. Relation to arterial blood pressure, weight and use of antihypertensive medicine. Sleep Res 14:170
6. Lavie P (1983) Incidence of sleep apnea in a presumably healthy working population: a significant relationship with excessive daytime sleepiness. Sleep 6:312–318
7. Peter JH, Köhler U, Mayer J, Podszus T, Penzel T, v. Wichert P (1985) The prevalence of sleep apnea activity (SAA). Sleep Res 14:197
8. Peter JH (1985) Holter monitoring technique in a comprehensive approach: ambulatory monitoring of sleep apnea. In: Hombach V, Hilger HH (eds) Holter monitoring technique. Schattauer, Stuttgart, pp 127–149

Part 5: Epidemiology III – Sleep-Related Breathing Disorders

Rediscovering Sleepy Patients: The Sleep Apnea Syndrome

P. Lavie

History

Recent studies have revealed that 4%–5% of the adult population complain of excessive daytime sleepiness [1, 17]. The sleepiness may vary in severity from chronic fatigue accompanied by feelings of drowsiness to unconquerable sleep episodes. The preponderance of sleepy patients among those referred to sleep clinics is supported by a recent comprehensive survey in 11 clinical sleep laboratories [5], showing that about 60% of the patients recorded complained of excessive daytime sleepiness. Among these patients, the most common diagnoses were sleep apnea syndrome (SAS), narcolepsy, periodic leg movements in sleep, and idiopathic hypersomnia.

The phenomenon of the "sleepy patient", who is constantly fighting sleep, is so pervasive, and apparently so preponderant, that it is difficult to explain how this symptomatic complaint was overlooked for so long.

In light of several literature reviews and epidemiological surveys [14, 26] the complaint of excessive daytime sleepiness appears to be unique to the seventh and eighth decades of the twentieth century. Kleitman's monumental book "Sleep and Wakefulness," first published in 1939 and then in 1963 [15] and containing a comprehensive bibliography of the early studies related to sleep and sleep disorders, cites only 298 publications out of 4337 (6.8%) related to excessive somnolence. Almost half of these (186, 62%) were specifically related to narcolepsy, 36 (12%) to encephalitis lethargica, and 67 (22%) to hypersomnia secondary to a proven central nervous system abnormality. Only a handful of these papers was published before 1900. Notwithstanding, each of these forms of pathological somnolence is distinctly different from SAS, which is the most preponderant finding among "sleepy patients" seen in clinical sleep laboratories nowadays.

Although medical literature from the turn of the century until the 1970s has been relatively silent regarding the "sleepy patient," a systematic historical review of the pre-1900 medical literature revealed a great awareness of this symptomatic complaint and its drastic effects on patients' lives and well-being. The Index Catalogue of the Chief Surgeon of the United States Army for the period 1881–1893, the nineteenth-century version of the Index Medicus, cited 867 publications related to sleep and sleep disorders [12]. Of these, 316 (36.4%) were related to various forms of excessive somnolence, which is three-fold more than the number of citations related to insomnia (106, or 12.2%). It is a point of interest that pre-1900 accounts of "sleepy patients" were much more colorful than those of our time. In MacNish's "Philosophy of Sleep" [27], sleepy patients are described as follows:

> They have a disposition to sleep on every occasion. They do so at all times, and in all places. They sleep after dinner; they sleep in the theater; they sleep in church. It is the same to them in what situation they may be placed: sleep is the great end of their existence - their occupation - their sole employment. Morpheous is the deity at whose shrine they worship - the only god whose inference over them is omnipotent . . . Let them sail, or ride, or sit, or lie, or walk, sleep overtakes them; binds their faculties in torpor . . . These are one dull, heavy-headed, drowsy mortals, those sons and daughters of phlegm - with passion as inert as a clutch fog, and intellects as sluggish as the movements of the hippopotamus or leviathan (p 211–212).

MacNish blamed the persistent drowsiness on a constitutional phlegmatic temperament, but added that in general these drowsy mortals are "great eaters." (For more details of the historical accounts of sleepy patients and the reasons for overlooking them see [23].)

Impact of Sleepiness

Although maintaining an adequate level of vigilance during working hours is an essential prerequisite for safety at work and for the prevention of occupational accidents, there is very little information on the impact of excessive daytime sleepiness (EDS) on the quality of life of working people.

In recent years we have investigated the prevalence of sleep disorders, including excessive daytime sleepiness, among industrial workers, and how they affect the workers' quality of life and safety at work [17].

We interviewed 1502 workers, 84% males and 16% females, all permanent day workers, individually about their sleep. Based on their responses to a detailed sleep questionnaire, five exclusive sleep complaint groups were formed to investigate the relationships of sleep complaints to work-related factors:

1. "difficulties falling asleep" included all the workers who claimed that sleep latencies of at least 45 min occurred "often" or "many times;"
2. "midsleep awakenings" included all workers who reported frequent midsleep awakenings;
3. the combination of 1 and 2;
4. "EDS" included all workers who reported falling asleep in at least two out of five passive and undemanding activites; and
5. the combination of 1, 2, and 4.

Some 119 workers met the criterion of EDS (groups 4 and 5). Excessive sleepiness was unrelated to age, sex, years of education, family status, or to height/weight ratio. The average age of the EDS workers was 37.9 ± 14.53 years as compared to the average of 36.97 ± 13.68 for the rest of the workers. The complaint of EDS was significantly related to various life style-, work-, and health-related factors, and to safety at work.

Workers complaining of EDS (groups 4 and 5) more frequently reported a multitude of presleep symptoms, including tension, body pains, sweating and feeling hot, difficulty in breathing, and feelings of suffocation. They also noted more frequent awakenings and greater difficulty falling back to sleep. Complaints of excessive movements in sleep and snoring were also more common in these workers.

Furthermore, about 50% of the workers complaining of EDS also reported difficulties at work due to interpersonal tensions and work pressure. A third of them complained of working conditions, particularly factors related to ventilation (smoke, gases, climate).

Most importantly, safety at work was significantly linked with EDS complaints. Workers complaining of EDS had the highest percentage of work accidents in the 2 years prior to the study. This was particularly prominent for the multiple work accidents category. The percentage of workers having three or more work accidents in the preceding 2 years was 9.1% in the group complaining of the combination of nocturnal sleep disturbances and EDS. This was 530% higher than in workers with no complaints about sleep. In the group complaining of EDS alone it was 5.3%, 310% higher than in noncomplainers. Also, the number of sick days per work accident was twice as many in the EDS workers as in noncomplainers.

In the first paper summarizing these data [17], it was noted that the cluster of pre- and postsleep complaints, as well as the disturbing midsleep phenomena, show a remarkable resemblance to the type of complaints presented by sleep apnea patients. This close resemblance strongly implicated sleep-related breathing disorders as the main underlying etiology in the complaint of EDS among the workers investigated in that study. That surmise was subsequently confirmed in sleep laboratory recordings of these workers [19].

Sleep Apnea Syndrome

In spite of the apparently brief modern history of SAS, it has become clear in recent years that the incidence of the syndrome is much higher than was considered just 15–20 years ago when the first laboratory-documented cases were reported. The accumulated data indicate that it affects a sizeable portion of the middle-aged male population. The first epidemiological study designed to assess the incidence of SAS in the adult population was based on the survey of sleep disturbances in industrial workers previously described [19]. According to their complaints, three groups of workers were invited for further sleep laboratory recordings: an insomnia group, consisting of workers who complained of either difficulties falling asleep or difficulties staying asleep, or of both; an EDS group; and a control group that had no sleep-related complaints.

Whole-night sleep laboratory recordings revealed that 35% of the EDS group had more than ten apneas per hour of sleep vs. 5.8% of the insomnia group and 7.3% of the control group. The majority of the apneas in the EDS group were of the obstructive or mixed types, while in the control group they were of the central type. Apneic workers complained significantly more of excessive sleepiness, loud snoring, morning fatigue, chronic fatigue, and morning headaches than nonapneic workers. Also, they suffered significantly more from various forms of airway obstructions and had more previous ear, nose, or throat operations. Extrapolating these findings to the general industrial working population in Israel resulted in an estimated sleep apnea incidence of 1%–1.5% in adult men older than 21 years. Since all the apneic workers were within the 35–60 age group, it can be safely assumed that the incidence increases considerably with age and may reach 5%–6% in the 40–60 age group.

Evidence that sleep apnea is a preponderant finding among patients complaining of daytime sleepiness was also provided by the data accumulated in diagnostic sleep laboratories mentioned before [5]. In a survey of nearly 5000 patients seen in 11 clinics dealing with sleep–wake disorders, SAS was the most common diagnosis. It accounted for 22% of all the diagnoses made. As expected, it was particularly prevalent (43%) among patients complaining of EDS. Similarly, in our sleep laboratory, sleep apnea was diagnosed in more than one-third of the patients seen during 1982–1985, and in more than two thirds of the patients who complained of EDS.

The incidence of the syndrome rises in several high-risk populations. Morbid obesity constitutes a definite risk factor for SAS, particularly in males. Based on our experience with such patients [2], we estimated that one out of every three adult, morbidly obese male patients suffers from severe SAS. In some of those patients, sleep apnea is complicated by arrhythmias and hypertension [32]. Although the prevalence of SAS among patients with obstructed airways has not been formally investigated, the link demonstrated between airway obstructions and breathing disorders in sleep makes it safe to assume that the prevalence of the syndrome among obstructed patients is much higher than in the general population.

A recent study from our laboratory provided preliminary evidence that the link between increased airway resistance and disordered breathing in sleep may be genetically determined [20]. We have shown previously that mechanical nasal occlusion in apnea-free young adults causes an increase in the number of sleep-related apneas in a few of the subjects [18]. These effects were much more dramatic, however, in sons of symptomatic sleep apnea patients. Mechanical occlusion of the nasal passages in patients' sons caused a ten-fold greater increase in the number of apneas during sleep in comparison to a group of age-matched controls without a familial history of sleep apnea. The fact that anesthesizing the nasal passages without an increase in resistance also caused an increased number of apneas during sleep (unpublished data) suggests that nasal receptors may also play a role in the regulation of breathing during sleep or in the adaptation of the breathing regulatory mechanism to the wake–sleep transition.

Hypertension and Sleep Apnea

Data accumulated in recent years in different laboratories have indicated that there is a significant association between SAS and hypertension (HT). Previously, several case series showed that about 60%–80% of SAS patients suffer from HT [9, 11, 21, 25]. In our own epidemiological study investigating the frequency of SAS among industrial workers, there was a significant association between SA and HT. The incidence of essential HT among the apneic workers was five-fold higher than in the rest of the workers (36.3% vs. 7.4%). Significant association was also found between HT and EDS [17], and snoring [24], two of the most typical complaints of SAS patients.

In a recent publication, Koskenvuo et al. [16] confirmed and extended these findings. They reported that snoring is a significant risk factor for both HT and angina pectoris. The relative risk of HT between habitual snorers and those who never snored was 1.94 in men and 3.19 in women. This association was also found after adjusting for body mass index. The relative risk of angina pectoris for habitual snorers, which was significant only for men, was 2.22.

Three independent studies directly investigated the incidence of SAS among HT patients. Lavie et al. [22] interviewed 50 HT patients about their sleep habits and sleep complaints, and suspected SAS in 16 of them, based on their responses to a sleep questionnaire. Whole-night sleep laboratory recordings revealed that 13 of the 16 patients had more than five apneas per hour of sleep, 11 had more than ten apneas per hour and eight had more than 30 apneas per hour. Almost identical results were reported by Kales et al. [13] and by Fletcher et al. [6]. In the first study, the incidence of sleep apnea among a group of 50 nonselected HT patients was 30%. The criterion for SAS was the occurrence of at least five apneas per hour of sleep. Most importantly, patients with the most severe sleep apnea had the highest initial blood pressure levels and were more refractory to treatment. Fletcher et al. [6] studied the prevalence of SAS in a group of 46 middle-aged and older men with essential HT, in comparison with 34 age- and weight-matched normotensive men. Using a cutoff point of an apnea index greater than 10, they defined 30.4% (14/46) of the HT and 8.8% (3/34) of the controls as sleep apneics. However, they could not distinguish between the apneic and nonapneic men by their answers to a sleep questionnaire.

Coincidental Association or Causal Relationship?

Although the association between SAS and HT does not necessarily prove causality, there is supportive evidence that SAS may indeed play an important role in the etiology of HT. First, while 60%–80% of the SAS patients suffer from HT, only 30% of the HT patients suffer from SAS. Secondly, successful treatment of SAS results in blood pressure normalization. This was particularly impressive in HT apneic adolescents who underwent tracheostomy [8] and in superobese patients who underwent gastric bypass surgery [28]. The mechanism by which SAS causes chronic systemic HT is not known. The fact that during sleep systemic and pulmonary pressure of SAS patients was shown to rise, sometimes dramatically, led to the suggestion that the nightly occurrence of alveolar hypoventilation, combined with the transient increases in blood pressure, caused irreversible disturbance of the cardiorespiratory system in some patients [4].

Diagnosis of the SAS Patient

It is clear from the above findings that the diagnosis of SAS should be taken into consideration in the clinical evaluation of HT patients, particularly if they are overweight males in their midlife. Although a definite diagnosis of SAS can only be made by monitoring respiratory activity during sleep, a preliminary diagnosis and a decision regarding the necessity of sleep recording can be made in the physician's office. SAS patients have typical complaints which make such a preliminary diagnosis a relatively easy task. Based on our accumulated experience with SAS and on the results of the epidemiological study described previously, we designed a seven-item minisleep questionnaire (MSQ) to assist the clinician in reaching a decision regarding the necessity of sleep laboratory evaluation (Table 1).

The MSQ proved to be most efficient for a preliminary screening of large populations [34] for suspected sleep apnea patients. Patients indicate, on a scale of 1 (never) to 7 (always), the severity of each of the items. Figure 1 displays the mean scores for each of the seven items and the overall mean score based on all seven items for 1617 normal adults aged 20–60 years, and for 480 laboratory-diagnosed SAS patients. The data was divided into three 15-year age groups, 20–34, 35–49, and 50–65 years. Outstanding stability of the mean score is demonstrated for each of the items for both patients and controls. The complaint profile is essentially identical for the three age groups for both patients and controls. The mean total MSQ scores for the three age groups were 4.1 ± 2.1, 4.2 ± 2.1, and 4.3 ± 2.2 for the 20–34, 36–49, and 50–64 groups, respectively, compared to mean scores of 2.3 ± 1.4 for the normal population.

Although the majority of the controls were males, a similar mean MSQ of 2.4 $\pm$ 1.5 was found for a group of 177 normal females (Fig. 2). Calculating the complaint profile of the female SAS patients separately ($n = 27$) did not alter the profile.

Table 1. Mini sleep questionnaire for preliminary diagnosis of sleep apnea syndrome

1. Do you fall asleep during the day, particularly when you are not busy (not including planned naps)?
2. Do you suffer from morning fatigue (on awakening)?
3. Do you snore during sleep?
4. Do you frequently wake up during sleep?
5. Do you suffer from headaches on awakening?
6. Do you suffer from chronic unexplained fatigue?
7. Do you suffer from restless sleep?

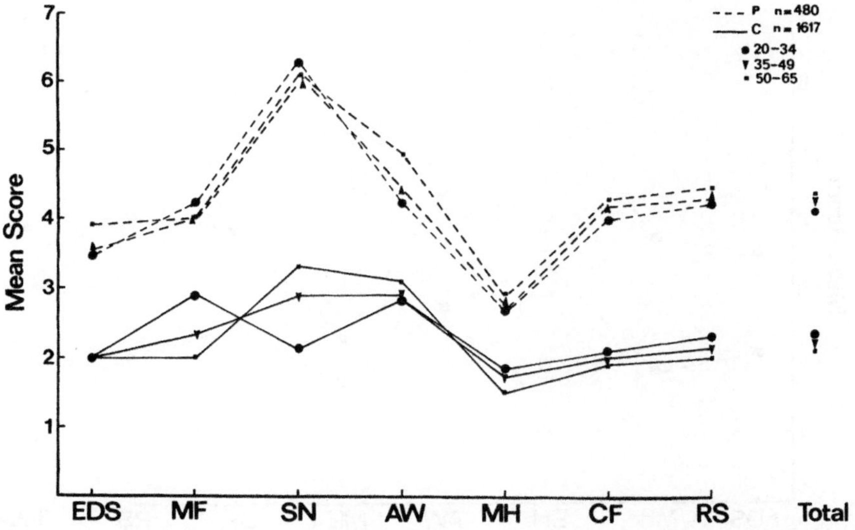

Fig. 1. Profile of complaints for three age groups of SAS patients *(broken lines, n* = 480) and controls *(straight lines, n* = 1617). *EDS,* excessive daytime sleepiness; *MF,* morning fatigue; *SN,* snoring; *AW,* frequent midsleep awakenings; *MH,* morning headaches; *CF,* chronic fatigue; *RS,* restless sleep; *total,* mean of all items. ●, 20–34 years of age; ▼, 35–49; ■, 50–65

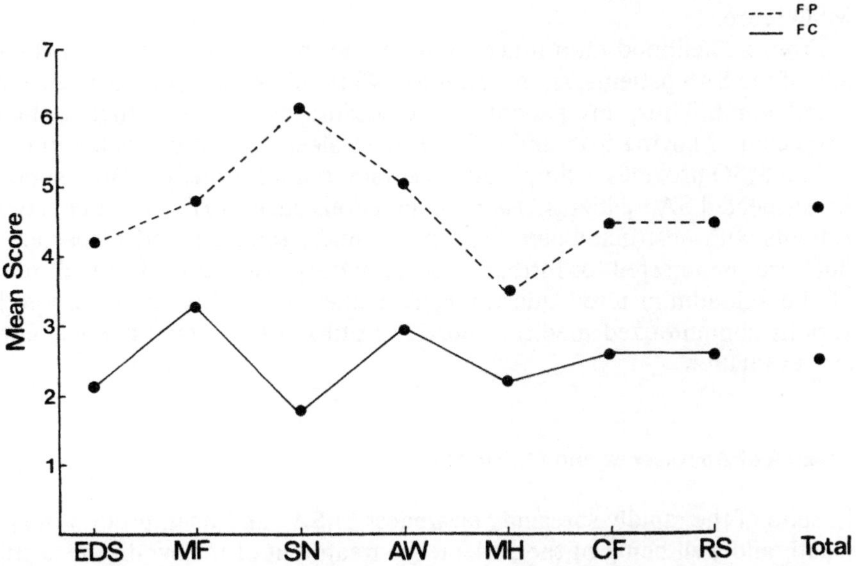

Fig. 2. Profile of complaints for female SAS patients *(broken line)* and female controls *(straight line).* Abbreviations as in Fig. 1

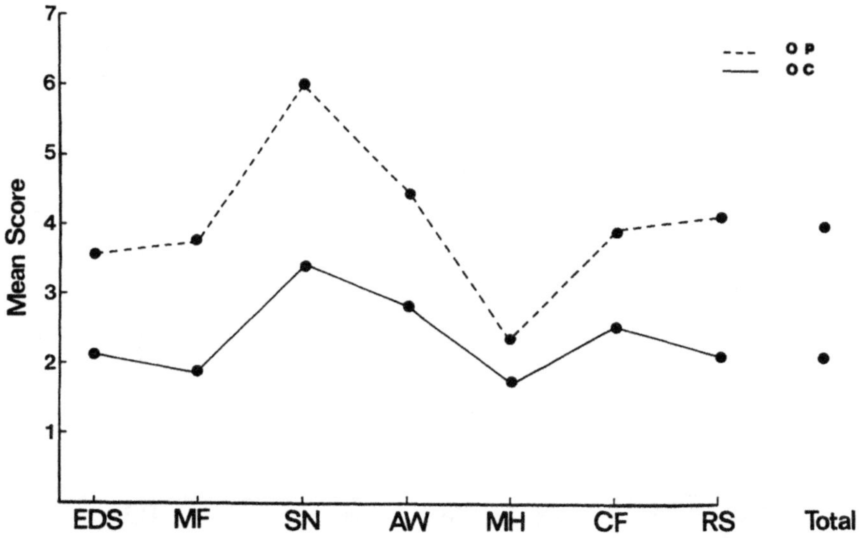

Fig. 3. Profile of complaints for obese SAS patients *(broken line)* and obese controls *(straight line)*. Abbreviations as in Fig. 1

A separate comparison made for patients and normal persons weighing over 100 kg revealed similar profiles (Fig. 3). The mean MSQ score for the obese SAS patients was 4.2 ± 2.2, 1.7 times higher than that of the 29 normal obese males (2.5 ± 1.6). Thus it appears that obesity per se does not have a major effect on the MSQ score.

From a likelihood ratio function, based on the scores of the normal controls and of the SAS patients, an overall mean score of 3.9 was selected as the criterion cutoff point. Thus, any patient whose mean score is 3.9 or higher should be suspected of having SAS and referred for a sleep laboratory evaluation.

The MSQ provides a simple and accurate tool for screening large populations for suspected SAS patients. Target populations such as HT or obese patients, or patients with obstructed airways, can be rapidly screened and suspected individuals can be referred for further sleep laboratory evaluation. The high reliability of the self-administered questionnaire makes it suitable for incorporation in various computerized medical interviews utilized for annual medical checkups and evaluation.

Treatment Approaches and Outcome

In spite of the rapidly spreading awareness of SAS and its impact on the general health and well-being of the patient, the treatment of the syndrome is still controversial. The early enthusiasm for tracheostomy as the treatment of choice [10] has been replaced by a more conservative and cautious approach. At the present time there are four different types of treatment: surgical, pharmacological, dietetic, and continuous positive air pressure (CPAP). The surgical treatments include various sorts of interventions in the upper airway regions such as adenotonsillectomy [29], nasal surgery [30], and uvulopalatopharyngoplasty (UPPP) [7]. But these surgical treatments provide only partial relief of the apneas. Any conclusions regarding the efficacy of the surgical treatments are hindered by the lack of long-term follow-up studies. From the various drug treatment attempts in sleep apnea patients, the choice has been narrowed down to trycyclics such as imipramine and protriptyline [3, 31]. These were reported to be effective in only a few of the patients. Here, too, the longest follow-up period is no more than 2 years and only partial relief has been reported.

There is general agreement that weight reduction is obligatory in massively overweight sleep apnea patients. But to remain apnea-free, the patient must not only lose weight, but should also keep his/her weight down - a condition which appears impossible for most superobese patients. In such patients who were unable to keep their weight down, we resorted to gastric surgery. This resulted in a remarkable reduction of apneas and symptomatology [28]. Although CPAP, first introduced by Sullivan in 1981 [33], has been shown to be highly effective in preventing sleep apneas, approximately 40%–50% of the patients are unable to tolerate the nose mask during long-term use. When given a choice between CPAP and surgical treatment, the majority of patients prefer the latter.

In view of the controversies surrounding the treatment of SAS patients, much more information is required, particularly on the long-term outcomes of the different treatments, before definite recommendations can be made.

Preliminary Follow-up Data

We have recently conducted a follow-up study of SAS patients diagnosed in the Technion Sleep Laboratory up to December 1984 (Wollman, Pollack and Lavie, in preparation) in order to assess treatment efficacy. Patients were sent a detailed questionnaire in which they were asked to indicate the type of treatment they had received and its efficacy, their subjective assessment of their present condition, usage of medication, present weight, and any significant changes in their health and life style since the sleep laboratory recordings.

Only the highlights of this study, based on the responses of 200 adult patients, will be presented here. Table 2 presents the patients' assessment of their condition in comparison with the pretreatment condition for each of the treatment groups. The age distribution of these patients is presented in Table 3.

After the laboratory diagnosis of SAS, 137 patients (66.5%) received some kind of medical treatment. The treatments were as follows: nasal surgery - 32, tonsillectomy - 8, UPPP - 12, obesity surgery - 18, minor weight loss ($<$ 5 kg, achieved by dietetic means) - 13, moderate weight loss ($>$ 5 kg, $<$ 20 kg) - 12, great weight loss ($>$ 20 kg) - 9, and pharmacological treatment - 31. In cases of multiple treatment, the table indicates the last treatment received. Patients who were treated for their sleep disorder tended to judge their condition as "better" or "completely recovered" more often than patients who did not receive any treatment. Overall,

Table 2. Patients' assessment of their present condition as a function of treatment

Treatment	Present condition								
	"Worse"		"Same"		"Better"		"Recovered"		Total
	(n)	(%)	*(n)*	(%)	*(n)*	(%)	*(n)*	(%)	*(n)*
UPPP	0		4	36.4	4	36.4	3	27.3	11
Tonsillectomy	2	28.6	2	28.6	2	28.6	1	14.3	7
Nasal surgery	3	9.4	11	34.4	13	40.6	5	15.6	32
Obesity surgery	0		2	11.1	5	27.8	11	61.1	18
Medication	5	16.1	21	67.7	4	12.9	1	3.2	31
Minor weight loss	2	15.4	7	53.8	3	23.1	1	7.7	13
Moderate weight loss > 5 kg, < 20 kg	1	8.3	8	66.7	2	16.7	1	8.3	12
Great weight loss > 20 kg	0		1	11.1	4	44.4	4	44.4	9
No treatment	10	14.9	45	67.2	7	10.4	5	7.5	67
Total	23	11.5	101	50.5	44	22	32	16	200

Table 3. Patients' ages in each treatment group

Treatment	Age group						
	20–39		40–59		60–79		Total
	(n)	(%)	*(n)*	(%)	*(n)*	(%)	*(n)*
UPPP	1	9.0	3	27.3	7	63.6	11
Tonsillectomy	1	14.3	6	85.7	0		7
Nasal surgery	11	33.3	12	36.4	9	27.3	32
Obesity surgery	11	61.1	5	27.8	2	11.1	18
Medication	3	9.4	17	53.1	11	24.4	31
Minor weight loss	1	7.7	8	61.5	4	30.7	13
Moderate weight loss > 5 kg, < 20 kg	2	16.7	9	75	1	8.3	12
Great weight loss > 20 kg	3	33.3	5	55.6	1	11.1	9
No treatment	7	10.4	39	58.2	21	31.3	67
Total	40		104		56		200

50% of the treated patients assessed their condition as "better" or "completely recovered," as compared to 6% of the nontreated patients.

Among the treatments, obesity surgery and nonsurgical weight reduction of more than 20 kg were the most effective treatments: 88% of the patients treated by both methods assessed their present condition as "better" or "completely recovered," in comparison to about 50% of the patients treated by upper airway surgery. Notwithstanding, 61% of the patients who were treated by obesity surgery and 44% of the patients who drastically reduced their weight by other means assessed their condition as "completely recovered."

Table 4. Patients' ages as a function of present condition for those treated by surgery

Age group	Present condition				
	"Worse" (n) (%)	"Same" (n) (%)	"Better" (n) (%)	"Recovered" (n) (%)	Total (n)
20–39	2 7.4	5 18.5	6 22.2	14 51.8	27
40–59	2 6.9	10 34.5	13 44.8	4 13.8	29
60–79	1 8.3	4 33.3	5 41.7	2 16.7	12
Total	5	19	24	20	68

In contrast with the above treatments, which were beneficial to at least 50% of the patients, there were no noticeable differences between the responses of patients treated by drugs and by minor or moderate weight loss, and those who did not receive any medical treatment. In each of these groups the majority of the patients (75%–85%) assessed their present condition as "the same" or "worse."

Patients' age interacted significantly with treatment outcome. Table 4 presents the assessment of patients who were treated by either upper airway surgery or obesity surgery as a function of three age groups: 20–39, 40–59, and 60–79 years old.

Of the patients aged 20–39, 51% assessed their condition as "completely recovered," as compared to 13% and 17% in the older age groups. The reverse was found for the "no improvement" categories, approximately 40% of the patients in the 40–59 and in the 60–79 groups assessed their condition as either the "same" or "worse" in comparison to 25% in the youngest age group. Age, on the other hand, did not interact with the outcomes of nontreated patients or of patients who were treated with drugs. In each of the age groups, 70%–80% assessed their condition as "worse" or the "same."

Table 5 presents the number of patients in each of the treatment groups who were forced into early retirement (before the obligatory retirement age of 65

Table 5. Working and retiring patients (< 65 years) in each treatment group

Treatment	Early retirement (n) (%)	Working (n) (%)	Total (n)
UPPP	1 11.1	8 88.9	9
Tonsillectomy	1 12.5	7 87.5	8
Nasal surgery	7 28	18 72	25
Obesity surgery	0	12 100	12
Medication	5 20	20 80	25
Minor weight loss	4 36.4	7 63.6	11
Moderate weight loss > 5 kg, < 20 kg	1 8.3	11 91.7	12
Great weight loss > 20 kg	3 37.5	5 62.5	8
No treatment	12 24.5	37 75.5	49
Total	34 21.4	125 78.6	159

years) because of their daytime symptoms. Overall, one out of every five patients (21.4%) was forced to retire. The highest rates of early retirement were in the group of patients who lost more than 20 kg by nonsurgical methods (37%), in the group which was treated by nasal surgery (28%), in the nontreatment group (26%), and in the drug-treated group (20%). In view of the controversy regarding the necessity of obesity surgery in order to achieve a substantial weight reduction, it is important to emphasize that none of the SAS patients who underwent surgery was forced into early retirement. This is in sharp contrast to the high rate of retirement among those who achieved massive weight loss by nonsurgical methods. As yet we have no explanation for this difference.

Although preliminary, the data analyzed so far allow some tentative conclusions regarding treatment approaches to SAS. First, surgical treatment of SAS, either in the upper airways region, or obesity surgery is much more effective than drug treatment or minor and moderate weight reduction. Secondly, younger patients generally responded more favorably to treatment than older patients, which emphasizes the importance of early diagnosis of the syndrome. And thirdly, for obese patients, the present data clearly indicate that massive weight reduction is obligatory. Although it appears drastic, obesity surgery is highly effective in superobese SAS patients.

The high percentage of patients who were forced into premature retirement among the untreated patients and among the patients who were treated ineffectively clearly emphasizes the impact of SAS on patients' life and well-being.

Summary

SAS is a preponderant disease affecting, almost exlusively, males in their midlife. It is significantly associated with upper airway obstructions and obesity and constitutes a definite risk factor for the development of HT. The fact that most of the SAS patients suffer from HT, and only 30% of all patients with essential HT suffer from SAS, and that successful treatment of SAS normalizes blood pressure, suggests that the syndrome plays an important role in HT etiology. The typical presenting symptoms of the SAS patients, EDS, chronic fatigue, loud snoring, and restless sleep, make the preliminary diagnosis of SAS a relatively easy task. Patients suspected of having the syndrome should be evaluated in a diagnostic sleep laboratory to determine the type and severity of the syndrome in order to decide upon the appropriate treatment approach. Most importantly, early diagnosis of the syndrome is essential to ensure effective treatment.

References

1. Bixler ED, Kales A, Soldatos CR, Kales JC, Healey S (1979) Prevalence of sleep disorders in the Los Angeles metropolitan area. Am J Psychiatry 136:1257–1262
2. Charuzi I, Ovnat A, Peizer J, Saltz H, Weitzman S, Lavie P (1985) The effect of surgical weight reduction on sleep quality in obesity-related sleep apnea syndrome. Surgery 97:535–538

3. Clark RW, Schmidt HS, Scaal SF, Boudoulas H, Schuller DE (1979) Sleep apnea: treatment with protriptyline. Neurology 29:1287-1292
4. Coccagna, G, Mantovani M, Brignani F, Parchi G, Lugaresi E (1972) Tracheostomy in hypersomnia with periodic breathing. Physiopathe Respiv 8:1217-1221
5. Coleman RM, Roffwarg HP, Kennedy SJ et al. (1982) Sleep-wake disorders based on polysomnographic diagnosis. JAMA 247:997-1003
6. Fletcher EC, Debehnke RD, Lovo MS, Govin AB (1985) Undiagnosed sleep apnea in patients with essential hypertension. Ann Intern Med 103:190-195
7. Fujita S, Conway W, Zorick F, Roth T (1981) Surgical correction of anatomic abnormalities in obstructive sleep apnea syndrome: uvulopalatopharyngoplasty. Otolaryngol Head Neck Surg 89:923-934
8. Guilleminault C, Eldridge FL, Simmons FB, Dement WC (1976) Sleep apnea in eight children. Pediatrics 58:23-27
9. Guilleminault C, Tilkian A, Dement WC (1976) The sleep apnoea syndromes. Annu Rev Med 27:465-484
10. Guilleminault C, Simmons FB, Motta J et al. (1981) Obstructive sleep apnea syndrome and tracheostomy: long term follow-up experience. Arch Intern Med 141:985-988
11. Guilleminault C, Cummisky J, Dement WC (1980) Sleep apnea syndromes: recent advances. Adv Intern Med 26:347-372
12. Index catalogue of the library of the Surgeon General's Office (1880-1893) United States Army (eds) Government Printing Office, Washington
13. Kales A, Bixler E, Cadieux RJ et al. (1984) Sleep apnoea in hypertensive population. Lancet 2:1005-1008
14. Karacan I, Thornby JI, Anch M, Holzer CE, Warheit GJ, Schwabb JJ, Williams RL (1976) Prevalence of sleep disturbance in a primarily urban Florida county. Soc Sci Med 10:239-244
15. Kleitman N (1963) Sleep and wakefulness, Ind edn. University of Chicago Press, Chicago
16. Koskenuo M, Kaprio J, Partinen M et al. (1985) Snoring as a risk factor for hypertension and angina pectoris. Lancet 1:893-895
17. Lavie P (1981) Sleep habits and sleep disturbances in industrial workers in Israel: main findings and some characteristics of workers complaining of excessive daytime sleepiness. Sleep 4:147-158
18. Lavie P, Fischel N, Zomer J, Eliaschar I (1983) The effects of partial and complete mechanical occlusion of the nasal passages on sleep structure and breathing in sleep. Acta Otolaryngol 95:161-166
19. Lavie P (1983) Incidence of sleep apnea in a presumably healthy working population. A significant relationship with excessive daytime sleepiness. Sleep 6:312-317
20. Lavie P, Rubin A (1984) Effects of nasal occlusion on respiration in sleep: evidence for inheritability of sleep apnea proneness. Acta Otolaryngol 97:127-130
21. Lavie P, Alroy G, Halpern E (1982) Apneic and nonapneic breathing disorders in sleep. Isr J Med Sci 18:523-533
22. Lavie P, Ben-Yosef R, Rubin AE (1984) Prevalence of sleep apnea snydrome among patients with essential hypertension. Am Heart J 108:373-376
23. Lavie P (1984) Nothing new under the moon. Historical accounts of sleep apnea syndrome. Arch Intern Med 144:2025-2028
24. Lugaresi E, Coccagna G, Cirignotta F (1978) Snoring and its clinical implications. In: Guilleminault C, Dement WC (eds) Sleep apnea syndromes. Liss, New York, pp 13-21
25. Lugaresi E, Coccagna G, Mantovani M (1978) Hypersomnia with periodic apneas. Advances in sleep research series, vol 4. Spectrum, New York
26. McGhie A, Russell SM (1962) The subjective assessment of normal sleep patterns. J Ment Sci 108:642-654
27. MacNish R (1830) The philosophy of sleep. M'phun, Glasgow
28. Peiser J, Ovnat A, Uwyyed K, Lavie P, Charuzi I (1985) Cardiac arrhythmias during sleep in the morbidly obese sleep apneic patients, before and after gastric bypass surgery. Clin Cardiol 8:519-521
29. Orr WC, Martin RJ (1981) Obstructive sleep apnea associated with tonsillar hypertrophy in adults. Arch Intern Med 141:990-992

30. Rubin AE, Eliaschar I, Joachim Z, Alroy G, Lavie P (1983) Effects of nasal surgery and tonsillectomy on sleep apnea. Bull Eur Physiopathol Respir 19:612–615
31. Rubin AE, Alroy G, Peled R, Lavie P (1986) Preliminary experience with imipramine HCl in the treatment of sleep apnea syndrome. Eur Neurol 25:81–85
32. Peiser Y, Lavie P, Ovnat A, Charuzi I (1985) Sleep apnea syndrome in the morbidly obese as an indication for gastric bypass surgery. Ann Surg 199:112–116
33. Sullivan CF, Issa FG, Berthon-Jones M, Eves L (1981) Reversal of obstructive sleep apnea by continuous positive airway pressure applied through the nares. Lancet 1:862–865
34. Zomer J, Peled R, Rubin AE, Lavie P (1985) Mini sleep questionnaire for EDS complaints. In: Koella WP, Ruther E, Schulz H (eds) Sleep 84. Fischer, Stuttgart, pp 467–470

The Prevalence of Increased Pulmonary Arterial Pressure Among Sleep Apneics

T. PODSZUS, and I. BECKER

Introduction

Alveolar hypoventilation is one of the factors in the pathogenesis of pulmonary hypertension [1–3]. Vasoconstriction of the precapillary pulmonary arteries due to hypoxia, a mechanism described by von Euler and Liljestrand [4], is regarded as the cause. This active form of precapillary pulmonary hypertension [2] is found in patients with chronic obstructive lung disease, pickwickian patients, and otherwise healthy subjects who exhibit pulmonary hypertension under conditions of high altitude.

Pulmonary hypertension related to alveolar hypoventilation has become widely known from the descriptions of the Pickwickian syndrome [5], which is characterized by obesity, polycythemia, and cor pulmonale. As the pickwickian syndrome is an extreme variant of the picture of sleep apnea [6], a disease which affects a much larger group of patients, it is not unimportant to ask how frequent pulmonary hypertension is among patients with sleep apnea, and which pathomechanisms can be recognized as possible causes of this disease.

Tilkian et al. [7] were able to show that five out of 12 patients with sleep apnea suffered from pulmonary hypertension after physical exercise. The present author demonstrated, in an earlier investigation, that 57% of patients with sleep apnea suffered from pulmonary hypertension without any indication of a primary pulmonary or cardiac disease [8]. In the present investigation we asked if patients with sleep apnea suffered from pulmonary hypertension during the day, and if the inclusion of a great number of hemodynamic parameters allowed specific pathomechanisms to be recognized.

Methods

Sixty male patients participated in the study. Their mean age was 52 ± 6, their relative weight 124% ± 18% of normal weight according to Broca. Prior to the hemodynamic measurements, sleep apnea activity was established by means of ambulatory nocturnal recordings by means of our portable unit [9, 10] including an ECG, inductive plethysmography of abdominal and thoracic respiratory activities, and transcutaneous measurement of the partial arterial oxygen tension. All patients more than fulfilled the criteria for a result of sleep apnea syndrome as described by Guilleminault [11]. The average apnea index in the study population was 18 ± 6 episodes per hour, and the mean duration of each patient's 30 longest apnea episodes was 26 ± 11 s.

Apart from the apnea measurements, all patients underwent careful clinical examinations. The main investigation included hemodynamic measurements by means of a flow-directed Swan-Ganz-catheter. Systemic arterial blood pressure was established noninvasively. The measurement were conducted during wakefulness at rest and on exertion. Ergometer exercise was carried out for 1 min at 50 W, 1 min at 75 W, and at 100 W for another 3 min as a minimum until steady-state values had been reached. In addition, there was arterial blood gas analysis during wakefulness. For the evaluation of the findings, the study population was split into three groups on the basis of the pulmonary artery pressure readings, distinguishing patients with normal findings at rest (< 22 mmHg) and on exertion (< 30 mmHg), patients with pathological findings on exertion (≧ 30 mmHg), and patients with pulmonary hypertension even at rest (≧ 22 mmHg). The statistical evaluation of the data included the analysis of linear regression, the *H* test according to Kruscal and Wallis, and the *U* test according to Wilcoxon.

Results

The clinical examinations did not show any relevant pathological results. The findings in the lung function tests were normal. All patients had normal blood count results, and none had a history of cardiac diseases which might result in cardiac myopathy. There was also no sign of a history of lung embolism. The blood gas condition during wakefulness, too, was normal in all patients.

Table 1 shows the results of the pulmonary artery pressure recordings, differentiating between patients with normal findings (group I, $n = 19$), patients with pulmonary hypertension under physical load (group II, $n = 31$), and patients with pulmonary hypertension during exercise as well as at rest (group III, $n = 10$). In terms of percentages, 68.3% suffered from pulmonary hypertension during exercise, including 16.7% with pulmonary hypertension even at rest. Figure 1

Table 1. Systolic, diastolic, and mean pulmonary artery pressure values in three groups of patients with sleep apnea, differentiating patients with normal findings (I), patients with elevated values under load (II), and patients with pathological values at rest and during exercise (III). Mean values per group at rest and during ergometer exercise at 100 W (steady state)

	Rest			Load		
	P_{PAs}	P_{PAd}	$\bar{P}_{PA}$	P_{PAs}	P_{PAd}	$\bar{P}_{PA}$
Group I ($n = 19$)	20	8	12	34	16	21
Group II ($n = 31$)	23	10	14	51	27	36
Group III ($n = 10$)	35	19	24	69	39	48

P_{PAs}, systolic pulmonary artery pressure (mmHg);
P_{PAd}, diastolic pulmonary artery pressure (mmHg);
$\bar{P}_{PA}$, mean pulmonary artery pressure (mmHg).

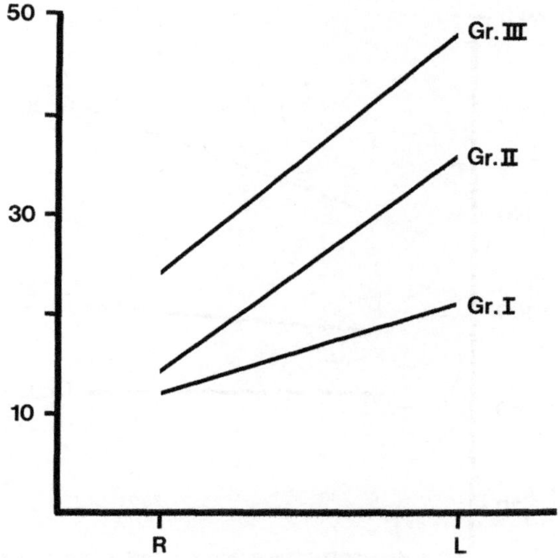

Fig. 1. Differences in $\overline{P}_{PA}$ at rest and during exercise in patients with normal values *(I)*, normal resting values *(II)*, and pathological values at rest and during exercise *(III)*. *R*, rest; *L*, load

shows the average increases in $\overline{P}_{PA}$ in the three groups. During physical load, this value increased by 9 mmHg on average in group I, by 22 mmHg in group II, and by an average 24 mmHg in group III. The pulmonary capillary wedge pressure ($\overline{P}_{PCW}$) during exercise increased by 4 mmHg in group I, 13 mmHg in group II, and 10 mmHg on average in group III, as compared with the initial values at rest, which were an average 6 mmHg higher in group III than in the other two groups (Fig. 2).

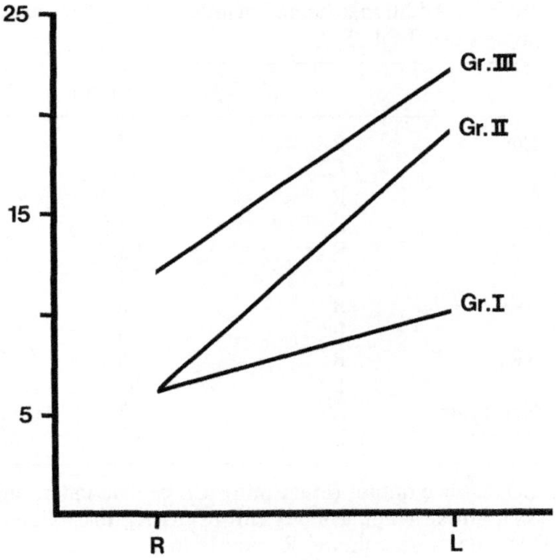

Fig. 2. Differences in $\overline{P}_{PCW}$ (mmHg) at rest and during exercise in patients with normal values *(I)*, normal resting values *(II)*, and pathological values at rest and during exercise *(III)*. *R*, rest; *L*, load

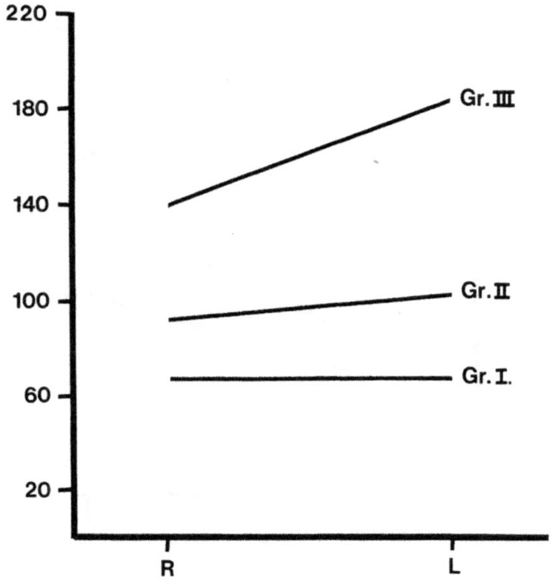

Fig. 3. Differences in PVR ($dyn \cdot s \cdot cm^{-5}$) at rest and during exercise in patients with normal values *(I)*, normal resting values *(II)*, and pathological values at rest and during exercise *(III)*. *R*, rest; *L*, load

The values of pulmonary vascular resistance (PVR) calculated at rest and on exertion also show a development towards higher values, with the highest values in group III. At the same time, the difference between the value at rest and the value on exertion steadily increases from group I to group III (Fig. 3).

Table 2 provides a synopsis of the remaining hemodynamic parameters in the three groups. There is a significantly lower increase of the cardiac index (CI), and

Table 2. Additional hemodynamic values of 60 patients with sleep apnea. For definition of groups, see Table 1

		Group I	Group II	Group III
CO	R	7.4	6.5	7.1
	L	13.8	14	11.4
CI	R	3.4	3.1	3.3
	L	6.5	6.8	5.4
SV	R	95	92	95
	L	134	135	111
SVI	R	46	46	46
	L	66	67	53
RR_d	R	86	86	96
	L	97	98	102
Heart rate	R	77	71	74
(bpm)	L	97	98	102

CO, cardiac output (liters/min); CI, cardiac index ($liters \cdot min^{-1}/m^2$); SV, stroke volume (ml); SVI, stroke volume index (ml/m^2); RR_d, diastolic systemic arterial blood pressure (mmHg); bpm, beats per minute; R, rest; L, load.

Table 3. Results of intergroup comparison

		Groups II/III	Groups I/II	Groups I/III
$\bar{P}_{PA}$	R	***	**	***
	L	*	***	***
P_{PCW}	R	***	NS	***
	L	NS	***	***
CO	R	NS	NS	NS
	L	*	NS	**
CI	R	NS	NS	NS
	L	**	NS	*
SVI	R	NS	NS	NS
	L	**	NS	*
PVR	R	*	NS	**
	L	**	**	***
RR_d	R	NS	NS	NS
	L	NS	NS	NS

$\bar{P}_{PA}$, mean pulmonary artery pressure (mmHg); P_{PCW}, mean pulmonary capillary wedge pressure (mmHg); CO, cardiac output (liters per minute); CI, cardiac index (liters · min $^{-1}$/m^2); SVI, stroke volume index (ml/m^2); PVR, pulmonary vascular resistance (dyn·s·cm^{-5}); RR_d, diastolic systemic arterial blood pressure (mmHg); R, rest; L, load, statistical significances are indicated as follows: NS, not significant; * $p < 0.05$; ** $p < 0.01$; *** $p < 0.001$

the stroke volume index (SVI) during exercise in group III as compared with groups I and II. Whereas the diastolic systemic arterial blood pressure measured in group III is higher than the comparable values in the other two groups, the statistical evaluation did not result in a significant difference between the values measured at rest and during exercise in the three groups. Table 3 shows the results of the statistical analysis for the hemodynamic parameters, indicating the different levels of statistical significance in the intergroup comparison.

The statistical analysis of all 60 patients' data showed a significant correlation between $\bar{P}_{PA}$ and $\bar{P}_{PCW}$ (coefficient of correlation $r = 0.66$ at rest, $r = 0.69$ on exertion), the same applies to the comparison of $\bar{P}_{PA}$ and PVR ($r = 1.0$ at rest, $r = 0.79$ on exertion).

Discussion

Several investigators have described the pulmonary hemodynamics during sleep in patients with sleep apnea [12–14]. Hemodynamic abnormalities coinciding with the occurrence of apneic episodes could be demonstrated. Pathophysiological studies have established an influence of alveolar hypoxia [8, 13, 16] and left ventricular dysfunction [15, 17] on the nocturnal hemodynamics in sleep apnea, as well as an influence of intrathoracic suction during episodes of obstructive apnea on the variations in cardiac output [8, 18]. As these phenomena are immediately associated with the occurrence of apnea, investigations into the hemodynamic situation of sleep apnea patients during the day can open up a new dimension of relevant information. The question if, and to what extent, patients suffer from cardiopulmonary complications during the day affects therapeutical decisions and has a bearing on the prognosis of the disease.

The present investigation in a large sample of sleep apnea patients shows that pulmonary hypertension is frequent among these patients. The occurrence of pathological alterations of the pressure conditions during the day is not linked with abnormal blood gas results: in spite of normal blood gas conditions, as many as 68.3% of the patients we investigated exhibited pathological increases in P_{PA} during exercise or even at rest.

The evaluation of the hemodynamic parameters suggests two mechanisms which can have a causal influence on the development of pulmonary hypertension:

- Especially during physical load, we found abnormal increases in left ventricular end-diastolic pressure indicating an impairment of the left ventricular function. It is known that hypoxia leads to myocardial rigidity [1]. Boysen [19] could show that intermittent hypoxia resulted in pulmonary hypertension. This could explain why patients with sleep apnea develop a left ventricular function impairment due to intermittent and recurrent hypoxia at night.
- Distinct differences in PVR among our patients may be due to interindividual differences in vascular reactivity.

Our results clearly indicate that sleep apnea leads to pathological changes in the cardiac and pulmonary hemodynamics even during wakefulness. The development of pulmonary hypertension and consecutive cor pulmonale must therefore be regarded as a serious complication in sleep apnea, the probability of which should not be underestimated.

References

1. Blount SG, Grover RF (1978) Pulmonary hypertension. In: Hurst JW (ed) The heart, arteries and veins. Mc Graw-Hill, New York, pp 1456–1472
2. Widimsky J (1981) Pulmonale Hypertonie. Thieme, Stuttgart
3. Grossman W, Braunwald E (1980) Pulmonary hypertension. In: Braunwald E (ed) Heart disease. Saunders, Philadelphia, pp 835–851
4. von Euler US, Liljestrand G (1946) Observations on the pulmonary arterial blood pressure in the cat. Acta Physiol Scand 12:301–320
5. Burwell CS, Rubin ED, Whaley RD, Bickelmann A (1956) Extreme obesity associated with alveolar hypoventilation: a pickwickian syndrome. Am J Med 21:811–818
6. Jung R, Kuhlo W (1965) Neurophysiological studies of abnormal night sleep and the pickwickian syndrome. In: Alkert K, Bally C (eds) Progress in brain research, vol 18. Elsevier, Amsterdam, pp 140–157
7. Tilkian AG, Guilleminault C, Schroeder JS, Lehrman KL, Blair-Simmons F, Dement WC (1976) Hemodynamics in sleep-induced apnea. Studies during wakefulness and sleep. Ann Intern Med 85:714–719
8. Podszus T, Bauer W, Mayer J, Penzel T, Peter JH, von Wichert P (1986) Sleep apnea and pulmonary hypertension. Klin Wochenschr 64:131–134
9. Peter JH, Becker E, Fuchs E, Meinzer K, von Wichert P (1982) Ambulante transkutane Langzeitregistrierung von arterieller Sauerstoffspannung und Herzrhythmusstörungen bei Patienten mit Schlafapnoesyndrom. Verh Dtsch Inn Med 88:390–393

10. Peter JH (1985) Holter monitoring technique in a comprehensive approach: ambulatory monitoring of sleep apnea. In: Hombach V, Hilger HH (eds) Holter monitoring technique. Schattauer, Stuttgart, pp 127–149
11. Guilleminault C, Tilkian A, Dement WC (1976) The sleep apnea syndromes. Am Rev Med 27:465–484
12. Schroeder JS, Motta J, Guilleminault (1978) Hemodynamic studies in sleep apnea. In: Guilleminault C (ed) Sleep apnea syndromes. Liss, New York, pp 177–196
13. Coccagna G, Mantovani M, Brignani F, Parchi C, Lugaresi E (1972) Continuous recording of the pulmonary and systemic arterial pressure during sleep in syndromes of hypersomnia with periodic breathing. Bull Physio-Pathol Respir 8:1159–1172
14. Guilleminault C, Eldridge F, Simmon FB, Dement WC (1975) Sleep apnea syndrome. Can it induce hemodynamic changes? West J Med 123:7–16
15. Buda AJ, Schroeder JS, Guilleminault C (1981) Abnormalities of pulmonary artery wedge pressures in sleep-induced apnea. Int J Cardiol 1:67–74
16. Podszus T, Mayer J, Penzel T, Peter JH, von Wichert P (1986) Nocturnal hemodynamics in patients with sleep apnea. Eur J Respir Dis 69 (Suppl 146):435–442
17. Scharf SM (1984) Influence of sleep state and breathing on cardio-vascular function. In: Saunders NA, Sullivan CE (eds) Sleep and breathing. Dekker, New York, pp 221–240
18. Podszus T, Mayer U, Penzel T, Peter JH, von Wichert P (1985) Hemodynamics during sleep in patients with sleep apnea. Sleep Res 14:198
19. Boysen PG, Block AJ, Wynne JW, Hunt LA, Flick MR (1987) Nocturnal pulmonary hypertension in patients with chronic obstructive pulmonary disease. Chest 76:536–542

Sleep Apnea Activity and General Morbidity in a Field Study

J. H. PETER, U. HESS, H. HIMMELMANN, U. KÖHLER, J. MAYER, T. PODSZUS, J. SIEGRIST, and E. SOHN

Introduction

The sleep apnea syndromes (SAS) are complex diseases which are caused by an increased number of apneas during sleep. The symptoms and findings which are specific for SAS can be reversed via a successful therapeutic reduction of the apneas if the disease is diagnosed during its early stages.

The clinical symptoms are mainly psychophysiological signs such as altered sleep behavior with excessive daytime sleepiness (EDS) and reduced sleep latency combined with insomnia and snoring, morning headaches, sexual dysfunction, depression, and deterioration of the intellectual powers. The leading internal symptoms are signs of myocardial insufficiency (dyspnea, exercise intolerance, pedal edema). Cardiac arrhythmias including sinus arrhythmia and bradycardia, systemic arterial and pulmonary hypertension, polycythemia, and obesity are the common clinical features of SAS.

In spite of the fact that some of the features of SAS are quite common internal diagnoses, and in spite of the fact that only little is known on the etiology of some of the most widespread findings such as essential hypertension or certain cardiac arrhythmias, only few representative data have been reported, up to present, on the prevalence of sleep apnea activity (SAA) in unselected samples in the field and the coincidence rates with the related symptoms and findings.

Methods

SAA was measured in an unselected sample of blue-collar workers employed in an electrical power company. Of 106 employees, 95 consented to the investigation, which was supplemented by an anamnestic questionnaire and internal examinations in order to determine coincidence rates of SAA and other diseases and symptoms.

SAA was measured continuously during the night after a normal working day. The recordings were performed in the subjects' home by means of our portable four-channel recording unit, which measures respiratory activity (inductive plethysmography) and partial arterial oxygen tension (transcutaneously), and includes a long-term ECG. The unit has been described elsewhere [1]. We determined the apnea index (Ai, number of apnea episodes per hour of sleep), distinguishing physiologically normal SAA, slightly increased SAA, and significantly high SAA. Following the definiton given by Lavie [2], an apnea index of > 10 is regarded as critically high. Less than five episodes per hour can by regarded as an irrelevant finding according to Guilleminault [3]. In addition, each subject's 10-min period of maximum SAA was determined, and the duration of the episodes was measured.

On the morning following the recordings, the subjects were given a thorough internal investigation in our outpatients' department. The investigation included:

- Anamnestic questionnaire
- Clinical checkup
- Laboratory tests
- ECG at rest and during exercise
- Chest X-ray
- Lung function and blood gas analysis
- Cardiac echogram

Results

The 95 subjects who participated in this study were all males and aged between 20 and 62 years, mean age was 38 (Fig. 1). Body weight in the group ranged from

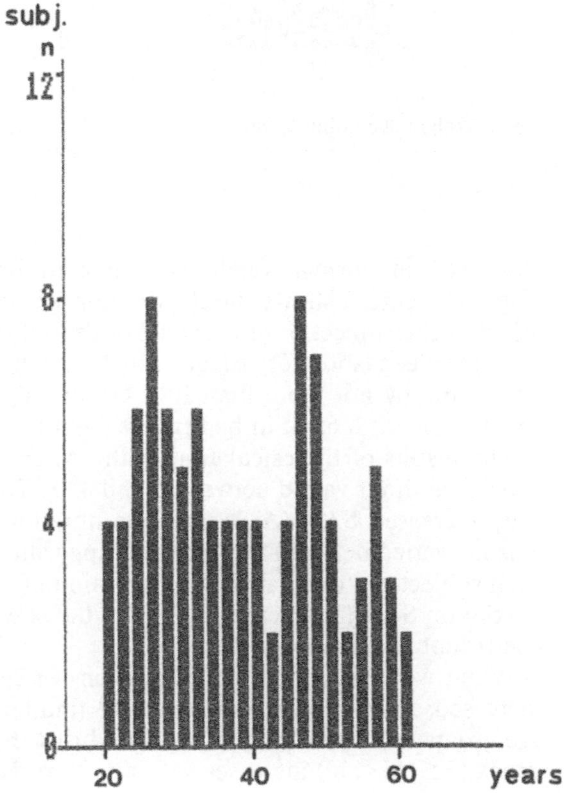

Fig. 1. Distribution of age (years)

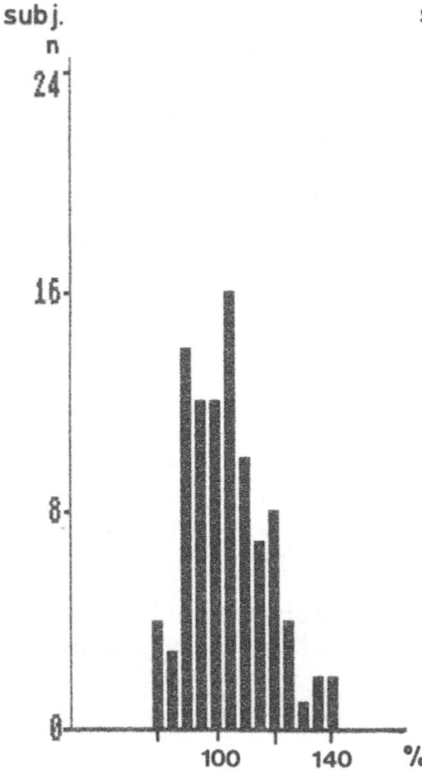

Fig. 2. Weight according to Broca

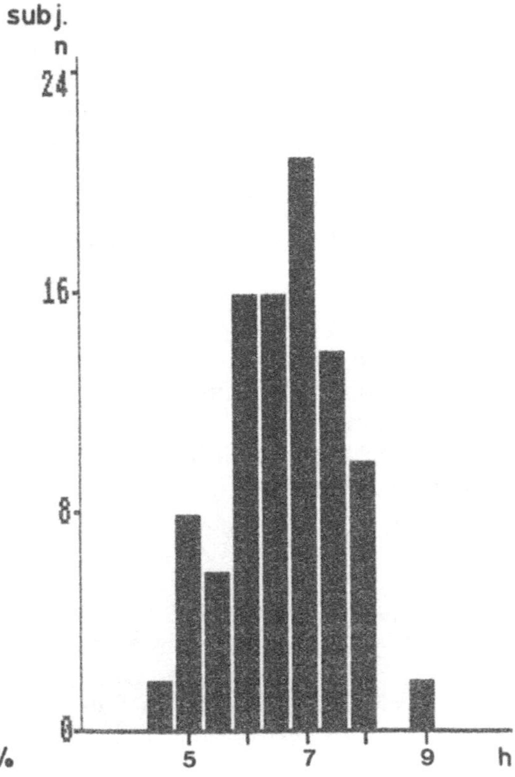

Fig. 3. Time spent in bed (hours), average 6.5 h, range 4–9 h

80%–144% of normal weight according to Broca, the mean index was 106% (Fig. 2). Figure 3 shows the distribution of "time in bed." This parameter was asked of the subject or, if possible, of the subject's bed partner. Our experience from the sleep laboratory suggests that time in bed usually exceeds EEG-defined sleep time by not more than 10%. On the night of the recording, our subjects spent an average 6.5 h in bed (range 4–9 h).

The results of the calculation of the Ai are shown in Fig. 4. The number of apneas per hour varied between 0 and 42.3. There were nine subjects with critically increased SAA (Ai > 10). The duration of each subjects' longest apnea episode varied between 10 s (the defining value for apnea) and 100 s (Fig. 5). For each subject, we calculated the proportion of apnea within the 10-min period of maximum SAA (as a percentage). The index was found to correlate with Ai, the coefficient of correlation was $r = .74$.

When we determined the proportions of significantly increased, moderately increased, and clinically irrelevant SAA findings in relation to age, distinguishing age groups in 10-year groups, we found that the proportion of slightly increased apnea ($5 \leqq \text{Ai} < 10$) increases with age. Surprisingly, however, the proportion of

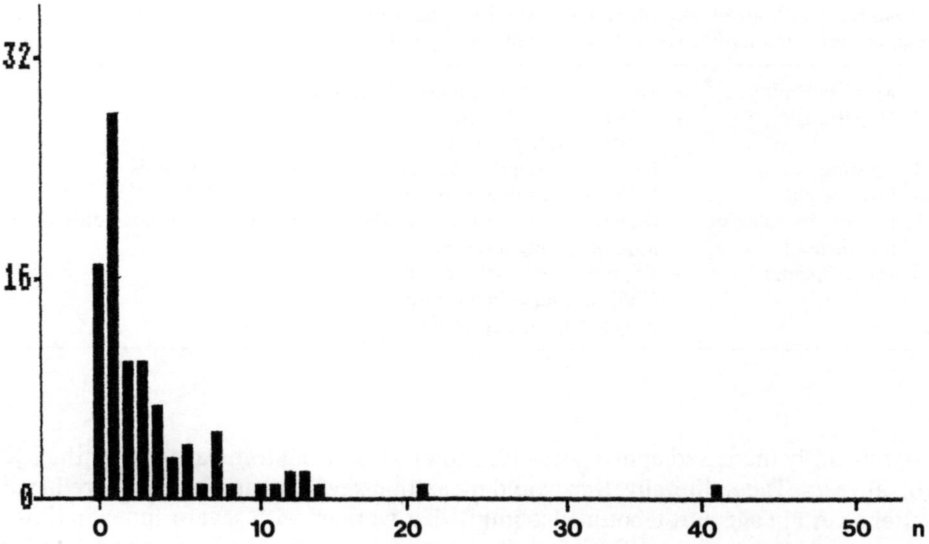

Fig. 4. Apnea index (number of apnea episodes per hour of sleep) *(n)* of all subjects. There were nine subjects with critically increased SAA (Ai > 10)

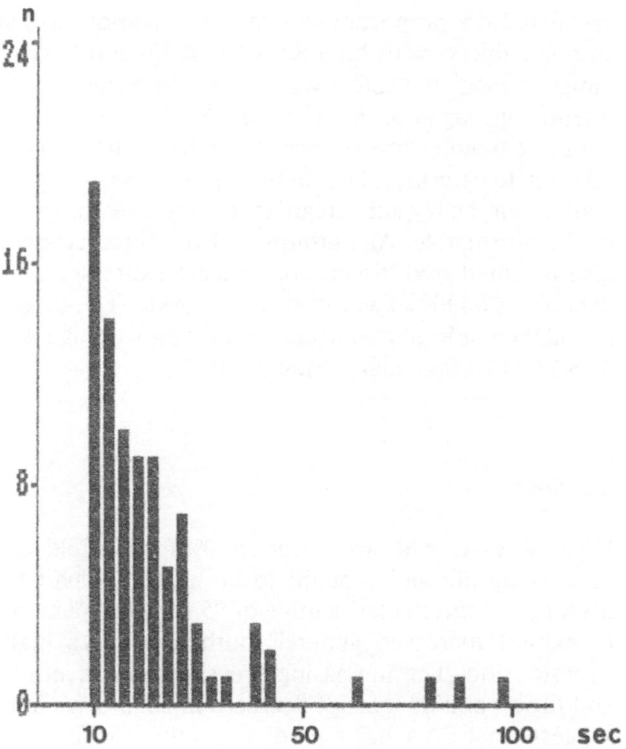

Fig. 5. Duration of each subject's longest apnea episode

Table 1. Definitions of additional diagnoses. Findings within all of these categories were significantly more frequent in subjects with high SAA ($p < 0.01$)

1. Multimorbidity	- More than three different diagnoses
2. Hypertension	- > 160 mmHg systolic > 95 mmHg diastolic
3. Snoring	- Loud and irregular, occurrence reported in anamnesis
4. Overweight	- > 115% according to Broca
5. Psychophysiological impairment	- Questionnaire: morning headaches, excessive sleepiness, difficulties in maintaining attention
6. Hyperlipemia	- Triglycerides > 200 mg/dl Cholesterine > 260 mg/dl or types according to Frederickson

significantly increased apnea (Ai > 10) shows a declining trend again after the age of 50 years. Taken literally, this would mean that severe apnea is actually reduced after a certain age, but it could also imply that workers with severe apnea in those upper age groups do not figure in the present study, due to increased mortality after a long history of SAA, or because they had to retire prematurely as a consequence of the incapacitating influence of SAA. The finding may therefore be an indirect expression of the elevated cardiovascular risk which is the consequence of severe SAA. This hypothesis will have to be tested by studying larger samples.

In order to correlate SAA with diagnoses and symptoms related to SAA, we calculated the proportions of various disorders, as listed and defined in Table 1, among subjects with high SAA (Ai ≧ 10) and lower SAA (Ai > 10). All the findings defined in Table 1 were found to occur significantly ($p < 0.01$) more frequently among subjects with high SAA.

Figure 6 represents the responses to the item in the anamnestic questionnaire relating to snoring. The figure shows the relative proportions of those who denied that heavy and irregular snoring ever occurred and those who responded in the affirmative. Age groups and the three classes of SAA results were again distinguished, and the proportions are expressed as a percentage of the number of subjects (= 100%) within each age group. The diagram illustrates the increasing prevalence of loud and irregular snoring with age as well as the high correlation of SAA with this anamnestic datum.

Conclusion

High SAA (Ai > 10) was found in 10% of this field sample of men, who are active in working life and thought to be healthy. Apart from the high prevalence of SAA in this unselected sample of 95 subjects, persons with SAA were also found to exhibit increased general morbidity and a higher prevalence of systemic hypertension. The increasing prevalence of severe SAA in men in their forties and fifties, and the abrupt decrease in such SAA in men beyond their midfifties suggests that SAA has a predictive value for fitness for work.

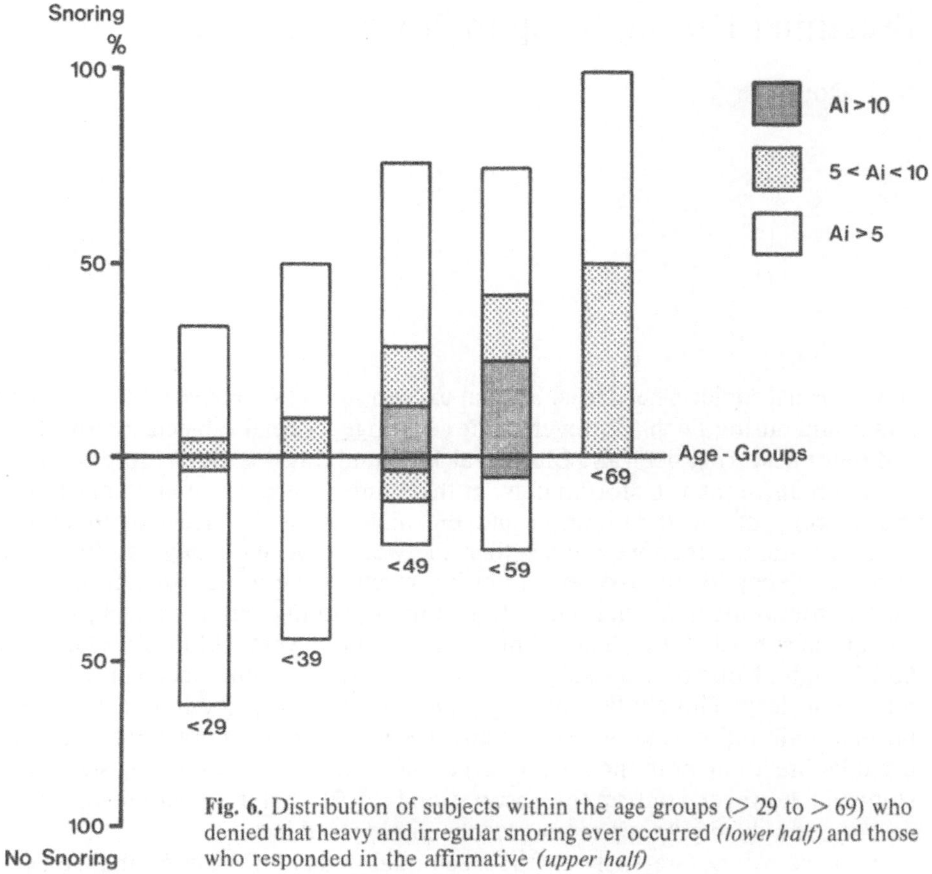

Fig. 6. Distribution of subjects within the age groups (> 29 to > 69) who denied that heavy and irregular snoring ever occurred *(lower half)* and those who responded in the affirmative *(upper half)*

In terms of epidemiology, these first results suggest that SAA plays an important part as a risk factor for general morbidity and, more specifically, the morbidity spectrum of cardiovascular diseases. As the present paper shows the preliminary data of an ongoing study, a future report, based on more comprehensive data, will include a detailed discussion of the full results and their implications.

References

1. Peter JH (1985) Holter monitoring technique in a comprehensive approach: ambulatory monitoring of sleep apnea. In: Hombach V, Hilger HH (eds) Holter monitoring technique. Schattauer, Stuttgart, pp 127–149
2. Lavie P (1983) Incidence of sleep apnea in a presumably healthy population: a significant relationship with excessive daytime sleepiness. Sleep 6:312–318
3. Guilleminault C, van den Hoed J, Mitler MM (1978) Clinical overview of the sleep apnea syndromes. In: Guilleminault C, Dement WC (eds) Sleep apnea syndromes. Liss, New York, pp 1–12

Breathing During Sleep in Normal Subjects

N. J. Douglas

Most normal subjects keep their arterial oxygen saturation above 90% both when awake and during sleep. However, some seemingly normal subjects intermittently desaturate during sleep and Block et al. [5] found this was much more common in men than women. Unfortunately, in that study four obese males contributed the majority of the desaturation and the majority of the irregular breathing. Furthermore, the men were older than the women in that study and there was also a tendency for the oxygen saturation when awake to be lower in the men than in the women. We therefore studied the breathing patterns during sleep of 40 normal subjects (21 women, 19 men), all of whom were within 12% of average body weight. None of these subjects described daytime somnolence or disturbed nocturnal sleep. This study showed [8] that there was no sex difference between normal men and normal women at any age in either the amount of nocturnal irregular breathing or in the lowest oxygen saturation achieved during sleep. The study did, however, confirm the observation [4, 7, 21] that irregular breathing and desaturation during sleep are commoner in older subjects.

We have recently re-analysed the sleep quality data in these normal subjects [8] and have found that arousals are relatively uncommon, no normal subjects having more than nine arousals per hour of sleep [14], despite the attached equipment (Hewlett Packard 47201A ear oximeter, EEG, EOG, EMG; oronasal thermocouples and thoracoabdominal inductance stethogram). This low arousal frequency contrasts markedly (Fig. 1) with that found in patients with the sleep apnoea syndrome or who have clinically important recurrent sleep hypopnoea [14] syndrome. This low rate of arousal in normal subjects during polysomnography should perhaps be used to clarify the definition of abnormal breathing sleep, as it is these recurrent arousals which are believed to result in the disabling daytime somnolence. There is a need for a new definition of the "sleep apnoea syndrome" and one possibility would be the co-existence of symptoms plus 15 apnoeas or hypopnoeas associated with arousals during each hour of sleep.

In normal subjects, breathing tends to be fairly regular in stable NREM sleep. However, at sleep onset and early in the night, breathing during stage 1 and stage 2 NREM sleep may be extremely irregular [6]. Bulow felt that this irregularity was due to laxity in the relationship between the ventilation/end tidal carbon dioxide tension set points during wakefulness and the hypercapnic ventilatory response slope during sleep. Nevertheless, we found no relationship between this laxity and irregular breathing and also found that increasing the carbon dioxide tension

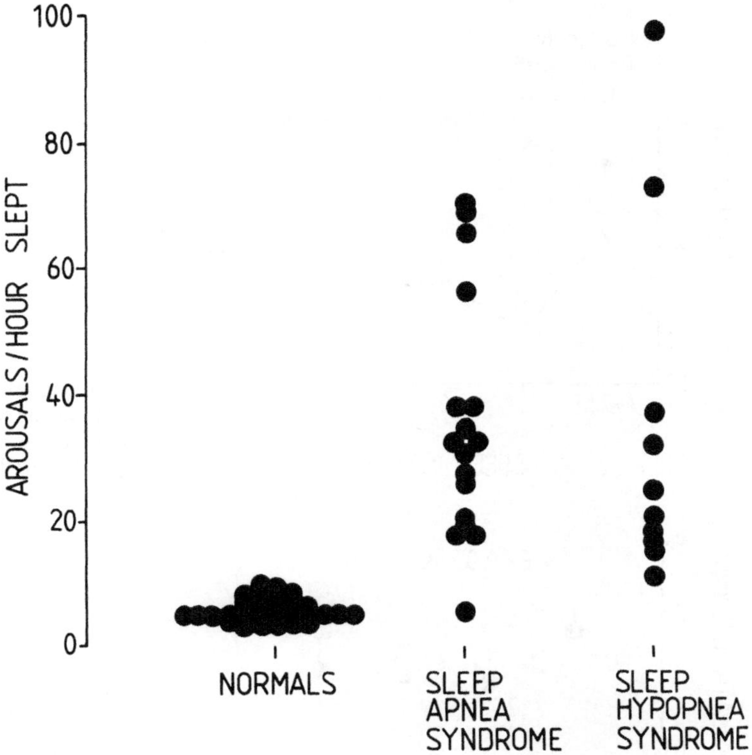

Fig. 1. Number of arousals per hour of sleep in normal subjects, subjects with sleep apnoea syndrome and subjects with clinically important sleep hypopnoea. (Data from [14])

during irregular breathing in NREM sleep did not regularise irregular breathing [11]. During REM sleep, breathing is extremely irregular, and this irregularity is such that consideration of a mean level of ventilation during REM sleep is of limited value.

My original interest in breathing during sleep was on the mechanism and consequences of nocturnal hypoxaemia in patients with chronic bronchitis and emphysema. Having observed [10] that desaturation in such patients occurred almost exclusively during REM sleep, we found that the breathing pattern during these hypoxaemic episodes was that of irregular hypoventilation. The prevailing dogma at that time was that ventilation increased during REM sleep and that the hypoxic drive was preserved during REM sleep, but these views were based exclusively on experiments in animals, mainly dogs, and our observations suggested that they were not applicable to man. I therefore measured ventilation and ventilatory responses to chemostimulation during sleep in normal subjects.

These studies, carried out at a height of 1600 m in Denver, Colorado, confirmed previous studies which had suggested that ventilation fell during NREM sleep, compared to wakefulness, in normal subjects [12]. They also showed that,

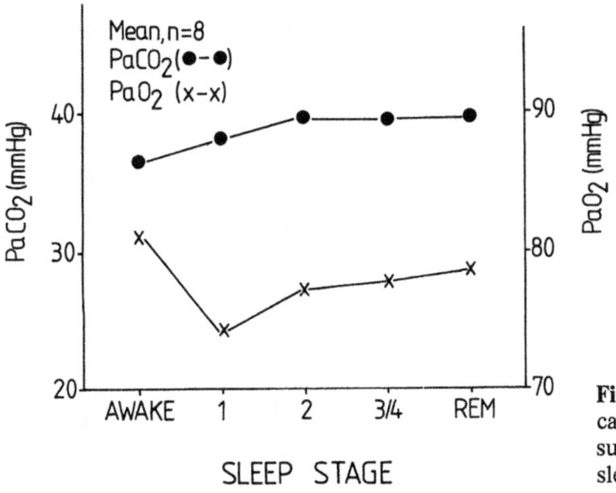

Fig. 2. Mean arterial oxygen and carbon dioxide tension in eight subjects during different stages of sleep. (Data from [9])

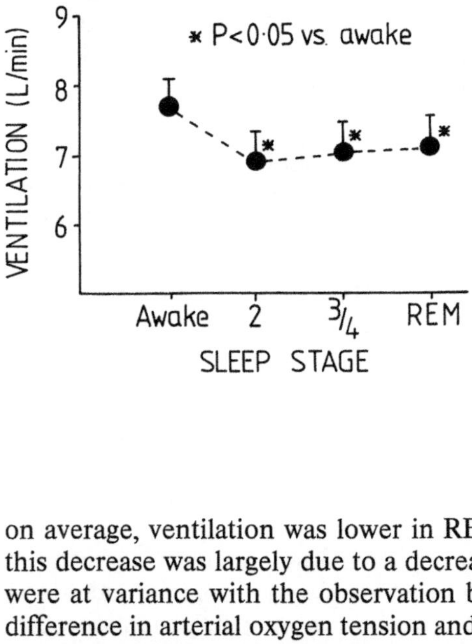

Fig. 3. Mean ± SEM minute ventilation during different sleep stages in 21 normal subjects. (Data redrawn from [33])

on average, ventilation was lower in REM sleep than during NREM sleep, and this decrease was largely due to a decrease in tidal volume. However, these data were at variance with the observation by Coccagna et al. [9] that there was no difference in arterial oxygen tension and arterial carbon dioxide tension between REM and NREM sleep (Fig. 2). Recent observations by White et al. [33] have shown no difference in ventilation between REM and NREM sleep (Fig. 3). I believe the discrepancy between these results and my own [12] is due to the fact that our own measurements of ventilation were recorded prior to studies of ventilatory control and that 1-min periods of re-breathing pattern were recorded "live" whenever we were sure that we were in stable REM sleep. In practice, one can only identify REM sleep in real time by the occurrence of eye movements, and thus the majority of the ventilation that we recorded in our 19 subjects was recorded during periods of fairly intense eye movements. Aserinsky [1] showed that ventilation decreases during periods of intense eye movements (Fig. 4) and

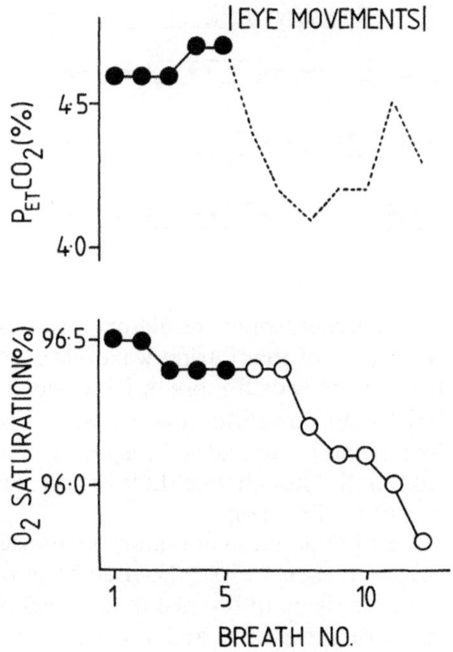

Fig. 4. Effect of eye movements on oxygen saturation *(below)* and end tidal carbon dioxide *(above)* during REM sleep. During the period of eye movements, end tidal plateaus were not achieved due to the shallow breathing, and thus spuriously low end tidal carbon dioxide readings were obtained. (Redrawn from [1])

this has recently been confirmed [23]. Thus I believe that ventilation during sleep is, on average, little different from that during NREM sleep, but that there is episodic marked hypoventilation during periods of intense eye movements.

Pulmonary resistance increases during sleep. This increase is maximal during NREM sleep, as has been shown by Lopes et al. [22]. Hudgel et al. [18] went on to partition this increase in resistance between the upper and lower airways. They found that the increase in pulmonary resistance was exclusively due to an increase in upper airways resistance and again observed that the increase in resistance was greater during stage 2 sleep than during REM sleep. The same workers [19] also found that the functional residual capacity decreases during sleep in normal subjects. They found that this decrease was similar in stage 3/4 sleep and NREM sleep.

The ventilatory response to hypoxia is blunted during sleep. During NREM sleep in men the response is around two-thirds of the level during wakefulness, falling to one-third of that level during REM sleep [13]. On the other hand, we found that women preserved their hypoxic ventilatory response during NREM sleep at around the level during wakefulness, but that their response was significantly depressed during REM sleep [31]. Other workers have also found the hypoxic ventilatory response to be decreased during sleep, and all have found the response to be lowest during REM sleep [2, 17]. The only study which has shown no decrease in the hypoxic drive during sleep is that of Gothe et al. [16]. It was performed on sleep-deprived subjects and without isocapnia, and both these features explain the markedly reduced ventilatory responses [30, 32].

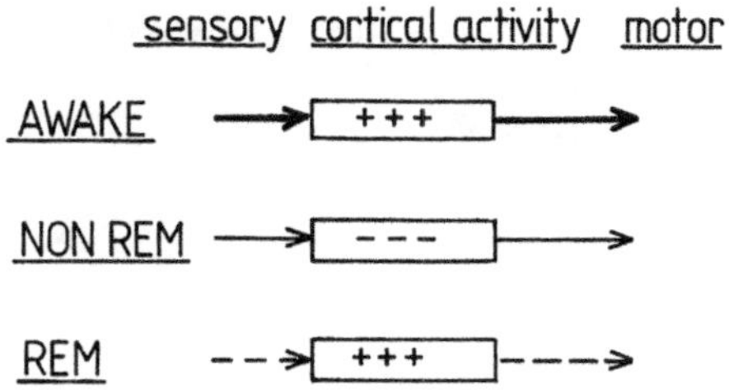

Fig. 5. Schematic diagram of afferent, cortical and efferent activity in wakefulness, during NREM and REM sleep

The hypercapnic ventilatory response is also reduced during sleep, to around two-thirds of that during wakefulnes in NREM sleep and to around one-third of that during wakefulness in REM sleep [11]. Although neither we nor Gothe et al. [15] found any difference between men and women in the effect of sleep on hypercapnic ventilatory response Berthon-Jones and Sullivan [3] found that women did not change their hypercapnic ventilatory responses to any significant extent during sleep.

Ventilation and ventilatory responses during sleep are probably depressed for several reasons. First, the metabolic rate falls during sleep by around 10%–15%, but there is no difference in the level of metabolic rate between sleep stages [33]. As both ventilation and ventilatory responses to chemostimulation are closely linked with metabolic rate, this will be one factor in their depression during sleep. Secondly, alterations in central nervous system function will contribute (Fig. 5). During NREM sleep there is inhibition of the reticular activating system which results in cortical suppression and functional cortical deafferentation. As cortical activity influences breathing, mental concentration increasing both ventilation and ventilatory responses [6], it seems likely that the hyperventilation and decreased responses during NREM sleep reflect decreased cortical activity and the loss of the "wakefulness" drive to ventilation [13]. In REM sleep, there is both pre- and post-synaptic inhibition of afferent neurons [25] and post-synaptic inhibition of motor neurons [24]. This combination of impaired sensory and motor function probably contributes to the markedly impaired ventilatory responses during REM sleep. Thirdly, brain blood flow increases during sleep, and this increase may be maximal during REM sleep [26]. In goats, the increase in blood flow during sleep is greater than can be accounted for by the increased carbon dioxide levels [27]. This increased brain blood flow/brain metabolism ratio would depress central chemoreceptor activity during REM sleep and this, if confirmed in man, might be a factor in reducing ventilatory responses during REM sleep. Fourthly, the increase in airways resistance during REM sleep [18, 22] may contribute to the decrease in ventilation and ventilatory responses, although it must be noted that these increases are maximal during NREM sleep, and thus the changes in airflow resistance cannot account for the lower levels of ventilatory responses during REM sleep.

The clinical significance of the above observations is largely in patients with hypoxic lung disease, as in such patients the decreases in ventilation, functional residual capacity and ventilatory responses during sleep may at least partially explain the REM-related desaturation. The above observations, however, are of limited applicability to the sleep apnoea syndrome. During the above studies of ventilatory responses, observations were also made on arousal responses which are relevant to sleep apnoea. Neither Berthon-Jones and Sullivan [2, 3] nor our own group [11, 13] could find any difference between sleep stages in the arousal response to isocapnic hypoxia or to hyperoxic hypercapnia. Indeed, neither was a very potent stimulus to arousal, many normal subjects staying awake even though their oxygen saturation was dropped to as low as 70% or their end tidal carbon dioxide was raised by 15 mmHg. Many patients with the sleep apnoea syndrome arouse at higher levels of oxygen saturation than this, and all arouse well before their carbon dioxide has risen by 15 mmHg, the average carbon dioxide elevation during an apnoea being <3 mmHg. It is thus not clear whether hypoxia or hypercapnia are major factors in arousal in sleep apnoea, although the above studies do not test their co-existence.

Issa and Sullivan [20] found that occlusion of the airway in normal subjects resulted in more rapid arousal from REM than from NREM sleep. This is contrary to the observation in patients with the sleep apnoea syndrome who tend to arouse more readily from NREM than from REM sleep [29]. However Issa and Sullivan [20] produced airway occlusion externally, and it is possible that the discrepancy between these two observations results from the fact that upper airway mechanoreceptors could sense respiratory effort in the normal subjects when the airway was occluded whereas this would not be the case in obstructive apnoea. Nevertheless, it is unusual for arousal to be more rapid to any stimulus during REM sleep, the classical pattern being that arousal is suppressed during REM sleep [28] .

I conclude that during sleep in normal subjects:

- Ventilation is reduced
- Ventilation is variable during REM sleep and may be further reduced particularly during periods of intense eye movements
- Ventilatory responses to chemostimuli are reduced, particularly during REM sleep
- Irregular breathing and hypoxia increase with age
- Normal men and normal women have similar breathing patterns and similar oxygenation during sleep.

References

1. Aserinsky E (1965) Periodic respiratory pattern occuring in conjunction with eye movements during sleep. Science 150:763–766
2. Berthon-Jones M, Sullivan CE (1982) Ventilatory and arousal responses to hypoxia in sleeping humans. Am Rev Respir Dis 125:632–639
3. Berthon-Jones M, Sullivan CE (1984) Ventilation and arousal responses to hypercapnia in normal sleeping adults. J Appl Physiol 57:59–67
4. Bixler EO, Kales A, Cadieux RJ, Vela-Bueno A, Jacoby JA, Soldatos CR (1985) Sleep apneic activity in older healthy subjects. J Appl Physiol 58:1597–1601
5. Block AJ, Boysen PG, Wynne JW, Hunt LA (1979) Sleep apnea, hypopnea and oxygen desaturation in normal subjects. N Engl J Med 300:513–517
6. Bulow K (1963) Respiration and wakefulness in man. Acta Physiol Scand 59 (Suppl 209):1–110

7. Carskaddon MA, Dement WC (1981) Respiration during sleep in the aged human. J Gerontol 36:420–423
8. Catterall JR, Calverley PMA, Shapiro CM, Flenley DC, Douglas NJ (1985) Breathing and oxygenation during sleep are similar in normal men and normal women. Am Rev Respir Dis 132:86–88
9. Coccagna G, di Donato G, Verucchi P, Cirignotta F, Mantovani M, Lugaresi E (1976) Hypersomnia with periodic apnoeas in acquired micrognathia. Arch Neurol 33:769–776
10. Douglas NJ, Calverley PMA, Leggett RJE et al (1979) Transient hypoxaemia during sleep in chronic bronchitis and emphysema. Lancet 1:1–4
11. Douglas NJ, White DP, Weil JV, Pickett CK, Zwillich CW (1982) Hypercapnic ventilatory responses in sleeping adults. Am Rev Respir Dis 126:758–762
12. Douglas NJ, White DP, Pickett CK, Weil JV, Zwillich CW (1982) Respiration during sleep in normal human. Thorax 37:840–844
13. Douglas NJ, White DP, Weil JV et al (1982) Hypoxic ventilatory response decreases during sleep in normal men. Am Rev Respir Dis 125:286–289
14. Gould GA, Rhind GB, White KF, MacFie J, Catterall JR, Douglas NJ (1986) The sleep hypopnoea syndrome? Am Rev Respir Dis 133:A234
15. Gothe B, Altose MD, Gotham MD et al (1981) Effect of quiet sleep on resting and CO_2 stimulated breathing in humans. J Appl Physiol 50:724–730
16. Gothe B, Goldman MD, Cherniack NS et al (1982) Effect of progressive hypoxia on breathing during sleep. Am Rev Respir Dis 126:97–102
17. Hedemark LL, Kronenberg RS (1982) Ventilatory and heart rate responses to hypoxia and hypercapnia during sleep in adults. J Appl Physiol 53:307–312
18. Hudgel DR, Martin RJ, Johnson B et al (1984) Mechanics of the respiratory system and breathing pattern during sleep in normal humans. J Appl Physiol 56:133–137
19. Hudgel DW, Devadatta P (1984) Decrease in functional residual capacity during sleep in normal humans. J Appl Physiol 57:1319–1322
20. Issa FG, Sullivan CE (1983) Arousal and breathing responses to airway occlusion in healthy sleeping adults. J Appl Physiol 55:1113–1119
21. Krieger J, Turlot JC, Mangin P, Kurtz D (1983) Breathing during sleep in normal young and elderly subjects: hypopneas, apneas and correlated factors. Sleep 6:108–120
22. Lopes JM, Tabachnik E, Muller NL et al (1983) Total airway resistance and respiratory muscle activity during sleep. J Appl Physiol 54:773–777
23. Millman RP, Knight H, Chung DC, Cola MF, Kline LR, Pack AI (1986) Changes in compartmental ventilation in association with eye movements during REM sleep. Am Rev Respir Dis 133:A308
24. Nakamura Y, Goldberg LJ, Chandler SH et al (1978) Intracellular analysis of trigeminal motor neuron activity during sleep in the cat. Science 199:204–207
25. Pompeiano O (1973) Mechanisms of sensorimotor integration during sleep. Prog Physio Psychol 3:1–179
26. Reivich M, Issaacs G, Evarts E et al (1968) The effect of slow wave sleep and REM sleep on regional cerebral blood flow in cats. J Neurochem 15:301–306
27. Santiago TV, Scardella AT, Edelman NH (1984) Determinants of the ventilatory response to hypoxia during sleep. Am Rev Respir Dis 130:179–182
28. Steriade M, Hobson JA (1976) Neuronal activity during the sleep-waking cycle. Prog Neurobiol 6:155–376
29. Sullivan CE, Issa FG (1980) Pathophysiological mechanisms in obstructive sleep apnoea. Sleep 3:235–246
30. Weil JV, Byrne-Quinn E, Sodal IE et al (1970) Hypoxic ventilatory drive in normal man. J Clin Invest 49:1061–1072
31. White DP, Douglas NJ, Pickett CK et al (1982) Hypoxic ventilatory response during sleep in normal women. Am Rev Respir Dis 126:530–533
32. White DP, Douglas NJ, Pickett CK et al (1983) Sleep deprivation and the control of ventilation. Am Rev Respir Dis 128:984–986
33. White DP, Weil JV, Zwillich CW (1985) Metabolic rate and breathing during sleep. J Appl Physiol 59:384–391

Sleep-Related Disordered Breathing, Daytime Hypertension, and Nocturnal Hypotension in Older Males

M. R. LITTNER, D. MCGINTY, and N. STERN

Introduction

A number of investigators, including ourselves, have described a high prevalence of apnea and hypopnea during sleep in males 55 years of age and older [1-6]. This sleep-related disordered breathing (SRDB) is often without obvious daytime symptoms. For this reason, it is not known if SRDB is benign or has potential clinical sequellae [7].

The symptomatic sleep apnea syndrome can produce acute episodes of nocturnal hypertension during apnea and is associated with sustained daytime hypertension as well [8]. It has been hypothesized, by analogy with this symptomatic sleep apnea syndrome, that systemic hypertension may be a consequence of occult SRDB [7, 9-13]. Recently, several studies have documented a high prevalence of sleep apnea in hypertensive subjects [10-13]. However, the subjects in these previous studies were not all older than 55 and systemic blood pressure was not monitored during sleep.

The purpose of our present study was to determine if SRDB is more prevalent in hypertensive males aged 55-70 and if hypertensive episodes occur during sleep in these subjects. Two unexpected findings were as follows:

a) SRDB is not more prevalent in hypertensive males as compared to matched normotensive males aged 55-70; and
b) episodes of hypotension occur during sleep in some of the normotensive older males with SRDB.

The potential consequences of this latter finding are unknown but it may have relevance to the known increase in prevalence of cerebral infarction in men who snore [14]. A preliminary report of these results has been published [15].

Methods

Subject Selection and Protocol

Male veterans, aged 55-70 years, were recruited from the local community after screening of 176 volunteers for medical problems by

a) clinical history;
b) complete pulmonary function testing including arterial blood gases;
c) physical examination with fasting blood chemistry and urinalysis; and
d) an ECG in clinically indicated cases.

Exclusion criteria included a forced expiratory volume in one second < 80% predicted or signs of cerebrovascular, neurologic, metabolic, cardiac, pulmonary, or cognitive disorders. Subjects admitting to regular drug or alcohol use were also excluded. A history of mild to moderate hypertension was permitted. Twenty-six subjects formed the final study population. Subjects signed informed consent statements approved by the hospital's human use committee.

Hypertensive and normotensive groups were established by seated blood pressures (BP) obtained in a series of 27 readings, three readings taken on alternate weekday mornings for 3 weeks using an automated monitor (Sentry 2000). All antihypertensive agents were withdrawn during this period. Hypertension was defined by systolic and/or diastolic BP levels > 140/90 mmHg. Subjects were then hospitalized in the Sepulveda Veterans Administration Medical Center for 4 days, placed on a 100 mEq sodium, 80 mEq potassium diet and furnished with noncaffeinated fluids on request.

The rebreathing method (7% CO_2 in 93% O_2) was used to determine hypercapnic ventilatory responsiveness, reported as liters min^{-1} mmHg CO_2^{-1} [16, 17]. Hypoxic responsiveness was established by an isocapnic rebreathing method [17–19] and reported as liters min^{-1} % SaO_2^{-1}. The posterior rhinometric technique [20] was used to measure nasopharyngeal airway resistance in cm H_2O/liter s^{-1}. Results of ventilatory response and airway resistance studies have been described in detail elsewhere [9].

Sleep Evaluation

Subjects underwent 3 nights of polysomnographic monitoring, including three channels of EEG, eye movements, ECG and chin and anterior tibialis EMG recordings; sleep parameters were obtained using standard criteria [21]. Nocturnal respiratory parameters were assessed by measuring nasal-buccal airflow, chest and abdominal wall respiratory movements, and oxyhemoglobin saturation (SaO_2) by ear oximetry. Apnea and hypopnea were identified as episodes of 10 s or longer in duration in which a complete cessation (apnea) or 50% reduction (hypopnea) in airflow accompanied a drop in SaO_2 of at least 4% below the nocturnal baseline. An SRDB rate (i.e., an apnea–hypopnea rate) was calculated as a function of EEG established sleep time in hours and thus adjusted for any differences among subjects in time asleep. For the purposes of determining the association of apnea to waking hypertension, subjects were divided into two groups, one having an SRDB rate of more than 12, and the other having an SRDB rate of less than eight. No subject had an SRDB rate between 8 and 12 inclusive.

Blood Pressure

BP and heart rate were measured on 3 nights from 2100–0800 at 30 min intervals using an automated monitor which was frequently compared to auscultatory readings to check its accuracy. A technician monitored the observations and recorded the clock time in conjunction with the sleep recording. A mean arterial pressure (MAP) was calculated as the diastolic BP plus one-third of the difference between systolic and diastolic BP. MAP levels that were reduced from baseline were included in analyses only if systolic and diastolic readings showed parallel shifts.

Statistics

When three or more groups were compared, a one-way analysis of variance (ANOVA) was used [22]. When two groups were compared, either a chi-square or unpaired *t* test was used as appropriate [22]. A *p* less than 0.05 was considered significant. A *p* value between 0.05 and 0.10 was considered a trend.

Results

Awake BP and SRDB

Normotensive and hypertensive groups of 13 subjects each are compared in Table 1. These subgroups did not differ in age, weight, or height. MAP was higher in the hypertensives.

Eight of the 13 hypertensive subjects and eight of the 13 normotensive subjects had SRDB rates of greater than 12 per hour of sleep. These two subgroups of subjects did not differ in age, height, weight, total sleep time, % REM sleep, or SRDB rates (Table 2)

BP During Sleep

During sleep, we observed episodes of both increases in blood pressure (data not reported) and decreases in BP. In five of the subjects, the lowest (i.e., the minimum) MAP during the 3 nights of sleep was 60 mmHg or less. This level of MAP

Table 1. Hypertensive and normotensive subjects ($\overline{X} \pm$ SEM)

Group	Hypertensive	Normotensive	*p* value
n	13	13	NS
Age (years)	64 ± 3	64 ± 1	NS
Weight (kg)	84 ± 3.5	84 ± 2.8	NS
Height (cm)	174 ± 1.5	176 ± 1.5	NS
Daytime MAP (mmHg)	120 ± 2.3	94 ± 2.3	< 0.05

Note: "hypertensive" is BP greater than 140 systolic and/or 90 diastolic as measured during the day while the subject is awake.
NS, not significant; MAP, mean arterial pressure equal to [(systolic minus diastolic) divided by 3] plus the diastolic BP.

Table 2. Hypertensive and normotensive SRDB subgroups ($\overline{X} \pm$ SEM)

Subgroup	Hypertensive	Normotensive	*p* value
n	8	8	NS
SRDB per hour of sleep	26 ± 4.8	31 ± 4.9	NS
Total sleep time (min)	363 ± 16	360 ± 9.6	NS
% REM sleep	12.4 ± 1.7	13.1 ± 1.1	NS
Age (years)	66.6 ± 2.1	63 ± 1.8	NS
Weight (kg)	82.4 ± 5.3	86.3 ± 3.9	NS
Height (cm)	172 ± 2.2	76 ± 2.0	NS

Note: for abbreviations see note to Table 1; SRDB groups are those with SRDB rates greater than 12 per hour of sleep; these 16 SRDB subjects are subgroups of the 26 in Table 1 which also includes 10 control subjects (SRDB rates less than 8 per hour of sleep)

is the lowest that is considered to be compatible with maintenance of steady levels of cerebral blood flow through autoregulation of this flow despite wide changes in MAP [23]. Each of these five nocturnally hypotensive subjects was normotensive during the day and each had more than 12 episodes of SRDB per hour of sleep. In addition, the minimum heart rate during sleep in these five subjects did not differ from the minimum heart rate in the other 11 SRDB subjects. This indicated that bradycardia did not contribute markedly to the hypotension during sleep.

Hypotensive versus Nonhypotensive Subjects

In order to further examine hypotension during sleep, we compared the five hypotensive subjects to other subjects with similar waking BP. Specifically, waking BP was obtained immediately prior to sleep in all subjects. These pressures were on average somewhat lower than waking BP obtained during the daytime. For this reason, MAP prior to sleep was less than 100 mmHg in 16 of the 26 subjects. This included 11 subjects with SRDB and five control subjects. The SRDB group included the five subjects previously noted with episodes of MAP during sleep of 60 mmHG or less (hypotensive SRDB subjects) and six subjects with minimum MAP during sleep of greater than 60 mmHg (nonhypotensive SRDB subjects). A comparison of these subjects as well as the five control subjects (nonhypotensive controls) is given in Tables 3 and 4; note that all 16 subjects had a MAP of less than 100 mmHg prior to sleep. The major differences between the hypotensive group during sleep and the two nonhypotensive groups during sleep is a lower minimum SaO_2 during sleep and a trend to a higher supine nasal airway resistance during the daytime while awake (Table 4). It should be noted that total sleep time and MAP just prior to sleep are similar in the three groups. This indicates that the lower MAP during sleep is not markedly influenced by the awake MAP just prior to sleep or by exposure to sleep in the comparison between these three groups of subjects. It should also be noted that the SaO_2 just prior to sleep in the five subjects with minimum MAP during sleep

Table 3. MAP during sleep (MAP < 100 presleep) ($\overline{X} \pm$ SEM)

Groups	Hypotensive SRDB (minimum MAP 60 or less)	Nonhypotensive SRDB (minimum MAP > 60)	Nonhypotensive controls (SRDB < 8 per hour)	*p* value
n	5	6	5	NS
MAP (mmHG) (presleep)	85.6 ± 2.3	90.7 ± 2.9	91.6 ± 2.7	NS
Minimum MAP (mmHg) (during sleep)	56 ± 2.0	70 ± 2.7	68.4 ± 3.0	< 0.05
Age (years)	62.4 ± 2.4	65.2 ± 1.9	65.6 ± 1.7	NS
Weight (kg)	88.6 ± 6.1	86.9 ± 6.0	79 ± 3.5	NS
Height (cm)	177 ± 2.6	175 ± 2.5	175 ± 2.4	NS

Note: presleep is while the subject is awake just prior to sleep; minimum MAP during sleep is the lowest MAP recorded during the 3 nights of sleep; MAP presleep is the value just prior to sleep on the night of the minimum MAP. For other abbreviations see notes to Tables 1 and 2

Table 4. SaO_2, nasal resistance, and sleep parameters (MAP < 100 presleep)

Groups	Hypotensive SRDB (minimum MAP 60 or less) during sleep	Nonhypotensive SRDB (minimum MAP > 60) during sleep	Nonhypotensive controls (SRDB < 8 per hour)	*p* value
n	5	6	5	NS
SaO_2 prior to sleep (% saturation)	93.6 ± 0.40	95.7 ± 0.42	95.4 ± 0.51	< 0.05
Minimum SaO_2 during sleep (% saturation)	71.2 ± 7.0	85.3 ± 1.3	89 ± 1.2	< 0.05
SNAR (cmH_2O per liter per second)	5.10 ± 1.2 (*n* = 4)	3.17 ± 0.30	2.86 ± 0.59	< 0.1
SRDB per hour of sleep	33.8 ± 5.1	25 ± 50	4.6 ± 0.98	< 0.05
Total sleep time (min)	352 ± 15	374 ± 17	400 ± 26	NS
% REM	13.9 ± 2.8	12.7 ± 1.2	18.6 ± 3.0	NS

Note: values are $\overline{X} \pm$ SEM; SNAR, supine nasal airway resistance while awake during the day; for other abbreviations, see notes to Tables 1 to 3

of 60 mmHg or less was slightly but significantly less than in the other two groups. This may have contributed to the lower minimum SaO_2 during sleep in the subjects who were hypotensive during sleep (Table 4).

Hypercapnic and hypoxia ventilatory responses and upright nasal airway resistance did not differ significantly between the three groups (data not reported).

Discussion

Our results demonstrate the following new information in male subjects aged 55–70 years: (a) SRDB is not predominantly confined to hypertensive subjects; and (b) episodes of hypotension during sleep occur in some normotensive subjects with SRDB.

In contrast to our results, previous studies indicate that subjects with systemic hypertension have a higher prevalence of apnea during sleep than normotensive controls. However, the hypertensive subjects with sleep apnea are in some studies, on average, older and weigh more when compared to hypertensive subjects without sleep apnea [10, 11]. In other studies, both weight and age are postively correlated with prevalence of sleep apnea [2, 5, 6]. In addition, while the relative risk of hypertension is greater in snorers (a marker of sleep apnea), this is true only in the 40–49 year age group in men. Indeed, the relative risk is as low as 1.16 to 1 in the 60–69 year male age group [24].

The above information suggests that previous results indicating a high prevalence of sleep apnea in hypertensive subjects may result, at least in part, from the following: (a) the independent influence of older age or greater weight in producing both sleep apnea and hypertension; and (b) the inclusion of younger subjects in whom sleep apnea and hypertension are likely to be associated for unknown reasons [24]. On the other hand, our results of no relationship of SRDB to hypertension in older males is consistent with a similar lack of correlation between snoring and hypertension in males aged 50–69 [24].

Speculatively, our results taken together with those of others [24] suggest that SRDB or sleep apnea are most consistently potential contributers to hypertension only in younger males. As the males become older, there is an increase in prevalence of SRDB or sleep apnea [1–6, 9] but, for unknown reasons, these do not contribute selectively to hypertension. This suggests that neither SRDB nor sleep apnea contribute to hypertension in older males or that the contribution is blunted by host factors (e.g., a reduction in adrenergic responsiveness) that are present in some older males and are not present in most younger males. Finally, it should be emphasized that there may be other explanations for our finding of a lack of correlation between SRDB and hypertension. For example, a hidden selection bias may be present in our process of selecting subjects; however, it should be noted that our selection procedures are similar to those of others who have studied sleep apnea and hypertension [10, 11].

We sampled SaO_2 continuously by ear oximeter and sampled BP at 30-min intervals. For this reason, we were unable to compare adequately and directly episodes of reductions in MAP during sleep to reductions in levels of SaO_2. However, a reduction in MAP to 60 mmHg or less during sleep occurred in those subjects with the lowest minimum SaO_2 during sleep (Table 4). In addition, those subjects with MAP of 60 mmHg or less during sleep had, as a trend, a higher supine nasal airway resistance while awake (Table 4).

There are several possibilities whereby MAP may be episodically reduced during sleep. These include the following: (a) periodic reductions from impairment in central nervous system control of BP; (b) a decrease in cardiac output during an increase in left ventricular afterload from a reduction in intrathoracic pressure during a Mueller maneuver produced by obstructive sleep apnea or obstructive hypopnea; and (c) a decrease in peripheral vascular resistance from hypoxemic peripheral vascular vasodilation without an appropriate sympathetic response via the baroreceptors in the carotid or aortic bodies [25–27].

Our results provide indirect evidence to support the latter two possibilities. Specifically, those subjects with the greatest reduction in MAP during sleep had the lowest SaO_2 during sleep and the highest awake supine nasal airway resistance. This would support the hypothesis that hypoxemic vasodilation and the increased afterload effects of a Meuller maneuver from obstructive apnea can contribute to reduction in MAP during sleep. In addition, it is possible that other factors, such as occult left ventricular dysfunction, may also contribute to a reduced MAP under the stresses of hypoxemia and increased left ventricular afterload.

Our results indicate that SRDB is highly prevalent in otherwise healthy elderly male veterans with or without systemic hypertension and that nocturnal hypotension is common in the normotensive SRDB subjects. It can be hypothesized that such decreases in nocturnal blood pressure can contribute to an increase in prevalence of stroke during sleep in snoring men.

Summary

Sleeping and awake BP and respiration during sleep were examined in otherwise healthy men aged 55–70 years who were either hypertensive or normotensive while awake. SRDB was similar in prevalence in these hypertensive and normotensive groups. During sleep, episodes of both hypertension and, surprisingly, hypotension were observed. Specifically, five of the normotensive males had a minimum MAP of 60 mmHg or less during sleep. This hypotension occurred in those subjects with greater than control rates of SRDB, with the lowest SaO_2 during sleep and with the highest supine nasal airway resistance while awake. We conclude that the presence of SRDB in older men is not selective for awake systemic hypertension and that hypotension can occur during sleep in some normotensive older males with SRDB. This latter may be the result of hypoxemic peripheral vascular vasodilation or an increase in left ventricular afterload during obstructive SRDB. The presence of hypotension during sleep in older SRDB males suggests the hypothesis that this hypotension may contribute to the known elevated prevalence of cerebral infarction in snoring males.

Acknowledgement. This research was supported by the Medical Research Service of the Veterans Administration (USA). We thank Carole Gingo and Lois Rubin for typing the manuscript.

References

1. McGinty D, Littner M, Beahm E, Ruiz-Primo E, Young E, Sowers J (1982) Sleep related breathing disorders in older men: a search for underlying mechanisms. Neurobiol Aging 3:337–350
2. Webb P (1974) Periodic breathing during sleep. J Appl Physiol 37:899–903

3. Carskadon MA, Dement WC (1981) Respiration during sleep in the aged human. J Gerontol 36:420–423
4. Ancoli-Israel S, Kripke DF, Mason W, Messin S (1981) Sleep apnea and nocturnal myoclonus in a senior population. Sleep 4:349–358
5. Smallwood RG, Vitiello MV, Siblin EC, Prinz PN (1983) Sleep apnea: relationship to age, sex, and Alzheimer's dementia. Sleep 6:16–22
6. Block AJ, Boysen PG, Wynne JW, Hunt LA (1979) Sleep apnea, hypopnea, and oxygen desaturation in normal subjects: a strong male predominance. N Engl J Med 300:513–547
7. Littner MR, McGinty D (1985) Asymptomatic disordered breathing during sleep in older persons: disease or not? Arch Int Med 145:233–234
8. Schroeder JS, Motta J, Guilleminault C (1978) Hemodynamic studies in sleep apnea syndromes. In: Guilleminault C, Dement WC (eds) Sleep apnea syndromes. Liss, New York, pp 177–196
9. Littner MR, Young E, McGinty D, Beahm E, Riege W, Sowers J (1984) Awake abnormalities of control of breathing and of the upper airway: occurrence in healthy older men with nocturnal disordered breathing. Chest 86:573–574
10. Fletcher EC, DeBehnke RD, Lovoi MS, Gorin AB (1985) Undiagnosed sleep apnea in patients with essential hypertension. Ann Intern Med 103:190–195
11. Williams AJ, Houston DH, Finberg S, Lam C, Kinney JL, Santiago S (1985) Sleep apnea syndrome and essential hypertension. Am J Cardiol 55:1019–1022
12. Kales A, Cacheux RJ, Shaw LC, Vela-Bueno A, Bixler EO, Schneck DW, Locke TW, Soldatos CR (1984) Sleep apnea in a hypertensive population. Lancet 2:1005–1008
13. Lavie P, Rachamin BY, Rubin AE (1984) Prevalence of sleep apnea syndrome among patients with essential hypertension. Am Heart J 108:1019–1022
14. Partinen M, Palomaki H (1985) Snoring and cerebral infarction. Lancet 1:1325–1326
15. McGinty D, Beahm E, Stern N, Sowers J, Littner MR, Riege W (1985) Occult nocturnal hypotension in older men with sleep related breathing disorder. Sleep Res 14:190
16. Read DJC (1966) A clinical method for assessing the ventilatory response to CO_2. Aus NZ J Med 16:20–32
17. Littner MR, McGinty DJ, Arand DL (1980) Determinants of oxygen desaturation in the course of ventilation during sleep in chronic obstructive pulmonary disease. Am Rev Respir Dis 122:849–857
18. Rebuck AS, Campbell EJM (1973) A clinical method for assessing the ventilatory response to hypoxia. Am Rev Respir Dis 109:345–350
19. Read DJC, Nicholls PM, Herisley MJ (1977) Instability of the carbon dioxide stimulus under the "mixed venous isocapnic" conditions advocated for testing the ventilatory response to hypoxia. Am Rev Respir Dis 116:336–339
20. Taylor G, Shivalker PR (1971) Changes in nasal airway resistance on antigenic challenge in allergic rhinitis. Clin Allergy 1:63–73
21. Rechtschaffen A, Kales L (eds) (1968) A manual of standard terminology, techniques and scoring system for sleep stages on human subjects. Public Health Service, US Government Printing Office, Washington DC
22. Hoel PH (1964) Introduction to mathematical statistics, 3rd edn. Wiley, New York, pp 27–283, 297–328
23. Strangaard S (1975) Autoregulation of cerebral blood flow in hypertensive patients. The modifying influence of prolonged antihypertensive treatment on the tolerance to acute, drug induced hypertension. Circulation 53:720–727
24. Kaskenvuo M, Partinen M, Sarna S, Kaprio J, Langinvainio H, Heikkila K (1985) Snoring as a risk factor for hypertension and angina pectoris. Lancet 1:893–896
25. Heisted DD, Abboud FM (1980) Circulatory adjustments to hypoxia. Circulation 61:463–470
26. Lugliani F, Whipp BJ, Warserman K (1973) A role for the carotid body in cardiovascular control in man. Chest 63:744–750
27. Gribbin B, Pickering TG, Slaight P, Peto R (1971) The effect of age and high blood pressure on basoreflex sensitivity in man. Circ Res 29:221–239

Part 6: Cardiorespiratory Disorders During Sleep and Hemodynamics

Nocturnal Hypoxemia and Pulmonary Arterial Blood Pressure

K. H. RÜHLE, and H. MATTHYS

Sleep apnea and chronic obstructive lung disease (COLD) are often paralleled by a decrease in oxygen partial pressure. Hypoxemia leads to pulmonary vasoconstriction and an increase in pulmonary arterial pressure (P_{AP}).

Sleep Apnea

In the following, the hemodynamic mechanisms during apnea and the development of daytime pulmonary hypertension will be discussed. The clinical implications of the periodical increase in P_{AP} during the night are unclear, especially the development of right heart insufficiency. During obstructive apnea highly negative intrathoracic pressures are generated and the absolute value of P_{AP} can decrease. But the transmural pressures i.e., the difference between pleural pressure and the pulmonary artery, increases. Immediately after the termination of apnea the highest P_{AP} is observed (Fig. 1). In this example, chest movement, nose and mouth flow show a typical obstructive apnea. At the end of the apneic event, P_{AP} increases parallel to the decrease in oxygen saturation (SaO_2). P_{AP} rises from

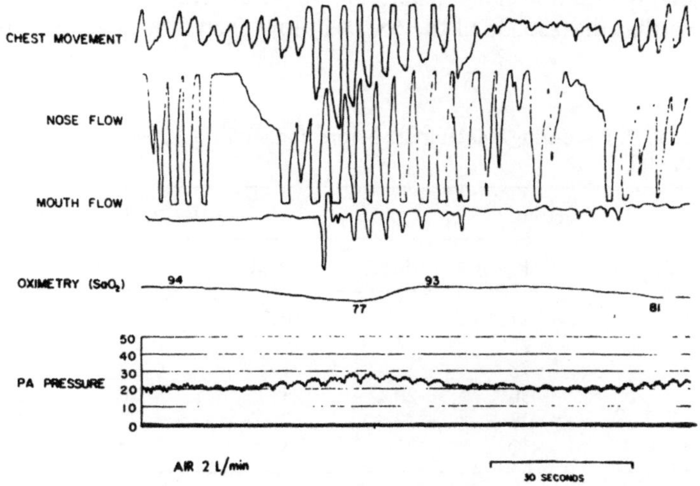

Fig. 1. OSA followed by a decrease of SaO_2 and an increase of $\overline{P}_{AP}$. Polygraphic tracing [2]

Table 1. P_{AP} in six patients during the night. After tracheostomy normalization of $\overline{P}_{AP}$ in four of six patients with OSA

Pat.	Before			After tracheostomy		
	P_{AP} syst	diast	mean	P_{AP} syst	diast	mean (mmHg)
1	38	24	27	39	26	29
2	60	40	47	30	18	22
3	70	50	57	38	14	22
4	80	54	63	28	15	19
5	60	48	52	22	10	14
6	38	22	27	40	18	25
			45±6			22±2

22 to 28 mmHg. The duration of the increase is about 30 s. After this period P_{AP} returns to the baseline value (22 mmHg), which means borderline pulmonary hypertension. Motta et al. [8] studied six male patients with predominant sleep-induced obstructive apnea before and after tracheostomy. During the obstructive episodes arterial PO_2 dropped and cyclic pressure elevations were observed. The abnormalities were heightened during REM sleep. The P_{AP} followed the pattern of systemic arterial pressure and tended to return to baseline after onset of ventilation. $\overline{P}_{AP}$ was 45 mmHg and returned after tracheostomy to 22 mmHg (Table 1). Baseline values, however, before tracheostomy where only slightly elevated in three patients with a mean value of 20 ± 5 mmHg. After tracheostomy there was no change in $\overline{P}_{AP}$ (Table 2).

Podszus et al. [10] of the Marburg working group performed right heart catheterization in 65 patients with sleep apnea. 40 patients showed either latent or manifest pulmonary hypertension. After eliminating patients with pulmonary or cardiac disease, 36 of the 65, i.e., more than 50% developed pulmonary hyperten-

Table 2. P_{AP} during wakefulness before and after tracheostomy. There is no increase of daytime P_{AP} [8]

Pat.	Before			After tracheostomy		
	P_{AP} syst	diast	mean	P_{AP} syst	diast	mean (mmHg)
1	17	7	10	22	16	18
2	28	4	19	28	18	21
3	28	18	21	28	14	19
4	30	20	23	30	16	21
5	28	12	17	22	10	14
6	32	26	28	40	20	27
			20±5			20±4

Table 3. Data of polysomnographic measurements in patients with RHF ($n = 6$) and those without RHF (from [3])

	Without RHF	With RHF	p Value
patients, n	44	6	
Apnea index, n per h sleep	33 ± 4	30 ± 10	NS
Apnea-hypopnea index, n per h sleep	60 ± 5	57 ± 9	NS
Duration apneas, s	20 ± 1	23 ± 3	NS
Total apnea time per h sleep, %	20 ± 7	22 ± 9	NS
Mean nocturnal SaO_2, %	90 ± 1	76 ± 3	<0.001

sion as a consequence of hypoxemia during sleep apnea. Right heart failure (RHF) in patients with obstructive sleep apnea (OSA) is a known complication of sleep apnea syndrome (SAS), but the percentage of patients developing decompensation with heart failure is not established. Bradley et al. [3] determined the incidence of RHF in 50 consecutive patients with OSA. The apnea index was about 33 per hour, the duration 20–23 s. The diagnosis of RHF was based on clinical criteria and required the presence of peripheral edema plus elevated jugular venous pressure, radiographic evidence of pulmonary hypertension, or standard electrocardiographic evidence of right ventricular hypertrophy. P_{AP} was not measured (Table 3). Of the 50 patients six satisfied the criteria for right heart insufficiency, but the apnea index, apnea hypopnea index, duration of apnea, and total apnea time per hour of sleep were not different when comparing the two groups. Only the mean nocturnal SaO_2 showed a difference of 14% during the night. When analyzing the factors which were involved in the pathogenesis of RHF, important differences between the groups with and without RHF could be detected. Patients with RHF were more obese. They had lower awake PO_2 and a higher PCO_2. Residual volume as a percentage of predicted values was increased and FEV 1.0 was significantly reduced. To demonstrate the importance of sustained hypoxemia during the day opposed to only nocturnal hypoxemia, eight patients without RHF but with the greatest degree of nocturnal oxygen desaturation were selected. The apnea and apnea/hypopnea index was even higher compared with the six patients with RHF. Lowest nocturnal SaO_2 reached 23% whereas patients with RHF demonstrated a higher SaO_2 (36%). There was again a difference of arterial PO_2 during wakefulness, and FEV 1.0 was significantly decreased compared with patients without RHF. It can be concluded that the development of RHF is related to the presence of daytime hypoxemia. It can be attributed to airway obstruction. FEV 1.0 was 1.8 liters in the patients with OSA and airway obstruction whereas patients with chronic obstructive pulmonary disease (COPD) alone and RHF usually show values smaller than 1 liter/s. The severe hypoxemia combined with hypercapnia may be attributed to the marked obesity of the patients with chronic obstructive lung disease (COLD).

Summarizing the presented data in patients with sleep apnea and increased P_{AP}, we hypothesize that the following stages can be observed (Table 4).

Table 4. Hypothetical development of daytime increase of P_{AP} and right heart insufficiency

Pap ↑ during apnoeic events 100%
⬇
Only nocturnal Pap ↑
⬇
Daytime Pap ↑ 58%
⬇
Right heart insufficiency (additionally airway obstruction and obesity)

The P_{AP} increased during each apneic event but after normalized ventilation the P_{AP} decreased to normal values. Repeated cyclical nocturnal events perhaps lead to a continuous increase of P_{AP} during the night but the P_{AP} returns to normal during wakefulness. The percentage is under current investigation. Daytime P_{AP} elevation could be observed in about 60% of patients with OSA. In about 12%, OSA can lead to RHF when airway obstruction and obesity are additionally present.

Chronic Obstructive Lung Disease

In contrast to SAS, hypoxemia in patients with COLD lasts longer. It often occurs during light and REM sleep. These episodes last as long as 20–30 min (Fig. 2) and are accompanied by increases of P_{AP}. In this patient (Fig. 2) with

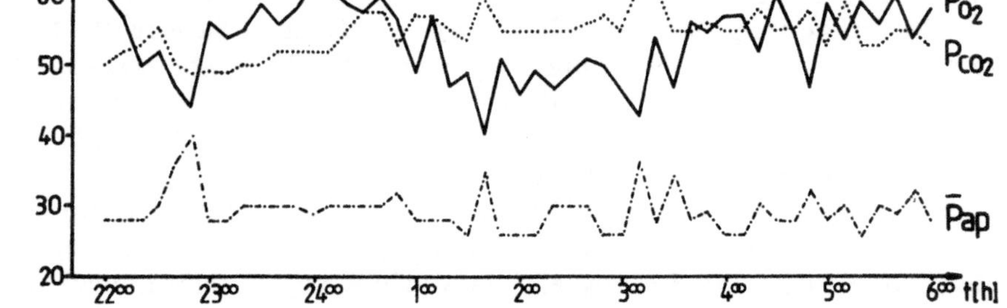

Fig. 2. Nocturnal polygraphic registration of a patient with COLD breathing room air. *Upper part,* sleep stages; *lower part;* transcutaneously measured PO_2, *dotted line,* PCO_2. $\bar{P}_{AP}$ during hypoxemia when the PO_2 falls below 50 mmHg. These hypoxemic episodes are also paralleled by REM sleep

Table 5. Factors influencing the increase of P_{AP} in patients with (COLD)

● Nocturnal hypoxemia	→	Pulmonary artery pressure ↑
- Hypopnoea (apnoea)		
- V'_A/Q' inequalities		
● Increase of cardiac output	→	

COLD breathing air, the first desaturation occurred in the 1st hour of sleep and was paralleled by REM sleep. Interestingly, PCO_2 did not increase during hypoxemia. This is in agreement with the literature. For instance Boysen et al. [2] found only minor increase of PCO_2 during these episodes. This example shows clearly that P_{AP} elevations are related to a fall of PO_2. Overall, four severe episodes during the night were observed with a decrease of PO_2 below 55 mmHg. The factors leading to P_{AP} elevation are nocturnal hypoxemia and an increase in cardiac output (Table 5).

Nocturnal Hypoxemia. The mechanism of nocturnal hypoxemia in patients with COLD is almost always caused by hypopnea and not apnea. In our patients with COLD we seldom found periods of apnea. The second cause of hypoxemia is ventilation/perfusion inequalities. The reason for the development of this ventilation/perfusion mismatching is unclear.

The desaturation occurring during hypoxemic episodes is also associated with a decrease of the esophageal pressure or abdominal respiratory movement, or an increase of esophageal pressure in association with snoring during NREM and REM sleep. Thus the added respiratory impairment of REM sleep or sleep-related partial upper airway obstruction is another cause of hypoxemia and increase of P_{AP} [6]. Koo et al. [7] studied arterial blood gases in 15 patients with COLD. In six patients alveolar hypoventilation could explain the increase of hypoxemia but in nine patients the ventilation perfusion mismatching contributed to the worsening of hypoxemia. When plotting PO_2 and PCO_2 on a O_2/CO_2 diagram there was a widening of the alveolar-arterial oxygen difference corresponding with a worsening of ventilation/perfusion mismatch.

Increase in Cardiac Output. The increase in cardiac output also leads to a change in P_{AP}. Fletcher et al. [5] examined the effect of arterial O_2 desaturation during NREM and REM sleep. All episodes of REM sleep were paralleled by an elevation of P_{AP}. During seven episodes there was only an increase in vascular resistance. During four episodes vascular resistance remained constant or increased, but cardiac index increased significantly from 2.7 to 3.8. In two cases cardiac index and vascular resistance showed an increase as a consequence of hypoxemia. Boysen et al. [2] recorded in patients with COLD the lowest level of SaO_2 and the corresponding P_{AP} during 4 h of sleep. Then P_{AP} was plotted against SaO_2. They found a very good linear relationship between these two variables.

For each patient an individual slope was calculated. Adding all data points, the mean slope of all patients was -0.97, i.e., if SaO_2 decreases 1%, the P_{AP} increases 1 mmHg.

Regarding the different sleep stages, there is a progressive nocturnal increase of P_{AP} from wakefulness to REM sleep (Table 6). In this stage P_{AP} reaches its highest value and therefore patients with COLD are perhaps predisposed to attacks of RHF in this stage [4].

Table 6. Increase in P_{AP} dependent on sleep stages in patients with COLD (mmHg) [4]

Stage	$\bar{P}_{ap}$	P_{ap} syst	P_{ap} diast	Normal
W	37	59.2	29.9	18/8
Stage 1	38	61.6	30.6	19/9
Stage 2	40.3	63.5	30.9	23/11
Stage 3/4	44.8	67.2	32.6	23/12
REM	55	79.3	37.7	23/11

We were especially interested in the integrated P_{AP} values during the night and whether this integrated value was higher than the baseline value [11] (Table 7). The integrated P_{AP} showed nearly the same value compared with the baseline value. The peak value of the mean P_{AP}, i.e., the highest value during the night, was about 10 mmHg higher than the baseline P_{AP}. These data also show that the temporarily increased P_{AP} was of no importance when calculating the integrated P_{AP} during the night. The integrated P_{AP} during the night can be predicted by awake PCO_2 values and even better by PO_2 baseline values (Fig. 3). Thus the functional impairment of gas exchange is a good predictor of the baseline level of P_{AP} during the night. The increase of P_{AP} in REM sleep during hypoxemic episodes can be better predicted by the PCO_2 characterizing alveolar ventilation during wakefulness (Fig. 4). Plotting PO_2 versus peak P_{AP} during the night, there is a wider scattering in a P_{AP}/PCO_2 diagram.

Table 7. P_{AP} at 10 p. m. and during sleep. There is no difference between baseline values and integrated values during the night. Increase of highest P_{AP} of about 10 mmHg during hypoxemic episodes ($n = 14$) [11]

Baseline values:	
$\bar{P}_{AP}$ 29.9 ± 11.1	P_{AP} syst 45.8 ± 18.1
	P_{AP} diast 17.1 ± 7.6
During sleep:	
P_{AP} 29.6 ± 10	$\bar{P}_{AP}$ max 41.2 ± 14.4

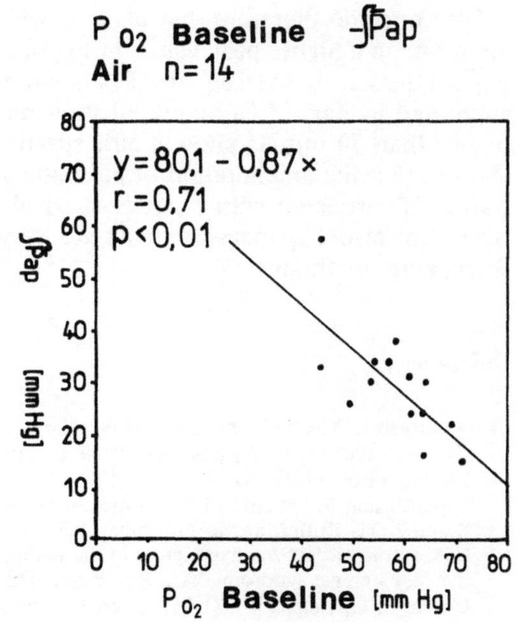

Fig. 3. Correlation between PO_2, baseline value at 10 p. m. and integrated $\overline{P}_{AP}$

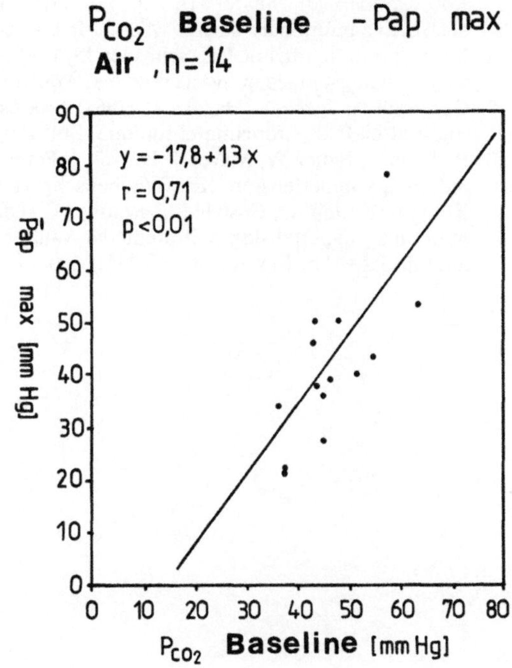

Fig. 4. Correlation between PCO_2 at 10 p. m. and highest P_{AP} during, the night. It correlates better with the PCO_2 than with PO_2 at 10 p. m. during wakefulness

We conclude therefore that patients with a higher PCO_2 during wakefulness are prone to a higher peak value during the night. The importance of measuring P_{AP} is stressed by the fact that P_{AP} is strongly correlated with survival. This is supported by data of Ourednik [9] showing that patients with COLD and a P_{AP} higher than 30 mmHg show a 50% survival of only 3 years. Ashutosh [1] also showed that the amelioration of pulmonary hemodynamics during O_2 administration is correlated with a better survival. We think, therefore, that not only SaO_2, but also P_{AP} measurements are very important to further improve our therapeutic methods.

References

1. Ashutosh K, Mead G, Dunsky M (1983) Early effects of oxygen administration and prognosis in chronic obstructive pulmonary disease and cor pulmonale. Am Rev respir Dis 127:399
2. Boysen PhG, Block AJ, Wynne JW, Hunt LA, Flick MR (1979) Nocturnal pulmonary hypertension in patients with chronic obstructive pulmonary disease. Chest 76:536
3. Bradley DT, Rutherford R, Grossman RF, Lue F, Zamel R, Moldofsky H, Philippson EA (1985) Role of daytime hypoxemia in the pathogenesis of right heart failure in the obstructive sleep apnea syndrome. Am Rev Respir Dis 131:835
4. Coccagna G, Lugaresi E (1978) Arterial blood gases and pulmonary and systemic arterial pressure during sleep in chronic obstructive pulmonary disease. Sleep 1(2):117
5. Fletcher EC, Levin DC (1984) Cardiopulmonary hemodynamics during sleep in subjects with chronic obstructive pulmonary disease. The effect of short- and long-term oxygen. Chest 85:6
6. Hudgel DW, Martin RJ, Capehart M, Johnson B, Hill P (1983) Contribution of hypoventilation to sleep oxygen desaturation in chronic obstructive pulmonary disease. J Appl Physiol 55(3):669
7. Koo KW, Sax DS, Snider GL (1975) Arterial blood gases and pH during sleep in chronic obstructive pulmonary disease. Am J Med 58:663
8. Motta J, Guilleminault Ch, Schröder JS, Dement WC (1978) Tracheostomy and hemodynamic changes in sleep-induced apnea. Ann Intern Med 89:454
9. Ourednik A, Jezek V, Bakova O (1968) Pronostic de l'hypertension pulmonaire chez les sujets atteints de bronchite chronique. Bull Physiopathol Respir 4:213
10. Podszus T, Bauer W, Mayer J, Penzel T, Peter JH, von Wichert P (1986) Sleep apnea and pulmonary hypertension. Klin Wochenschr 64:131
11. Rühle KH, Klein G, Costabel U, Matthys H (1986) Effect of oxygen breathing on nocturnal pulmonary hypertension and predictive value of blood gas analysis in chronic obstructive lung disease. Am Rev Respir Dis 133:A150

Interaction of Sleep Apnea and Chronic Lung Disease

E. C. Fletcher

Introduction

Oxyhemoglobin desaturation is probably the most significant pathophysiologic derangement associated with respiratory disease. In advanced stages, chronic lung disease may result in sustained hypoxemia. Severe obstructive sleep apnea syndrome (OSAS) may cause substantial episodic falls in oxyhemoglobin saturation resulting from transient upper airway occlusion. While both continuous and transient forms of desaturation may be deleterious by themselves, the consequences of their coexistence in a single patient can be profound. This paper describes the interacting pathophysiology of chronic obstructive pulmonary disease (COPD) and sleep apnea, and proposes theoretical mechanisms of potentially additive effects.

Additive Hypoxemia

Several reports have appeared in the literature describing the coexistence of sleep apnea syndrome with chronic lung disease [1–5]. Several more have paid particular attention to the possible interactions between these entities [6–10]. While the prevalence of such cases is unknown, there is no reason to associate these diseases with one another in any causal way [11]. There is, however, special reason for concern when sleep apnea and chronic lung disease coexist, because their combination may produce greater hypoxemia. The extreme hypoxemia produced by the interaction of these diseases is likely to have a more profound effect upon the brain, hematopoietic tissue, and the cardiovascular system than either disease alone.

Hypoxemia results from two basic mechanisms:

a) alveolar hypoventilation exemplified by apnea or breath hold; and
b) gas exchange abnormalities exemplified by ventilation/perfusion mismatch in pneumonia or chronic lung disease.

Figure 1 illustrates the additive effect of these two mechanisms of desaturation in the same patients. Slow speed (10 cm/h) ear oximetry tracings are shown for three patients with both COPD (diagnosed by clinical criteria and pulmonary function tests) and severe obstructive sleep apnea (diagnosed by polysomnogra-

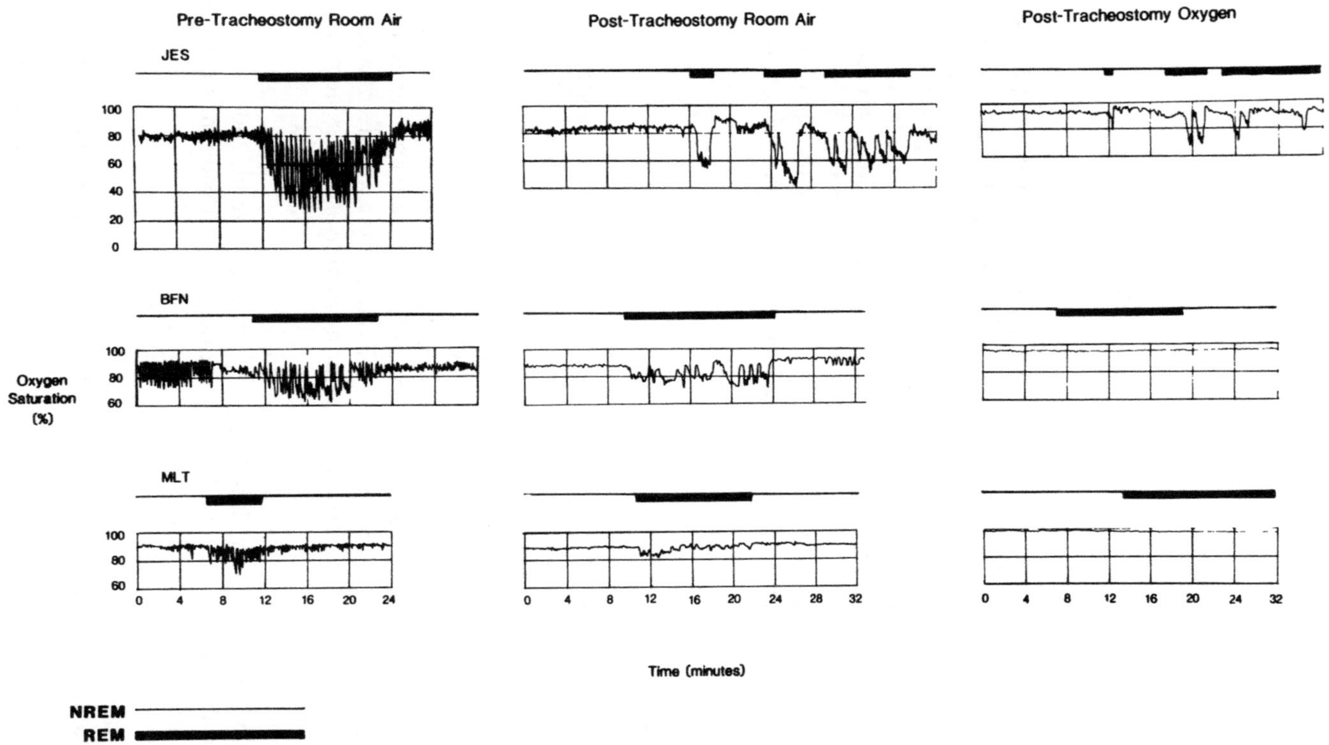

Fig. 1. Ear oximeter recordings (paper speed 10 cm/h) of three patients showing oxyhemoglobin desaturation during sleep before tracheostomy *(left panel)*, after tracheostomy with stoma open breathing room air *(center panel)*, and after tracheostomy, with stoma open, breathing supplemental oxygen (4 l/min) *(right)*. Solid bars and lines above the saturation curves represent rapid-eye-movement (REM) sleep and non-REM sleep, respectively. Apneic desaturation (most severe during REM sleep) for each of the three patients is characterized by rapid, sharp dips and recovery *(left panel)*. Elimination of the obstructive apneas by tracheostomy then reveals a more gradual fall and recovery in oxyhemoglobin saturation that uniformly corresponds to REM sleep and is attributed to a combination of hypoventilation and deterioration of gas exchange. The *right panel* shows amelioration of the desaturation using supplemental oxygen in the same three patients. (From [10])

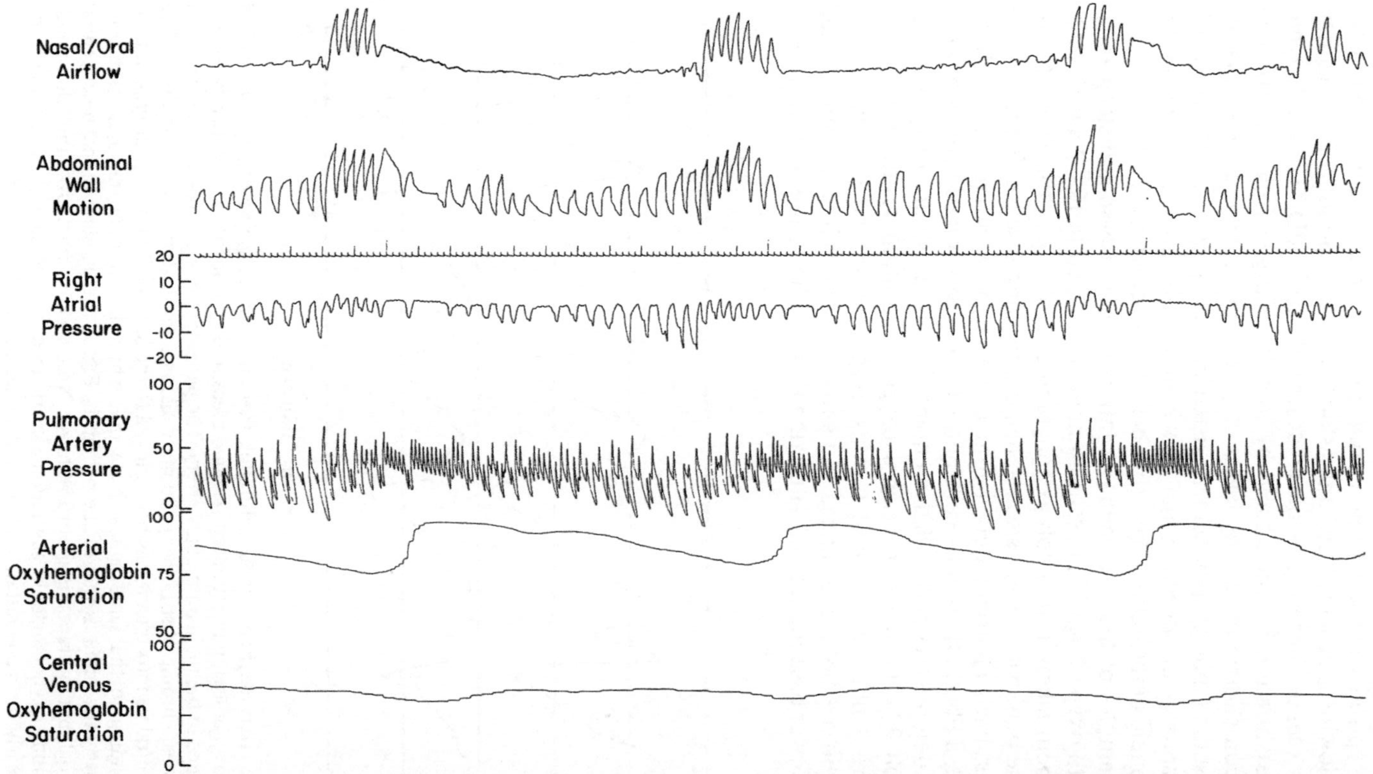

Fig. 2. Polysomnographic tracing of ventilatory, pulmonary hemodynamic, and oxyhemoglobin saturation parameters in an obese 64-year-old male with sleep apnea but no clinically obvious lung disease. The *top three panels* show mixed obstructive apneas of about 50 s duration characterized by cessation of air flow, continued abdominal wall motion, and progressive increase in negative intrathoracic pressure with each inspiratory effort, reflected in the right atrial pressure trace. The time scale in seconds appears just above the right atrial pressure trace. Systemic arterial oxyhemoglobin saturation (ear oximeter) is seen to fall about 20% with each apnea, while the baseline central venous saturation (fiberoptic bundle Swan–Ganz catheter) of 60% falls only about 4%–6%. (From [43])

phy). All three patients received tracheostomies. Transient desaturations on the pretracheostomy night (left panel) are illustrated by the rapid decrement and return to baseline seen at the onset and conclusion of each apneic episode. The most severe, episodic desaturations during rapid-eye-movement (REM) sleep disappear following tracheostomy, unmasking the more prolonged, nonapneic desaturations (center panel) previously described in COPD. The underlying, nonapneic desaturation is ameliorated by low-flow oxygen (right panel). This side-by-side comparison of varying levels of therapeutic intervention shows not only that episodic (apneic) hypoxemia existed in these patients, but that REM-related (nonapneic) desaturation may have played an important role in the severity of apneic desaturation occurring before tracheostomy.

Further examples of the interaction of intrinsic lung disease and sleep apnea with respect to oxyhemoglobin desaturation are presented in Fig. 2 and 3. Figure 2 is a segment taken from a polysomnographic recording of the sleep of a 64-year-old obese man with severe sleep apnea but no lung disease. It shows three mixed apneas, each approximately 1 min in duration. A Swan-Ganz catheter equipped with a fiberoptic bundle continuously monitors mixed venous oxygen. The catheter demonstrates 4%–6% decrements in central venous oxygen saturation with each 20% decrease in arterial oxygen saturation resulting from the apneas. Figure 3 illustrates central venous oxygen saturation in a 66-year-old obese man who has both sleep apnea and severe COPD. While this subject had only slightly lower baseline arterial saturation than the first subject (93% vs 89%),

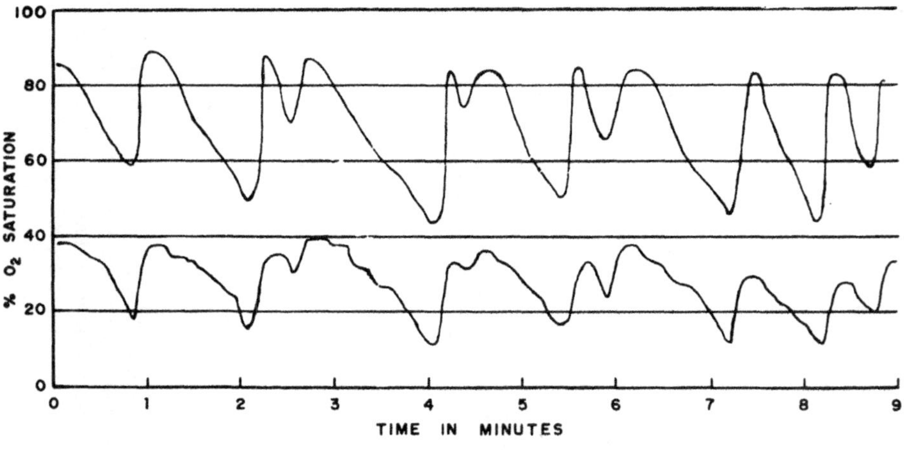

Fig. 3. Systemic artery oxyhemoglobin saturation measured by ear oximeter *(top tracing)* and central venous oxyhemoglobin saturation *(bottom)* measured by a fiberoptic bundle Swan-Ganz catheter positioned in the main pulmonary artery. The patient is an obese, 66-year-old male with severe sleep apnea, chronic obstructive pulmonary disease, and history of cor pulmonale. The timing of the central venous tracing has been moved to the left to fall under the arterial desaturation corresponding to the same apnea. Note that while the baseline (nonapneic) arterial saturation is nearly the same as that of the patient in Fig. 2, the baseline (nonapneic) central venous oxyhemoglobin saturation is about 20% lower. Note also the more profound falls in both arterial and venous oxyhemoglobin saturation experienced by this patient even though the apneas are of nearly the same duration as those depicted in Fig. 2. (From [43])

his baseline mixed venous saturation was markedly lower than that of the subject without COPD (62% vs 38%). More remarkable is the severe fall in central venous saturation to 15% during apneas of roughly the same duration as those in the patient without COPD. The marked difference in nadir central venous saturation between the apneic patients with and without COPD reflects the additive nature of hypoxemic effects present in coexistent apnea and chronic lung disease.

Pathophysiologic Implications of Coexisting Apnea and Chronic Lung Disease

The additive hypoxemic effects of coexistent COPD and sleep apnea are obvious from oximetry tracings. Recent research has given us new theories about apneic desaturation which may allow us to postulate mechanisms of its interaction with COPD.

Rate of Desaturation and Nadir Saturation

It is widely held that the arterial desaturation encountered in obstructive apnea is similar to the hypoventilation which occurs in voluntary breath holding. During a breath hold, alveolar oxygen tension decreases and alveolar carbon dioxide tension increases as capillary circulation interfaces with alveolar gas. Nadir saturation is a function of breath-hold duration and lung (i.e., alveolar) volume at onset. The greater the thoracic gas volume (TGV) at the onset of upper airway occlusion, the greater the alveolar oxygen store, and the longer the oxygen supply will last.

As alveolar capillary perfusion continues, the rate of fall of oxygen saturation during apnea is proportional to the level of saturation at the beginning of the apnea. This has been demonstrated by Strohl [13]. It is reasonable to assume that this is a function of both blood and alveolar oxygen stores at onset. Figure 4 illustrates the theoretical effect of initial TGV and degree of hypercarbia on breath-hold alveolar oxygen supply. Generally, at lower TGVs and higher levels of alveolar carbon dioxide, there is less oxygen available to returning central venous blood. A study by Findley [14] demonstrated a relationship between the magnitude of desaturation and starting lung volume for 30-s breath holds in healthy young males. Findley's subjects did not desaturate during 30-s trials starting at total lung capacity, but incurred moderate desaturation during breath holds beginning at functional residual capacity (FRC), and more severe desaturation with breath holds at 200 ml above residual volume. Figure 5 shows the rate of desaturation brought on by breath-hold periods at various lung volumes in a healthy male.

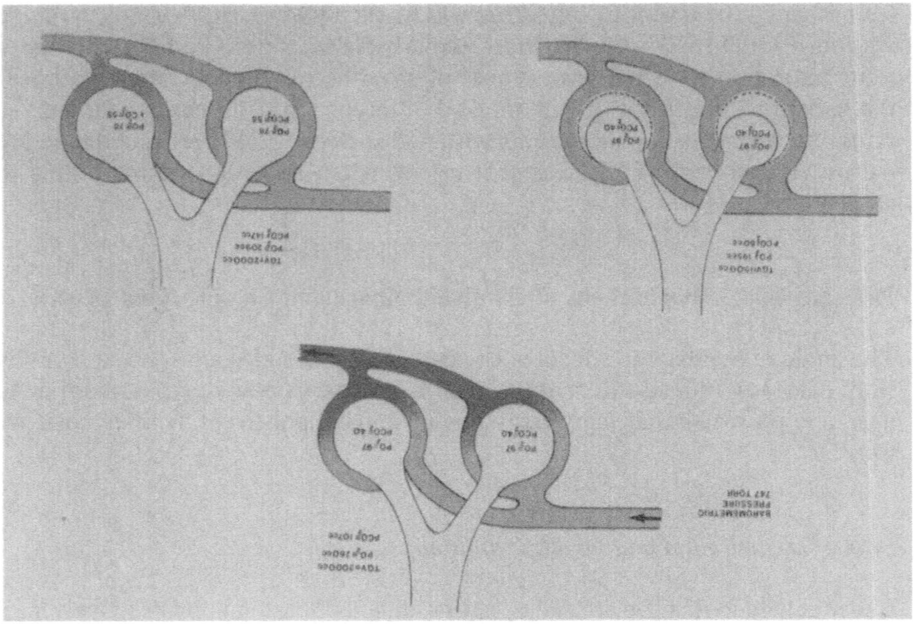

Fig. 4. The theoretical impact of thoracic gas volume *(TGV)* and degree of hypercarbia on capillary oxygenation in breath holding or apnea. The top alveoli assume a beginning breath hold of 2000 ml at a barometric pressure of 747 torr. The resulting alveolar PO_2 is 97 torr if the blood PCO_2 is 40 torr. If the TGV at breath-hold onset is lowered by 500 ml *(left alveoli)*, there is 65 ml less oxygen available for the alveolar capillaries to pick up, even though alveolar gas tensions remain the same as TGV - 2000 ml. If the blood PCO_2 is elevated to 55 torr *(right alveoli)*, the alveolar PO_2 is lower and only 209 ml oxygen is available to the alveolar capillaries compared with 260 ml with a normal PCO_2 at the same TGV

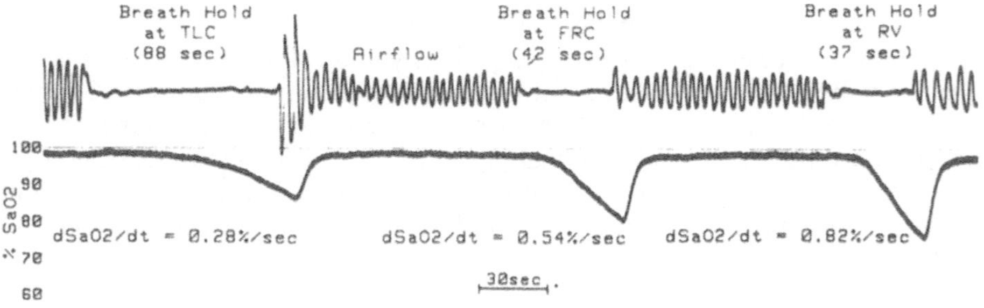

Fig. 5. The effect of breath holding at different lung volumes on the rate of oxyhemoglobin desaturation in a healthy young male. Breath holding at residual volume *(right)* produces a much steeper rate of desaturation than a breath hold at functional residual capacity *(FRC, center)* or total lung capacity *(TLC, left)*. (From [44])

Abnormal Gas Exchange

Recent theories about the pathophysiological interactions of the heart, lungs, and obesity with regard to desaturation indicate that conventional notions may be oversimplified. We have seen that Findley's [14] results account for apneic desaturation during the first 30 s in terms of simple alveolar hypoventilation. However, his data also show that, at intervals of longer than 30 s, or during apneas at low lung volume, there may be some additional mechanism at work. Using the Kelman digital computer algorithm and expired alveolar oxygen tension, Findley estimated pulmonary capilliary saturation. He then compared the estimated nadir oxyhemoglobin saturation with the actual value measured by ear oximetry. If the lung functioned as a one-compartment model, the estimated and actual values should have agreed. At all but the lowest lung volumes, actual saturations measured by ear oximetry did match the values predicted from expired gas concentrations. At low lung volumes and breath holds of long duration, however, the predicted values significantly underestimated the actual falls measured by the ear oximeter. This can be accounted for by postulating a multicompartment model: as some alveoli become gas-depleted (atelectatic) they allow mixed venous blood to be shunted. Atelectatic areas of this sort could exist at low lung volumes as dependent alveoli fall below closing volume (Fig. 6). The closure of these dependent alveoli prevents them from contributing hypoxic gases to the expiratory flow, resulting in a deceptively high oxygen concentration in expired gases on resumption of breathing.

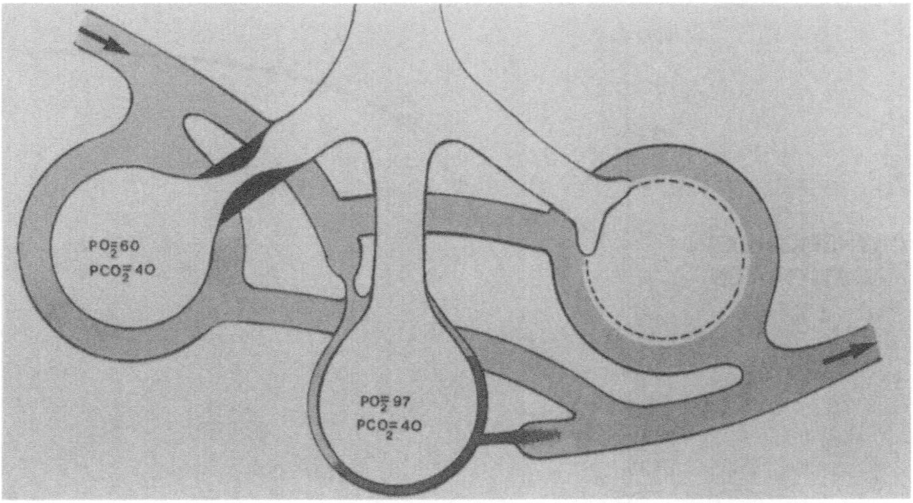

Fig. 6. Theoretical impact of low lung volume or long-duration breath hold on arterial oxyhemoglobin desaturation. Nondependent alveoli that are fully expanded and perfused will allow maximal oxygenation of capillary blood *(center alveolus)*. Partially collapsed *(left alveolus)* or completely atelectatic (right alveolus) alveoli will allow shunt or incomplete oxygenation of capillary blood. This will result in a more rapid fall and ultimately lower arterial oxyhemoglobin desaturation than in a breath hold or apnea starting at a higher TGV. The longer the duration of the breath hold, and the more oxygen removed from the alveolus, and the more likely that some alveoli may come near closing volume

Obesity is likely to have a profound effect upon gas exchange in apnea. While the lung volume at which apneic patients begin their breath hold is unknown, it is probably near FRC. Obesity is known to lower FRC, thereby placing more alveolar units near closing volume. A study by Emergil [15] found that FRC and FRC/total lung capacity ratio was increased in four obese subjects after their weight was reduced through starvation. Three of the subjects had abnormal venous admixture ($\dot{Q}_{va}/\dot{Q}_t$) before weight loss that improved after weight loss. Holey [16] examined regional lung ventilation distribution and blood perfusion with the use of ^{133}Xe in obese patients. This study found a reduction in ventilation of well perfused, dependent lobes in obese patients who had low FRCs.

Blood Oxygen Stores

In addition to the amount of alveolar oxygen, blood oxygen content at apnea onset may also influence the rate of oxyhemoglobin desaturation. This is due to the shape of the oxyhemoglobin dissociation curve. When blood oxygen tension is high, relatively small changes in pressure have little effect on percent oxygen saturation. However, when blood oxygen tension is low (e.g., 55 torr), relatively small changes in tension can have large effects on percent saturation. For example, at a PaO_2 of 95 torr, a 20 torr fall in pressure causes only a 3% decrease in saturation. At 55 torr PaO_2, the same 20 torr fall in pressure causes a 16% fall in saturation (Fig. 7).

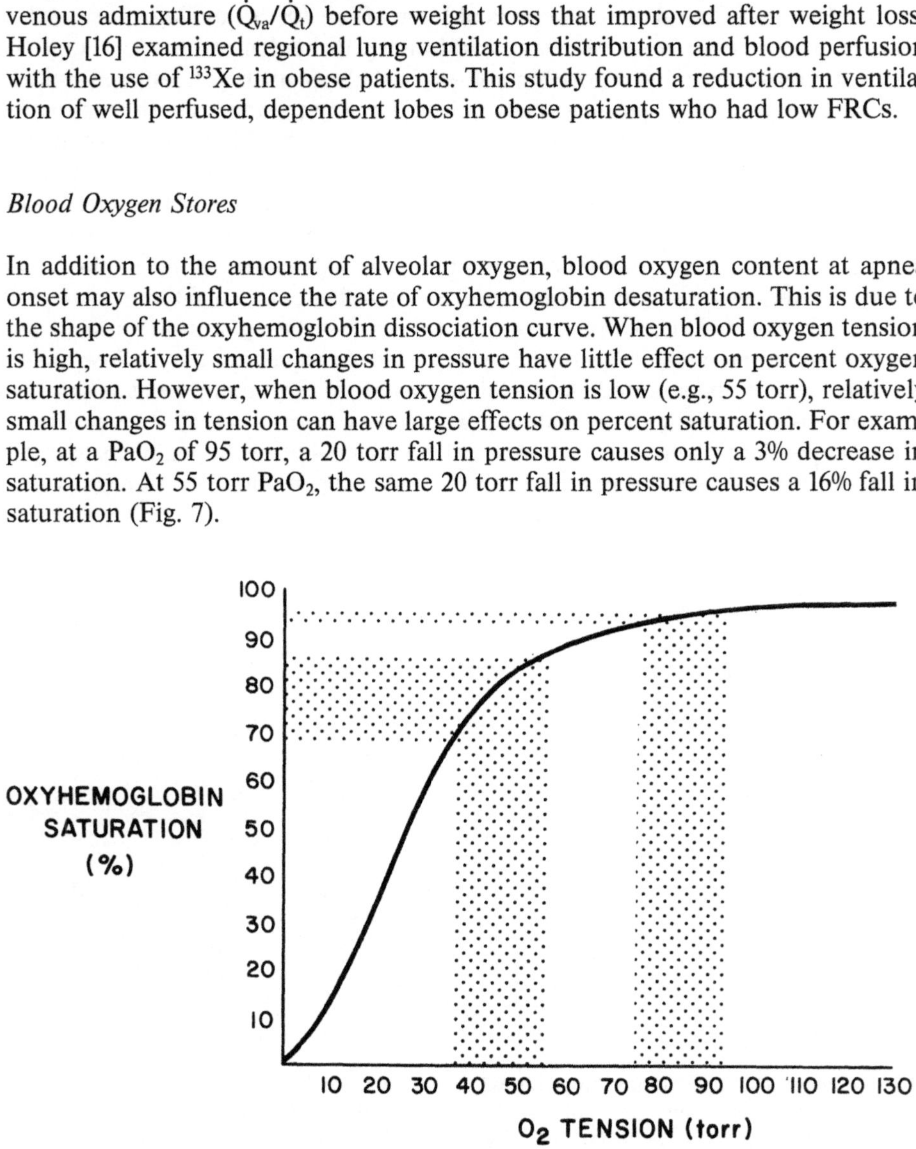

Fig. 7. Effect of blood oxygen tension on oxyhemoglobin saturation (see text for explanation)

Interaction of COPD and Apnea - Pathophysiology

The evidence gathered from breath hold studies in combination with what is known about the pathophysiology of COPD indicates the following interactions:

1. The lungs of patients with COPD may already have poor gas exchange due to ventilation/perfusion mismatch and shunt prior to the onset of apneas (Fig. 8).
   - Inadequate perfusion limits the pick up of alveolar oxygen (middle alveolus).
   - Alveolar oxygen stores may be low in underventilated and atelectatic units (left and right alveoli).
2. Patients who are carbon dioxide retainers because of decreased central drive or increased dead space will have lower oxygen stores (Fig. 4).
3. Patients who are hypoxemic prior to apnea onset will begin their apneic episodes at lower blood oxygen tension, and will desaturate more because of their position on the oxyhemoglobin dissociation curve.
4. Obese patients suffer from increased chest wall load, and may begin their apneas at lower thoracic gas volume. As we have seen, lower starting lung volume may place more alveolar units below closing volume, and may worsen desaturation. In our experience, most patients with combined COPD and obstructive sleep apnea are morbidly obese.

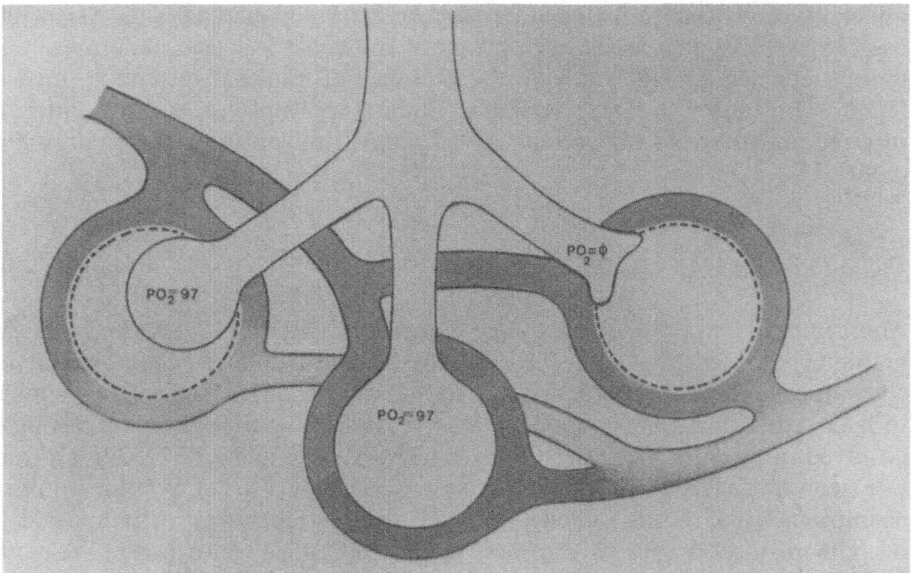

Fig. 8. The theoretical impact of the combination of ventilation/perfusion mismatch of chronic lung disease on capillary oxygenation in breath holding or apnea. The lower alveolus represents physiologic dead space in which the alveoli are ventilated but under-perfused. Very little well-oxygenated capillary blood is contributed to the arterial supply. Poorly ventilated *(left)* or nonventilated *(right)* but normally perfused alveoli also reduce the amount of capillary oxygenated blood reaching the arterial side

Respiratory Muscle Fatigue

Although sleep is typically held to be a restful time, it is probably the most stressful activity that patients with combined COPD and sleep apnea encounter. Patients with COPD breathe at a mechanical disadvantage that may impair diaphragmatic motion and that requires them to use accessory inspiratory muscles. Asynchronous abdominal and chest wall motion are commonly observed in severely impaired COPD patients [17–19], and respiratory muscle efficiency is compromised by the high work and energy demands placed upon them. Hypoxemia caused by hypoventilation and abnormal gas exchange could further impair respiratory muscle function [21]. Obesity alone and obesity-hypoventilation are also associated with either inspiratory muscle impairment or function at a much higher output than normal, allowing less reserve [20, 22]. Inspiratory occlusion pressure ($P_{0.1}$) is diminished in response to hypoxemic and hypercarbic loads in obese OSAS patients who have abnormal awake blood gases [23, 24]. Elevated inspiratory muscle loads in COPD patients with high lower airway resistance may be intensified further by increased upper airway resistance (pharyngeal relaxation?) observed during "nonoccluded" breaths in normals [25, 26] and apnea patients [27].

All these factors combine to indicate that obese sleep apnea patients with lung disease are likely to stress their inspiratory muscles to capacity during sleep. One could postulate that even a small aggravating factor, such as an upper airway infection, could lead to incipient respiratory failure in such patients. Staats [28] has observed asynchronous movements of the chest wall and abdominal wall during repeated apneas, implying the presence of transient respiratory muscle fatique. In theory, severely fatigued respiratory muscles could contribute to a reduced thoracic gas volume and decreased upper airway inspiratory diameter.

Control of Breathing

Another pathophysiologic interaction between COPD and OSAS may be the blunted chemosensitivity common to both disorders. Reduced chemosensitivity presents as lowered respiratory muscle output (neural or mechanical) in response to hypoxemia or hypercarbia. Decreased respiratory muscle function has been observed in patients with obesity [15], obesity-hypoventilation [22, 29], obstructive sleep apnea [23, 24, 30], and bronchitic type COPD [31–33]. Whether blunted chemosensitivity results directly from the disease (adaptive), or is allowed to become manifest because of a genetic predisposition [34] is unknown. Whatever the case, if coexisting diseases result in significant blunting of the body's ability to react to blood gas imbalances, more severe hypoxemia and hypercarbia than that seen in either disease alone is likely to develop. Such factors that blunt reactivity to hypoxia or hypercapnia may lower or raise respectively the arousal threshold required to terminate apneic episodes, thereby worsening apneic desaturation [35]. Blunted chemosensitivity may be a major factor in the development of apnea.

Additive Hemodynamic effects

Because of the additive hypoxemia and deleterious effects on pulmonary mechanics and control of breathing, interacting sleep apnea and chronic lung disease may produce more serious hemodynamic abnormalities [36]. Both sleep apnea and COPD are known to cause acute and/or chronic hypoxic vasoconstriction. Over time, right ventricular hypertrophy, strain, and decompensation can occur. In late stages of these diseases, right ventricular failure has been reported. It is reasonable to suspect that the additive effects of these diseases would hasten the onset of right heart failure, and that cardiac decompensation might occur well before it would be expected from either disease alone. In a study of 20 patients who had both COPD and OSAS [7], 15 had cor pulmonale (determined by clinical criteria, right ventricular gated ejection fractions, and right heart catheterization). By comparing the mean FEV_1 from this group with that of a group of patients with cor pulmonale (determined by similar criteria) but COPD only [12], it becomes apparent that the group with COPD and apnea developed right heart failure with less pulmonary dysfunction (evidenced by pulmonary function tests) than the group that had COPD alone.

The comparison is shown below:

Patients presenting with cor pulmonale

	FEV_1 S.D.	FEV_1/FVC S.D.	Reference
Apnea plus COPD	1.96 ± 0.53	64.8 ± 10.0%	[7]
COPD only	0.96 ± 0.53	45.0 ± 14.0%	[12]

Bradley et al. [8] propose that cor pulmonale does not occur at all in sleep apnea which is not accompanied by continuous hypoxemia resulting from chronic lung disease. In a study of 50 consecutive sleep apnea patients, these authors found only six who had cor pulmonale. These six patients were separated from eight apneic patients of equivalent age and weight with no cor pulmonale by two factors:

1. the presence of daytime hypoxemia (PaO_2: 52 versus 73 torr, respectively), and
2. restricted expiratory airflow (FEV_1% predicted: 57% versus 105%, respectively).

Prospective Evaluation of Cardiopulmonary Hemodynamics

In light of all the previous information, we developed the following hypotheses concerning patients with coexisting chronic lung disease and sleep apnea:

1. Hemodynamic disturbance would be more severe than in those patients with apnea alone.
2. Hemodynamic improvement following apnea cure would be slower or less complete than in those patients with apnea alone.

To test these hypotheses, we prospectively followed 24 patients with sleep apnea syndrome; 19 of them had COPD as well. Subjects were distributed into

Table 1. Clinical characteristics of all subjects at study entry

Subject	Age (yrs)	%IBW	Apnea Sympt. (yrs)	Lung Sympt. (yrs)	Pack Yrs Smoking	Apneas per hour	Cor Pulmonale	Ankle Edema (yrs)	RVEF/LVEF (%)	Sys/Dia PA pres. (mmHg)	Mean PA pres. (mmHg)	Pul Vas Resist (d/s/cm^{-5})
Group 1												
Mean	58.1	152	4.9	5.0	59	64.8	9	7.4	31/53	49/31	36.9	308
S.D.	(9.0)	(20.5)	(3.7)	(2.8)	(35)	(35)		(7)	(8/9)	(21/9)	(12.2)	(171)
Group 2												
Mean	59.2	156	5.4	7.3	66	51.3	7	4.1	37/55	35/19[c]	24.8[c]	132[c]
S.D.	(5.2)	(26.7)	(4.9)	(4.1)	(38)	(12)		(3.5)	(10/14)	(6/4)	(4.8)	(78)
Group 3												
Mean	52.2	163	2.5	0[a, b]	18[a, b]	97.2[a, b]	2	2.1	45/63[a]	30/17[a]	21.0[d]	116[a]
S.D.	(6.8)	(21.5)	(1.9)		(13)	(16)		(0.6)	(15/7)	(5/7)	(5.5)	(40)

[a] Group 3 varies from group 1 by $p < 0.05$ to $p < 0.001$
[b] Group 3 varies from group 2 by $p < 0.05$ to $p < 0.001$
[c] Groups 1 & 2 vary from each other by $p < 0.05$
[d] Group 3 varies from Group 1 but not Group 2 by $p < 0.05$
RVEF, right ventricular ejection fraction; LVEF, left ventricular ejection fraction

three nonrandomized groups. The first group was composed of nine subjects with both sleep apnea and COPD, who consented to curative tracheostomy. The second group consisted of ten subjects with both diseases who refused tracheostomy, but who consented to other, noncurative therapies. These included: nocturnal oxygen ($n = 9$), uvulopalatopharyngoplasty ($n = 2$), and protriptyline ($n = 4$). The third group consisted of five subjects who received curative tracheostomy for sleep apnea, but who did not have clinically significant lung disease. Follow-up was done at yearly intervals (mean follow-up 27.2 months) with radionuclide gated wall motion studies, and, in 15 of the 24 who consented, with right heart catheterization studies.

The three groups did not vary with regard to age, ideal percent body weight, or severity of apnea symptoms (Table 1). Group III actually had a higher apnea index than Groups I and II. Groups I and II did not vary with respect to measured pulmonary function (Table 2). The Group I daytime (nonapneic) PaO_2 values were significantly lower, and $PaCO_2$ values significantly higher than those of Group III patients. The severity of right heart hemodynamic compromise in Group III was less than that found in either Group I or Group II (Table 1 and Fig. 9).

Group I exhibited a substantial decrease ($p = 0.056$) in pulmonary artery pressure and significant improvement in right ventricular ejection fraction after tracheostomy (Fig. 9). Additionally, they exhibited marked improvement in daytime arterial blood gases (Fig. 10). The tracheostomy groups (I and III) showed marked postsurgical decrease in pulmonary vascular resistance. Two years

Table 2. Clinical data of all subjects at study entry and last follow-up

Subj	FEV_1 %pred	FEV_1/FVC	MMEF %pred	TLC %pred	RV %pred	PaO_2 (torr)	$PaCO_2$ (torr)
Group 1							
Mean	55 (43)	64 (61)	35 (31)	91 (100)	177 (179)	60 (73)	49 (41)
S.D.	13 (14)	12 (15)	14 (18)	16 (27)	49 (61)	10 (9)	6 (3)
	ns	ns	ns	ns	ns	$p < 0.005$	$p < 0.001$
Group 2							
Mean	56 (49)	59 (56)	29 (23)	96 (95)	167 (162)	67 (63)[b]	45 (45)
S.D.	11 (13)	9 (14)	13 (16)	8 (7)	27 (33)	7 (8)	5 (8)
	$p < 0.01$	ns	$p < 0.01$	ns	ns	ns	ns
Group 3							
Mean	89[a]	81[a]	101[a]	100	156	[c]73 (79)	[c]41 (41)
S.D.	13	6	35	10	45	12 (7)	4 (2)
						ns	ns

p values between entry and baseline columns represent differences determined by comparison of means using *t* test for paired values. Analysis of variance used to compare means for groups: [a] Group 3 varies from groups 1 and 2 by $p < 0.001$; [b] group 2 varies from Groups 1 and 3 by $p < 0.05$; [c] Group 3 varies from group 1 by $p < 0.05$. The numbers in parenthesis represent the value for that parameter at final follow-up

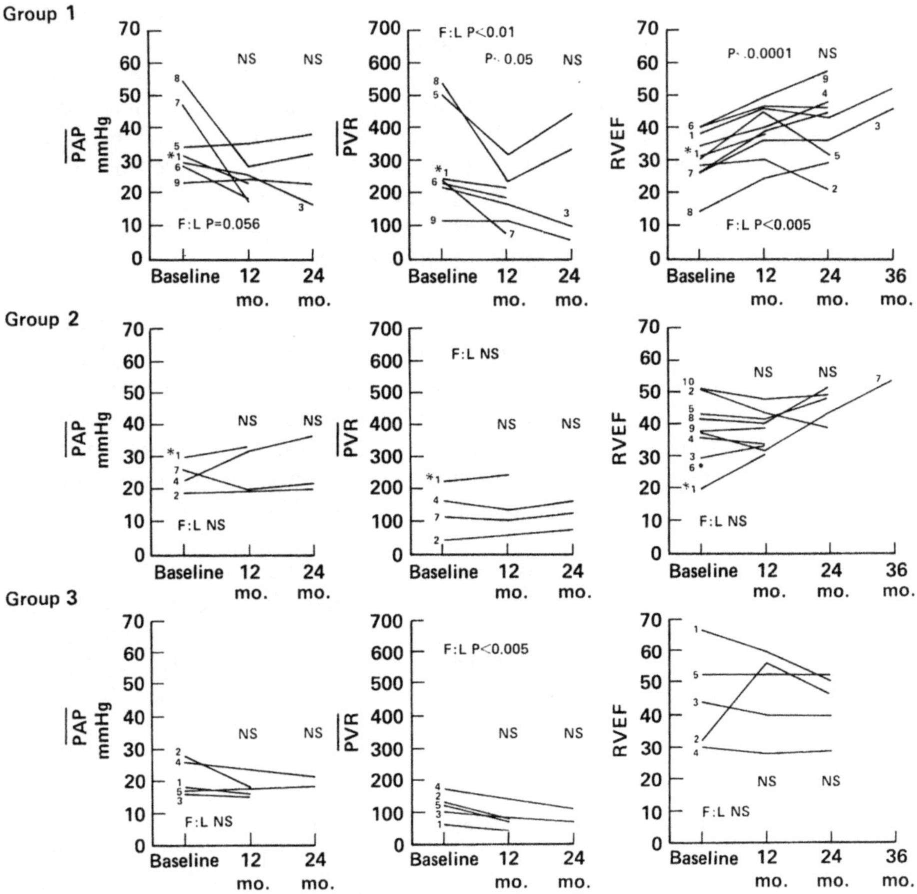

Fig. 9. Change in parameters of cardiopulmonary function from baseline to last follow-up measurements in 24 patients treated for severe obstructive sleep apnea. See text for explanation of treatment groups. The *left panel* shows change in mean pulmonary artery pressure ($\overline{PAP}$), the *center panel* shows change in pulmonary vascular resistance ($\overline{PVR}$), and the *right panel* shows change in right ventricular ejection fraction (RVEF) for the three groups. F:L stands for statistical change from first to last follow-up for each group. Group 1 had significantly lowered PVR and raised RVEF over 24 months of follow-up. The fall in PAP just missed statistical significance ($p = 0.056$). Group 2 showed no significant change in any parameter. Group 3 showed a significant reduction in PVR but was closer to normal to begin with (and thus had less room for improvement) in PAP and RVEF. (From [36])

after treatment, only the group of patients without lung disease who had received tracheostomy (Group III) showed normalization of hemodynamic values. The group that received noncurative therapy showed no appreciable change in pulmonary hemodynamics during the 3-year follow-up period.

The findings indicate that patients with coexistent COPD and obstructive sleep apnea have:

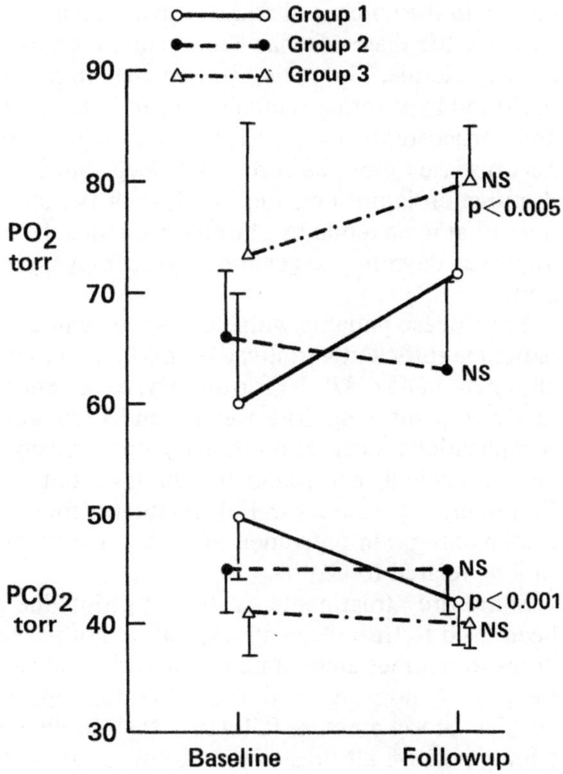

Fig. 10. Change in arterial blood gases following treatment of 24 apnea patients with various forms of therapy. Data at follow-up was gathered at 2 or 3 years after initiation of therapy. Group 1 patients (○) received tracheostomies and showed significant improvement in alveolar ventilation with a fall in $PaCO_2$ and a rise in PaO_2. The changes in group 2 (●; incomplete cure) and group 3 (△; tracheostomy but no obvious lung disease) were not significant

a) More severe cardiopulmonary dysfunction than those with sleep apnea alone
b) Less complete improvement in right heart hemodynamics following curative treatment than those with apnea alone
c) Little change in hemodynamics when treatment of apnea is incomplete
d) Improvement in ventilation following complete elimination of apnea.

Four patients died during the follow-up period. One patient in Group I died of adenocarcinoma of the lung with cerebral metastasis. Three patients in Group II died, and all had autopsies. One died from acute myocardial infarction, one from dilated cardiomyopathy, and one during sleep in the hospital while being treated for acute cor pulmonale and respiratory insufficiency. No particular cause of death was found in the latter case, but the pathologist listed visceral congestion (liver, spleen, intestine) and diffuse mucosal petechiae in the thorax typical of acute asphyxia as contributing factors.

Treatment

There is no question that timely diagnosis and treatment of these combined diseases is essential. As we have seen, clinical sequelae appear much more rapidly in the context of additive hypoxemia, and it must be dealt with effectively. Once the diagnosis has been made, the physician's primary goal is to correct the hypoxemia. The main thing to keep in mind is that one of the causes of this profound hypoxemia is eradicable, and the other is not. Though bronchodilators and corticosteroids are useful in improving airflow, chronic obstructive pulmonary disease cannot be cured. But sleep apnea can be cured. When hemodynamic dysfunction is present, the first line of therapy should be aimed at eliminating nocturnal hypoxemia by eliminating apnea. In many cases, elimination of apnea improves daytime oxygenation, so therapy aimed at one problem may improve both.

Most obese patients with sleep apnea will benefit from weight loss, and if the patient is sufficiently motivated, this benign therapy may be all that is required to eliminate apnea [37]. Unfortunately, experience shows that overweight patients rarely stop smoking, lose weight, and keep weight off over time. Furthermore, complications such as pulmonary hypertension and right heart failure do not permit gradual, controlled weight loss, but require more aggressive therapy. Extremely aggressive surgical treatments for obesity such as gastric resection or stapling are often precluded in these patients by potential perioperative complications related to COPD.

Some drug treatments, such as protriptyline and medroxyprogesterone, have been used to treat sleep apnea, but do not provide long term relief. While these drugs sometimes ameliorate apnea, they rarely eliminate it, and cure must remain the goal. A nonsurgical therapy that does appear promising is nasal continuous positive airway pressure (CPAP). CPAP facilitates upper airway patency by maintaining positive air pressure in the oropharynx. Patients treated with CPAP have been followed for up to 30 months with successful elimination of apnea and restoration of oxygenation [38, 39]. No reports of chronic administration of CPAP to patients with both COPD and apnea exist in the literature. Patient compliance could be a significant problem in COPD patients, because the tight-fitting mask required may make them feel as though they are suffocating. Additionally, the long-term effects of CPAP on hemodynamic improvement have not been studied, but there is no real reason to doubt that its conscientious use will improve pulmonary hemodynamics.

The value of nocturnal supplemental oxygen in apnea complicated by COPD remains controversial [6, 40]. The concerns of Guilleminault et al. [6] appear to be motivated by the prolongation of apneas characteristic of nocturnal oxygen administration. In their study, Guilleminault et al. administered 3 l/min supplemental oxygen over a period of 5 min to four of their 26 patients. They noted an increase in mean apnea duration from 21 to 42 s during NREM sleep and 37 to 73 s during REM sleep. Sinus bradyarrhythmia and atrioventricular block developed in one patient with the use of oxygen, so supplemental oxygen was discontinued and deemed hazardous in such patients. In an attempt to clarify this controversy, Alford [7] administered 4 l/min nocturnal supplemental oxygen to 20 patients with both severe apnea and COPD for an entire night. Data on apnea length, respiratory acidosis, and cardiac arrhythmias were collected on the oxygen night and compared to data collected in the same subjects on a sham night. In spite of the fact that mean apnea duration increased from 24.8 to 31.8 s with supplemental oxygen, mean whole night

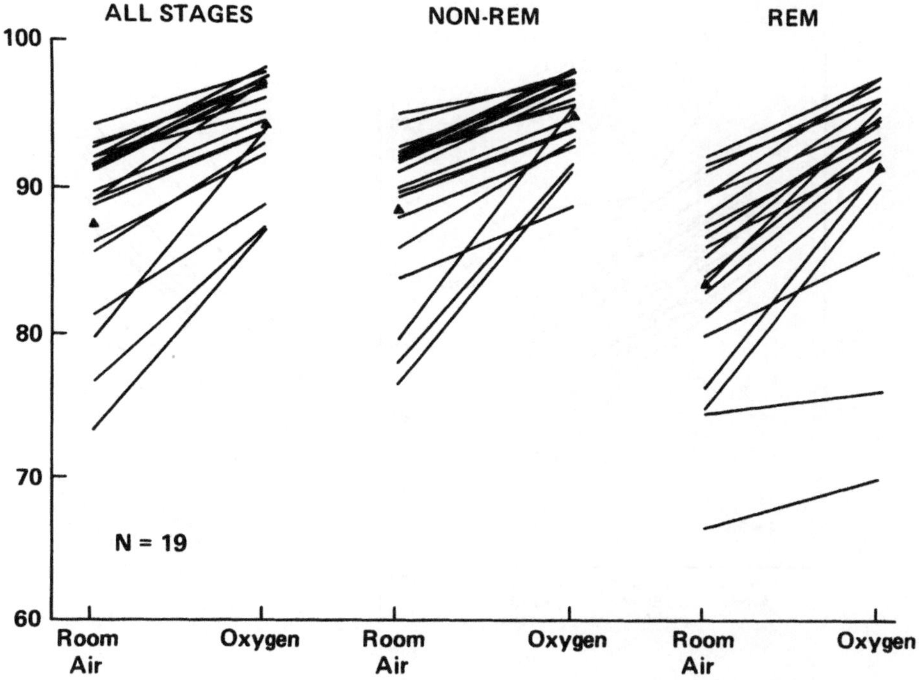

Fig. 11. Improvement in whole-night, non-REM, and REM sleep oxyhemoglobin saturation for 19 patients with combined obstructive sleep apnea and chronic obstructive pulmonary disease following treatment with supplemental oxygen 4 l/min via a face mask (From [7])

oxygen saturation improved from 87.7% to 94.6% (Fig. 11). End episode hypercarbia and acidosis were worse on the oxygen night (Fig. 12). The end apneic pH and $PaCO_2$ breathing room air were 7.34 and 52.5 torr, respectively, and 7.28 and 62.3 torr with supplemental oxygen (Fig. 12). Three subjects showed a small increase in the number of premature ventricular arrhythmias per hour, but the occurrence of complex ventricular extrasystoles and atrio-ventricular block either did not change or improved with oxygen administration. Thus, in the study by Alford et al., oxygenation improved with the use of low flow supplemental oxygen, and cardiac arrhythmias were essentially unchanged.

Most studies of the use of low flow oxygen in sleep apnea have found no immediate complications [3, 7, 41, 42]. All studies have, conversely, demonstrated improvement in mean nocturnal saturation (despite evidence of apnea prolongation), and reductions in both apnea frequency and mean sleep time spent in apnea [7, 41, 42]. The main question to be resolved in the future is that of whether supplemental oxygen will improve cardiopulmonary hemodynamics and mortality in this group of patients over time.

Conclusion

Even though the interaction of COPD with obstructive sleep apnea does not derive its significance from a vast proliferation of cases, it demands attention because of its

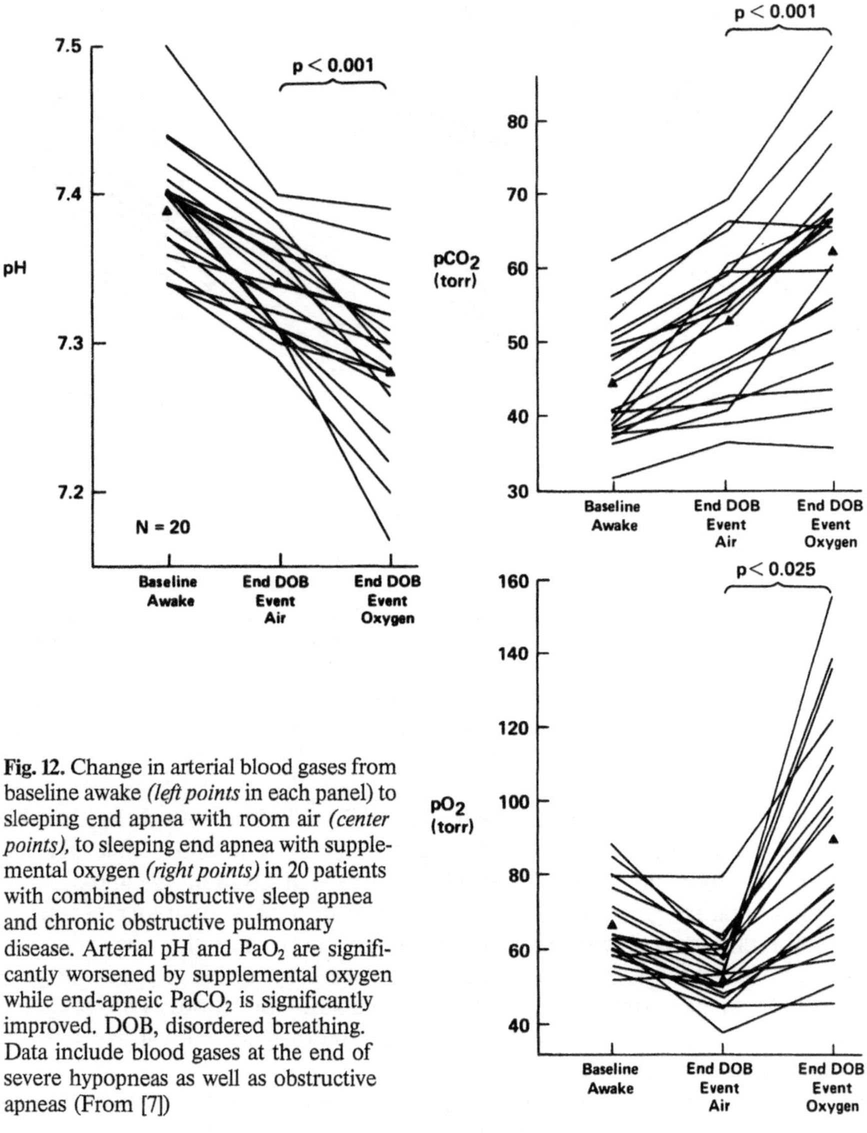

Fig. 12. Change in arterial blood gases from baseline awake *(left points* in each panel) to sleeping end apnea with room air *(center points),* to sleeping end apnea with supplemental oxygen *(right points)* in 20 patients with combined obstructive sleep apnea and chronic obstructive pulmonary disease. Arterial pH and PaO_2 are significantly worsened by supplemental oxygen while end-apneic $PaCO_2$ is significantly improved. DOB, disordered breathing. Data include blood gases at the end of severe hypopneas as well as obstructive apneas (From [7])

impact on a subset of the apnea population. As the significance of this interaction becomes recognized, and signs of one disease begin to be watched for in documented cases of the other, an increase in the recognition of cases of these coexisting diseases is certain to occur. Such cases may be recognized by the clinician by the following characteristics: The patients will be predominantly male and will complain of severe dyspnea upon exertion, along with other standard symptoms of COPD. If questioned, they will admit to being hypersomnolent during the day, and to having disturbed sleep and powerful snoring. The patients will nearly always have a positive smoking history. Obesity, cyanosis, expiratory wheezing, and peripheral edema may be present. They may have had recent respiratory failure that required the use of a mechanical ventilator. The degree of pulmonary dysfunction on objective testing may seem mild in respect to the patient's degree of dyspnea and hemodynamic dysfunction. Sleep polysomnography is an essential test for patients of this type once interactive COPD and apnea are suspected.

When the initial diagnosis is confirmed by objective test results, the focus of treatment should be the elimination of apnea and restoration of the best possible oxyhemoglobin saturation. Though nasal continuous positive airway pressure may be used effectively in some moderately ill patients, tracheostomy should still be considered for severe cases in which cor pulmonale is evident. The effectiveness of supplemental oxygen therapy, especially for the long run, remains unproven.

References

1. Hensley MJ, Read DJC (1976) Intermittent obstruction of the upper airway during sleep causing profound hypoxemia. A neglected mechanism excerbation chronic respiratory failure. Aust N Z J Med 6:481–486
2. Aubert-Tulkens G, Willems B, Veriter C, Coche E, Stanescu DC (1980) Increase in ventilatory response to CO_2 following tracheostomy in obstructive sleep apnea. Bull Eur Physiopathol Respir 16:587–593
3. Kearley R, Wynne JW, Block AJ et al (1980) The effect of low flow oxygen on sleep disordered breathing and oxygen desaturation. Chest 78:682–685
4. Goldstein RS, Ramcharan V, Bowes G et al (1984) Effect of supplemental nocturnal oxygen on gas exchange in patients with severe obstructive lung disease. N Engl J Med 310:425–429
5. Sullivan CE, Berthon-Jones M, Issa FG (1983) Remission of severe obesity-hypoventilation syndrome after short-term treatment during sleep with nasal continuous positive airway pressure. Am Rev Respir Dis 128:177–181
6. Guilleminault C, Cummiskey J, Motta J (1980) Chronic obstructive airflow disease and sleep studies. Am Rev Respir Dis 122:397–406
7. Alford NJ, Fletcher EC, Nickeson D (1986) Effects of acute oxygen in patients with sleep apnea and chronic obstructive lung disease. Chest 89:30–38
8. Bradley TD, Rutherford R, Grossmann RF et al (1985) Role of daytime hypoxemia in the pathogenesis of right heart failure in the obstructive sleep apnea syndrome. Am Rev Respir Dis 131:835–839
9. Onal E, Leech JA, Lopata M (1985) Relationship between Pulmonary Function and Sleep-Induced Respiratory Abnormalities Chest 87:437–441
10. Fletcher EC, Brown D (1985) Nocturnal oxyhemoglobin desaturation following tracheostomy for obstructive sleep apnea. Am J Med 79:35–42
11. Catterall JR, Douglas NJ, Calverley PMA et al (1983) Transient hypoxemia during sleep in chronic obstructive pulmonary disease is not a sleep apnea syndrome. Am Rev Respir Dis 128:24–29
12. Ashutosh K, Mead G, Dunsky M (1983) Early effects of oxygen administration and prognosis in chronic obstructive pulmonay disease and cor pulmonale. Am Rev Respir Dis 127:399–404
13. Strohl KP, Altose MD (1984) Oxygen saturation during breath-holding and during apneas in sleep. Chest 85:181–186
14. Findley LJ, Ries AL, Tisi GM, Wagner PD (1983) Hypoxemia during apnea in normal subjects: mechanisms and impact of lung volume. J Appl Physiol 55:1777–1783
15. Emirgil C, Sobol BJ (1973) The effects of weight reduction on pulmonary function and the senitivity of the respiratory center in obesity. Am Rev Respir Dis 108:831–842
16. Holley HS, Milic-Emili J, Becklake MR et al (1967) Regional distribution of pulmonary ventilation and perfusion in obesity. J Clin Invest 46:475–481
17. O'Connell JM, Campbell AH (1976) Respiratory mechanics in airways obstruction associated with inspiratory dyspnoea. Thorax 31:669–677
18. Rochester DF, Braun NMT, Arora NS (1979) Respiratory muscle strength in chronic obstructive pulmonary disease. Am Rev Respir Dis 119:151–154

19. Ashutosh K, Gilbert R, Auchincloss JH Jr, Peppi D (1975) Asynchronous breathing movements in patients with chronic obstructive pulmonary disease. Chest 67:553–557
20. Fritts HW Jr, Filler J, Fishman AP, Cournand A (1959) The efficiency of ventilation during voluntary hyperpnea: studies in normal subjects and in dyspneic patients with either chronic pulmonary emphysema or obesity. J Clin Invest 38:1339–1348
21. Jardim J, Farkas G, Prefaut C et al (1981) The failing inspiratory muscles under normoxic and hypoxic conditions. Am Rev Respir Dis 124:274–279
22. Rochester DF, Enson Y (1974) Current concerpts in the pathogenesis of the obesity-hypoventilation syndrome. Am J Med 57:402–420
23. Garay SM, Rapoport D, Sorkin B et al (1981) Regulation of ventilation in the obstructive sleep apnea syndrome. Am Rev Respir Dis 124:451–457
24. Lopata M, Onal E (1982) Mass loading, sleep apnea, and the pathogenesis of obesity hypoventilation. Am Rev Respir Dis 126:640–645
25. Lopes JM, Tabachnik E, Muller NL, Levison H, Bryan AC (1983) Total airway resistance and respiratory muscle activity during sleep. J Appl Physiol 54:773–777
26. Hudgel DW, Martin RJ, Johnson B, Hill P (1984) Mechanics of the respiratory system and breathing pattern during sleep in normal humans. J Appl Physiol 56:133–137
27. Anch AM, Remmers JE, Bunce H (1982) Supraglottic airway resistance in normal subjects and patients with occlusive sleep apnea. J Appl Physiol 53:1158–1163
28. Staats BA, Bonekat HW, Harris CD, Offord KP (1984) Chest wall motion in sleep apnea. Am Rev Respir Dis 130:59–60
29. Zwillich C, Sutton F, Pierson et al (1975) Decreased hypoxic ventilatory drive in the obesity-hypoventilation syndrome. Am J Med 59:343–348
30. Sullivan CE, Issa FG (1980) Pathophysiological mechanisms in obstructive sleep apnea. Sleep 3:235–246
31. Lorenco RV, Miranda JM (1968) Drive and performance of the ventilatory apparatus in chronic obstructive lung disease. N Engl J Med 279:53–59
32. Sorli J, Grassino A, Lorange G, Milic-Emili J (1978) Control of breathing in patients with chronic obstructive lung disease. Clin Sci Mol Med 54:295–304
33. Altose MD, McCauley WC, Kelsen SG, Cherniack NS (1977) Effects of hypercapnia and inspiratory flow-resistive loading on respiratory acitivity in chronic airways obstruction. J Clin Invest 59:500–507
34. Mountain R, Zwillich C, Weil J (1978) Hypoventilation in obstructive lung disease. N Engl J Med 298:521–525
35. Douglas NJ, White DP, Weil JV et al (1982) Hypercapnic ventilatory response in sleeping adults. Am Rev Respir Dis 126:758–762
36. Fletcher EC, Schaaf JW, Miller J, Fletcher JG (1986) Long-term cardiopulmonary sequellae in patients with sleep apnea and chronic lung disease. Am Rev Respir Dis 1987; 135:525–533
37. Browman CP, Sampson MG, Yolles SF et al (1984) Obstructive sleep apnea and body weight. Chest 7:79–82
38. Firth RW, Cant BR (1985) Severe obstructive sleep apnoea treated with long term nasal continuous positive airway pressure. Thorax 40:45–50
39. Sullivan CE, Issa FG, Berthon-Jones F, McCauley VG, Costas LJV (1984) Home treatment of obstructive sleep apnoea with CPAP applied through a nose mask. Bull Eur Physiopathol Respir 20:49–54
40. Motta J, Guilleminault C (1978) Effects of oxygen administration in sleep-induced apneas. In: Guilleminault C, Dement WC (eds) Sleep apnea syndromes. Liss, New York, pp 137–144
41. Martin RJ, Sanders MH, Gray BA, Pennock BE (1982) Acute and long-term ventilatory effects of hyperoxia in the adult sleep apnea syndrome. Am Rev Respir Dis 125:175–180
42. Smith PL, Haponik EF, Bleeker ER (1984) The effects of oxygen in patients with sleep apnea. Am Rev Respir Dis 130:958–963
43. Fletcher EC (1986) Chronic lung disease in patients with sleep apnea. In: Fletcher EC (ed) Abnormalities of respiration during sleep. Grune and Stratton, Orlando Florida, pp 181–202
44. Shepard JW Jr (1985) Gas exchange and hemodynamics during sleep. Med Clin North Am 69:1243–1264

The Role of Sleep-Related Breathing Disorders in Cardiorespiratory Disease: Hemodynamics

R. J. MARTIN

Introduction

Today's physician is fortunate to be associated with a time of rapid development in information on cardiorespiratory disorders during sleep. We are living in a time where knowledge in the area of respiration and sleep is mounting in such a way that we can transcribe it to the clinical setting and to treatment. It is interesting that investigators such as Robin stated over a quarter of a century ago: "A sleeping patient is still a patient. His disease not only goes on while he sleeps, but indeed may progress in an entirely different fashion from its progression during the waking state." As we can see from this symposium and medical publications of recent years, Robin and other investigators were very aware of the potential problems of sleep and its relationship to the cardiopulmonary system as well as other systems.

Of importance is the knowledge that mortality occurs on a circadian basis. Overall, for the entire population, the highest mortality is between 0500–0600 [1]. For postsurgical patients the peak mortality is at 0100. For cardiovascular diseases of all types it is between 0600–0830. For pulmonary diseases the peak mortality time is between 0230–0430. This exemplifies the importance of understanding the cardiorespiratory system during sleep. It was not until approximately 10 years ago that the medical literature recognized the importance of this area to any great extent. Figure 1 shows the overall publications on respiratory sleep disorders over the past 20 years. From 1966 until 1975 relatively few publications were sited in the literature. Since 1976 there has been a progressive and steep increase in the amount of publications on respiratory sleep disorders. This will undoubtedly continue to increase in the future. However, our knowledge in regard to hemodynamic changes during sleep is not well-established. This is for obvious reasons, as the study of hemodynamic change is an invasive procedural process. What follows in this text is an overview between normal and pathologic disease entities in regard to alteration in hemodynamics during sleep. Other chapters in this publication will go more specifically into certain details about the individual processes.

If we look at the population of normal subjects during sleep, various interesting respiratory patterns and hemodynamic changes occur. First, upper airway resistance increases slightly [2]. This potential for increasing upper airway resistance can lead to true obstructive apneas [3]. With apneas, oxygen desaturation

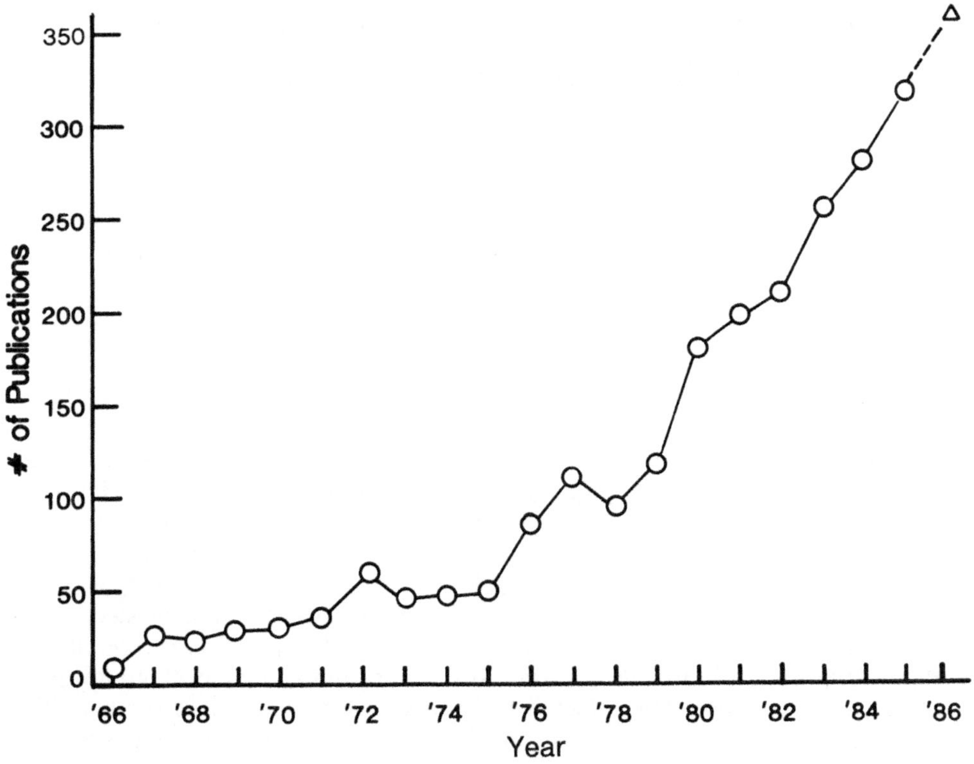

Fig. 1. Explosion of information over the last 10 years, in regard to respiratory disorders during sleep. Prior to 1976 only a relatively small number of publications per year were presented to the medical literature

can occur as well as cardiac rhythm disturbances. Secondly, cardiac output, as will be discussed below, has been shown to decrease during sleep in the normal population. Lastly, if normal nonsnoring subjects are compared to chronic snorers who are otherwise considered to be normal and these groups are compared to sleep apnea patients (Fig. 2), we see that there is a continuum. The very interesting group is the snorers. Awake, they tend to have minimally increased systemic artery pressure (SAP), pulmonary artery pressure (PAP), and carbon dioxide tension ($PaCO_2$), while the arterial oxygen tension (PaO_2) is slightly decreased compared to nonsnoring normals. Asleep, these factors increase to an even greater extent although the question remains if these are physiologically significant. Further studying needs to be done to really ascertain whether this group has any higher morbidity or mortality than nonsnoring normals. If that conclusion is reached, then, obviously, treatment intervention should be started. However, until it is proven in appropriately controlled research studies, treatment intervention on a medical basis is not indicated just for snoring.

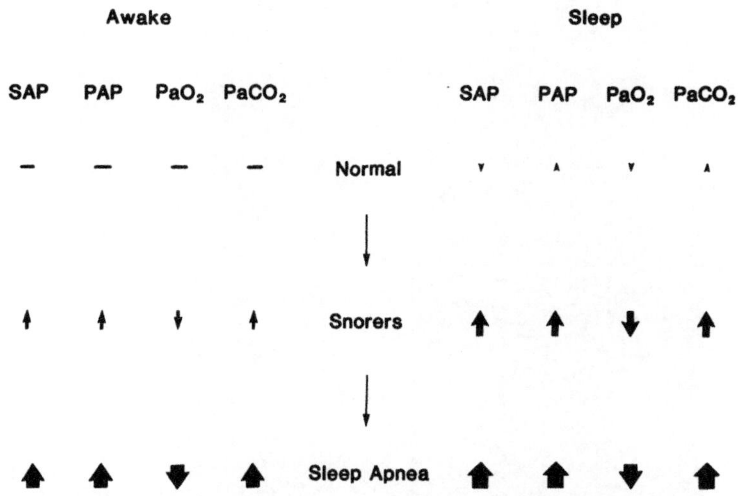

Fig. 2. Continuum from normal persons to habitual snorers to sleep apnea patients. There is a progressive worsening of hemodynamic and gas exchange variables. *Size of arrow,* degree of involvement. (Reproduced from [31])

Systemic Artery Pressure

The mean SAP decreases 5%–9% from awake values during stages 1 and 2 sleep. During stages 3 and 4 sleep the SAP decreases to about 8%–14% below baseline [4, 5]. Rapid eye movement (REM) sleep has fluctuations in the blood pressure but overall the pressure tends to increase 3%–6% from the preceding NREM values [5, 6]. There have been cyclical oscillations in the SAP noted in the literature [7]. The SAP will oscillate by 15–20 mmHg with a periodicity of 20–30 s. These are associated with oscillations in respiratory flow and heart rate and could represent either an underlying oscillation of the central neural control system [8] or partial upper airway obstructive episodes in the normal population.

In the sleep apnea patient the systolic and diastolic blood pressure increases during the apneic episode [9–13]. The systolic blood pressure increases more than the diastolic value and this suggests that stroke volume is increased. The elevation in systolic and diastolic pressures is associated with the nadir of the oxygen desaturation and also with apnea termination. The change in systolic pressure per change in saturation is approximately 2.4 ± 1.3 mmHg/% change, while the diastolic pressure per change in oxygen saturation is approximately 1.4 ± 0.8 mmHg/% [13]. It is felt that the reason the SAP increases further at apnea termination is due to an increasing stroke volume caused by increasing venous return during the apneic episode associated with increasing negative intrathoracic pressure. Additionally, there is probably an increase in sympathetic neural tone at this point. Figure 3 shows an unusual response during an upper airway obstruction. In this particular patient with severe obstructive apnea there was actually a slight fall in the pressure most likely related to a decrement in cardiac output.

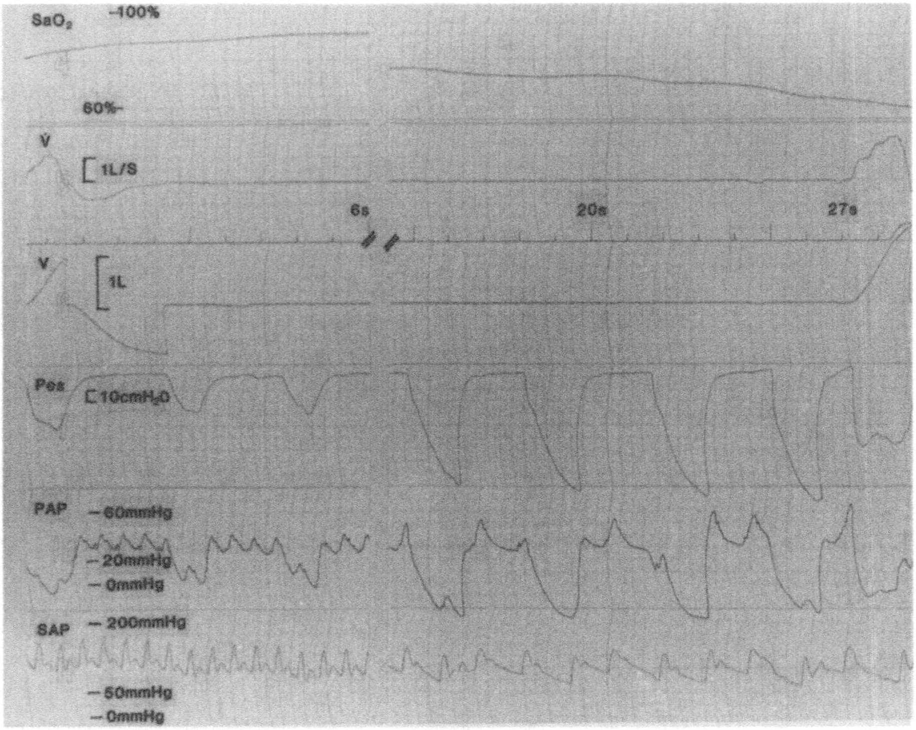

Fig. 3. As oxygen saturation (SaO_2) decreases during an upper airway obstruction, PAP progressively increases. Also note that the SAP is decreasing, most likely due to a decreasing cardiac output. A bradycardia is also developing. The intrapleural pressure swings measured by the esophageal pressure *(Pes)* tremendously alters the PAP reading, which needs to be analyzed during relaxation of respiratory muscle activity. $\dot{V}$, flow; *V, volume.* (Reproduced from [49])

In patients with essential hypertension their SAP during sleep follows the trend of normal subjects, i. e., the percentage fall in blood pressure [14]. Other disease processes have not been evaluated fully.

Heart Rate

Normal heart rate decreases 5%–8% during NREM sleep and increases to the awake level during REM sleep [5, 6, 15, 16]. In patients with sleep apnea the most common arrhythmia during the apnea is bradycardia. This is vagally mediated and can be aborted either with atropine or oxygen [17–19]. The bradycardia may be a protective mechanism in that myocardial oxygen demand will be decreasing as oxygen desaturation is occuring. In patients with chronic obstructive pulmonary disease there is a tachycardia seen during nonapneic oxygen desaturation which would tend to increase myocardial oxygen demand.

Cardiac Output

Cardiac output is poorly defined during sleep. Different ways of looking at cardiac output have shown progressive falls from awake to REM sleep [5, 20]. One study showed that a 7%–12% fall in cardiac output during NREM sleep was due to a decrease in the heart rate [5]. Another study estimated that as much as a 25% decrement during REM sleep was due to a decrease in stroke volume [20]. On the other hand, a third study estimated no change in cardiac output during normal sleep [15]. Miller et al. [20] showed additionally that not only is the cardiac output stage-dependent but also sleep-dependent. That is, a stage 2 decrement in cardiac output is more pronounced as the night goes on than at the beginning of the night. REM sleep shows the maximum decrease in cardiac output. This can perhaps help to explain the increase in mortality for all diseases during sleep as cardiac output tends to fall most when irregular breathing and oxygen desaturation are at their peak early in the morning. There is even less information known about cardiac output in the various disease states. In patients with chronic obstructive pulmonary disease, the cardiac output appears to be maintained during episodes of oxygen desaturation [21]. However, this may represent an abnormally blunted response.

Pulmonary Artery Pressure

As with the other cardiovascular hemodynamic variables, our knowledge in regard to PAP is limited. An appropriate question would be: where does pulmonary hypertension first develop in most disease states? One hypothesis would be that pulmonary hypertension develops initially during sleep. Then, with time, the elevated PAP becomes fixed and is seen during the waking intervals. The known cause for elevations in PAP during sleep is hypoxemia. However, other possibilities need investigation. These would be neurogenic reflexes activated by distension of the main pulmonary artery, arachidonic acid metabolites such as thromboxine, prostaglandin F_2 alpha, and leukotrine C_4; or perhaps lack of active vasodilatation again with arachidonic acid metabolites such as prostacyclin and PGE_1. Lack of beta adrenergic receptor activity in vasodilatation is also a potential mechanism. In normal man both the systolic and diastolic PAP increase during sleep from the awake state, however, the PAP does not exceed the physiologic range [14].

In sleep apnea the PAP increases progressively during the apnea (see Fig. 3) and is linked to oxygen desaturation [9–12]. Maximum PAP elevation is seen immediately post apnea. PAP differs in sleep apnea from the SAP in that post apnea, PAP does not return to baseline whereas SAP does. In sleep apnea, cor pulmonale apparently seldom occurs in the absence of lung disease and/or obesity associated with increased daytime CO_2 and hypoxemia [22]. Significant pulmonary hypertension with cor pulmonale can be a devastating event of sleep apnea. Figure 4a shows a pretreatment chest radiograph of a patient with classic obstructive sleep apnea. This patient had cardiomegaly, bilateral pleural effusions and exceedingly large pulmonary arteries. Figure 4b is 3 weeks post treat-

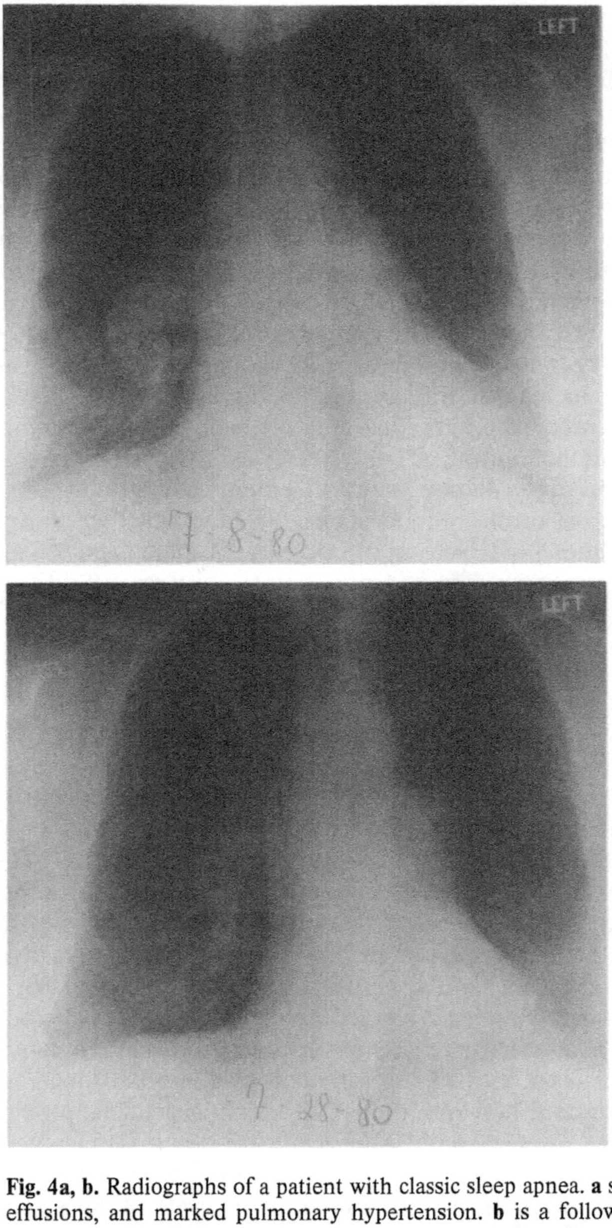

Fig. 4a, b. Radiographs of a patient with classic sleep apnea. **a** shows biventricular heart failure, effusions, and marked pulmonary hypertension. **b** is a follow up 3 weeks post therapy with resolution of heart failure and pulmonary hypertension. (Reproduced from [31])

ment and shows a dramatic reduction in heart size, pulmonary artery size, and clearing of the effusions.

In chronic obstructive pulmonary disease the alterations in PAP are again associated with hypoxemia ([21, 23], see Fletcher's chapter in this volume). There

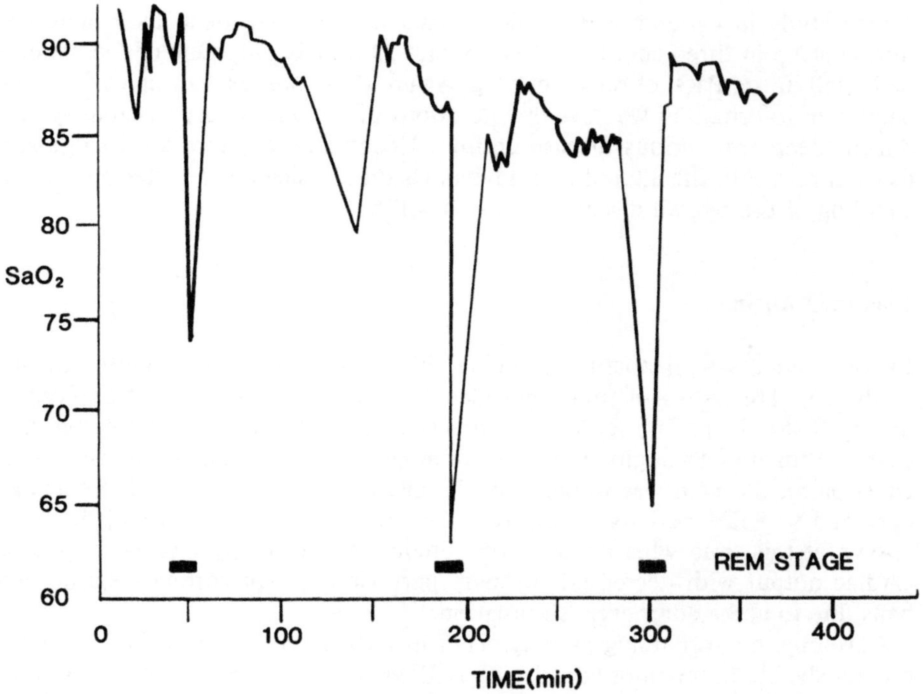

Fig. 5. Common pattern of oxygen desaturation over a night's sleep in a patient with chronic obstructive pulmonary disease. As the night progresses, the amount of desaturation becomes more severe. Also, REM sleep exhibits the most pronounced desaturation. (Reproduced from [31])

is an approximate relationship of a decrease in oxygen saturation of 1% causing an increase in mean PAP of 1 mmHg. Figure 5 shows the amount of oxygen desaturation that can occur in patients with chronic obstructive pulmonary disease during one individual sleep study. As occurs with most entities, oxygen desaturation during REM sleep is the greatest. However, elevations in PAP do not always correlate with hypoxemia, taking into account unaltered cardiac output. This change may represent the other variables hypothesized initially as potential additional causes of pulmonary hypertension during sleep.

Very little is known about other disease processes and alterations in PAP during sleep. Primary pulmonary hypertension may be worsened by sleep. We have seen four patients with the initial diagnosis of primary pulmonary hypertension who had histories of restless sleep, snoring and/or morning headaches. These patients had polysomnographic evaluations. In one patient the diagnosis was changed to obstructive sleep apnea. However, the other three patients had primary pulmonary hypertension. One had associated central apneas with moderate oxygen desaturation. The other two showed nonapneic oxygen desaturation to the 75% range. The exact relationship between primary pulmonary hypertension and abnormalities in the cardiorespiratory system during sleep needs further evaluation.

One study in patients with cystic fibrosis showed that mean PAP increased during sleep in three children by 14, 15, and 23 mmHg [24]. One of the patients had a fall in the PaO_2 of only 1 mmHg. Again, these are just examples from the paucity of information we have on alterations of the pulmonary vascular system during sleep and various disease entities. Eventually, as more knowledge surfaces in regard to the altered hemodynamics during sleep, the better our understanding of the overall disease processes will be.

Nocturnal Angina

In four patients with nocturnal angina, 39 episodes were documented in one study [25]. Thirty-two of these episodes occurred with ST segment depression during REM sleep. The REM stage preceded the ST segment alterations. In a case of Prinzmetal's angina (a variant of angina with ST segment elevation and chest pain), the pain was initiated in the awake state by emotional events and confined to REM periods during two 12-h nocturnal recordings [26]. It is not known at this time whether nocturnal angina is due to hypoxemia, decreased cardiac output with decreased coronary perfusion and/or coronary spasm perhaps due to alpha adrenergic stimulation.

Certainly, nocturnal angina may occur in NREM sleep stages [27]. As stated previously, blood pressure falls during NREM sleep. Depending on the diastolic pressure, which is the coronary artery filling force, there may be a significant decrement in flow. In addition, patients with congestive heart failure may develop angina at any time during sleep. In patients who were hospitalized for myocardial infarction, nocturnal angina prior to admission occurred with congestive heart failure and correlated with anterior infarction [28]. In 12 patients who were studied nightly after acute myocardial infarction there was poor, fragmented sleep with a reduction in REM periods until slow normalization of sleep stages occurred by the 9th day [29]. Twelve anginal attacks were also noted, with only two occurring during REM sleep.

In a simple but important study, Mohr et al. [30] showed that a 10° reverse Trendelenburg position (feet down, head up) was effective in relieving refractory nocturnal angina pain. This position was compared to the semiorthopnic position which elevates the head of the bed. They also found that the reverse Trendelenburg position significantly reduced the central venous pressure, diastolic PAP, and the number of isosorbide dinitrate tablets needed for chest pain. This information suggests that with increased left ventricular filling pressure during sleep, a rise in cardiac oxygen consumption occurs, resulting in angina. When this is reversed, the nocturnal angina is improved.

Mechanisms of Hemodynamic Alterations During Sleep

Figure 6 shows a very complex interaction between the various vascular beds, neurogenic tone, and cardiac output during sleep [31]. Redistribution of blood flow to various organ systems is an important aspect of medicine. Again, little is

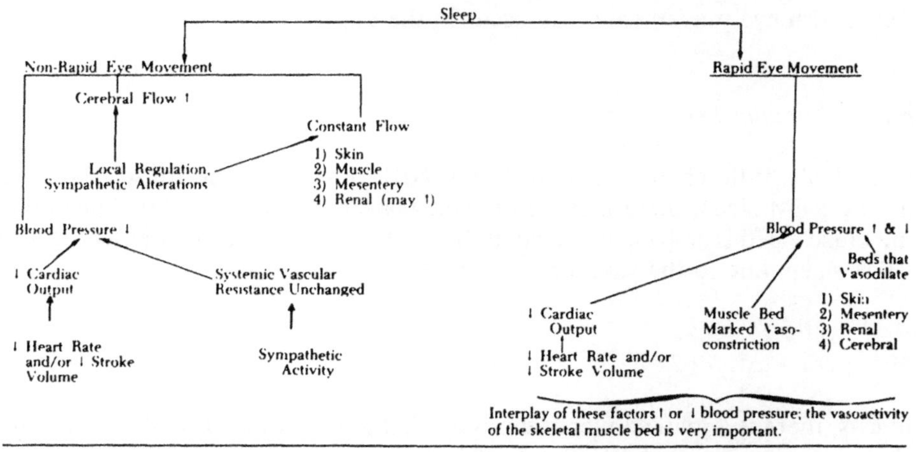

Fig. 6. Some of the mechanisms of hemodynamic alterations during sleep (based on human and animal data). The different physiologic sleep stages, i.e., NREM versus REM, have somewhat different hemodynamic variations. See text for explanation. (Reproduced from [31])

known about this aspect in man during sleep. There is a potential for changes to occur in the blood flow pattern during sleep which could alter the physiologic status of the ill patient. The discussion of events in this section is based both on animal and human work and will complement the above general discussions.

Peripheral Resistance

In the cat, peripheral resistance was found to be essentially unchanged or slightly decreased during NREM sleep [32, 33]. However, in REM sleep, the conductance increased by about 10%. This indicates a decrease in the total peripheral resistance due to vasodilatation, at least in some vascular beds. The NREM sleep results have been shown to hold true for man as well [5]. Relating this knowledge to the blood pressure changes seen during NREM sleep, the fall in pressure results from a decrease in cardiac output. The changes in blood pressure during REM sleep are dependent on alterations in total peripheral resistance as well as cardiac ouput.

Cutaneous Vascular Bed

Skin temperature and hand volume during NREM sleep show little change from the waking values. During REM sleep, however, there is a definite increase in skin temperature and hand volume suggesting a vasodilatory pattern and increased blood flow to the skin [5, 34, 35]. In man, phasic vasoconstriction associated with eye movements may occur in the digits.

Muscle Vascular Bed

In animals, little change is seen during NREM sleep in the muscle bed, but during REM sleep, there may be marked vasoconstriction [33, 36]. Apparently, the muscle bed is actively involved in the blood pressure increments seen during REM sleep, due to the vasoconstriction.

Mesenteric Vascular Bed

In cats, there is a marked increase in vasodilatation during REM sleep, but little change is seen during NREM sleep [33].

Renal Vascular Bed

Different animal models show that renal blood flow remains constant or increases even when blood pressure drops [36, 37]. This maintenance of flow is related to local autoregulation and changes in sympathetic nerve activity. In man, measurement of plasma renin will indirectly reflect changes in renal blood flow with an increase in renin activity indicating a decrease in blood flow. During REM sleep, there is a decrease in plasma renin levels, suggesting an augmented blood flow [38].

Cerebral Vascular Bed

Precise measurements of cerebral blood flow during natural sleep in animals is difficult to obtain. In the cat, blood flow is increased up to 70% during NREM sleep. Additionally, different brain regions receive different degrees of blood flow. During REM sleep, the brain blood flow increases further [39].

Sympathetic Nervous System Control

The sympathetic nervous system plays a major role in control of the cardiovascular system. Coote and Futuro-Neto [40, 41] performed measurements on unanesthetized cats that were decerebrated at the intercollicular level. In this type of preparation, REM sleep-like periods revealed inhibition of cardiac, renal, and splanchnic sympathetic nerve activity. Additionally, there was facilitation of vasoconstrictor fiber activity to the skeletal muscle. This reveals direct evidence in a cat model that there is a differential pattern of sympathetic nerve activity to the heart and blood vessels during sleep. These investigators found additionally that particular neurons in the brain stem were responsible for producing the differential pattern of sympathetic activity as compared to those observed during sleep [42, 43]. This leads to the conclusion that the pattern of changes seen during sleep in the cardiovascular pattern is the result of a central nervous system sympathetic pattern generator that is activated mainly during REM sleep [44].

The hemodynamically compromised patient in the intensive care unit has not been properly evaluated during sleep. Receiving a certain amount of vasoactive drugs to maintain a level of blood pressure and/or cardiac output during the waking hours may not be sufficient to maintain the pressure during sleep. Additionally, we do not know if the same blood flow distribution during sleep is maintained. Perhaps there is less cerebral blood flow, renal blood flow, etc. We know that coronary blood flow can be reduced to levels significant enough to cause nocturnal angina.

Obesity-Induced Complications Which Alter Cardiopulmonary Status

Obesity in and of itself is a significant disease entity which has tremendous effects on the cardiorespiratory system both upright, recumbent, and asleep [31]. Figure 7 shows the alterations that occur in obese patients in regard to the work of breathing, oxygen consumption, carbon dioxide production, respiratory muscle activity, ventilation to perfusion mismatching, altered lung volume, chemosensitivity, and cardiovascular status.

Concentrating on the cardiovascular effects of the obese patient in Fig. 7, several problems arise. The cardiovascular effects of obesity add additional problems for the physician dealing with these patients. Obesity is associated with an increased blood volume and cardiac output [45]. This state of hypervolemia and increased output produces an increase in left ventricular work and causes an increase in heart weight which is proportional to the degree of obesity [46]. This

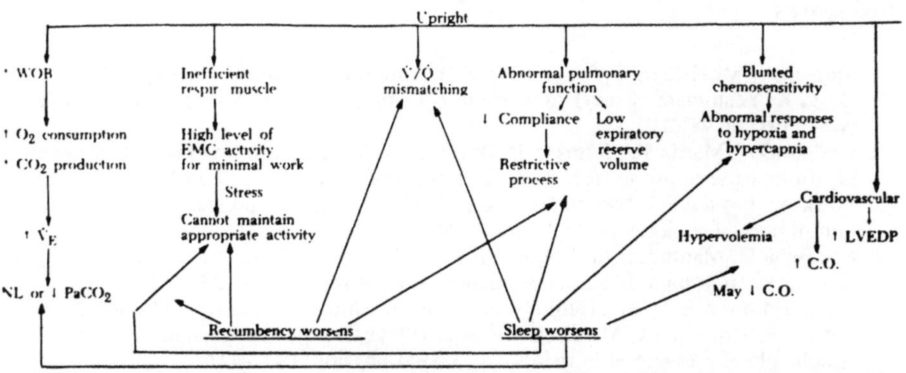

Fig. 7. The significant amount of complications induced by obesity. See text for explanation. *WOB*, work of breathing; V_E, minute ventilation; *NL*, normal; *CO*, cardiac output; *LVEDP*, left ventricular end-diastolic pressure. (Reproduced from [31])

increased heart weight is due to hypertrophy of the left, and to some extent, the right ventricles rather than to epicardial or myocardial fat. Left ventricular end-diastolic filling pressure is most commonly at the upper limits of normal in subjects who are over 100 kg in weight [47]. This becomes abnormal when venous return is increased by passive leg raising or exercise. The elevations in pressure are associated with high resting central blood volumes which are further increased by exertion. As weight is lost, the filling pressure to the left side is decreased and blood volume returns to normal.

In the patient with the obesity-hypoventilation syndrome where hypoxia and hypercapnia play a role in pulmonary hypertension and cor pulmonale, the pulmonary blood volume is further increased [48]. The pulmonary hypertension may increase lung water and thereby worsen lung compliance, increasing respiratory muscle work, worsen ventilation-to-perfusion matching, and further deteriorate gas exchange. Since ischemic and hypertensive cardiac diseases are both increased in obesity, they will further compromise the circulatory status.

As stated for normal persons, the cardiac output may fall significantly during sleep [5, 20]. If this is also true in the obese patient, the increased metabolic needs will not be met. Any obese patient in the coronary or intensive care unit must be carefully evaluated for worsening of cardiac function, arrhythmias, and blood gases during sleep.

Conclusion

As repeated numerous times throughout this chapter, the whole area of cardiorespiratory disorders during sleep is relatively new. In particular, the hemodynamic alterations in normal persons and in the different abnormal disease processes need to be further delineated. This is a relatively uncharted area for physicians. Forthcoming information will help the clinical aspects of treatment for hemodynamic problems during sleep.

References

1. Smolensky M, Halberg F, Sargent F (1972) Chronobiology of the life sequence. In: Itoh S, Ogata K, Yoshimara H (eds) Advance in climatic physiology. Springer, Berlin Heidelberg New York, pp 281–318
2. Hudget DW, Martin RJ, Johnson B, Hill P (1984) Mechanics of the respiratory system and breathing pattern during sleep in normal humans. J Appl Physiol 56:133–137
3. Block AJ, Boysen PG, Wynne JW et al (1979) Sleep apnea, hypopnea and oxygen desaturation in normal subjects. N Engl J Med 300:513–517
4. Coccagna G, Mantovani M, Brignani F et al (1971) Arterial pressure changes during spontaneous sleep in man. Electroencephalogr Clin Neurophysiol 31:277–281
5. Khatri IM, Freis ED (1967) Hemodynamic changes during sleep. J Appl Physiol 22:867–873
6. Snyder F, Hobson JA, Morrison DF et al (1964) Changes in respiration, heart rate, and systolic blood pressure in human sleep. J Appl Physiol 19:417–422
7. Andersson B, Kenney RA, Neil E (1950) The role of the chemoreceptors of the carotid and aortic regions in the production of Mayer waves. Acta Physiol Scand 20:203–220
8. Lugaresi E, Coccagna G, Mantovani M et al (1972) Some periodic phenomena arising during drowsiness and sleep in man. Electroencephalogr Clin Neurophysiol 32:701–705

9. Coccagna G, Mantovani M, Brignani F et al (1972) Continuous recording of the pulmonary and systemic arterial pressure during sleep in syndromes of hypersomnia with periodic breathing. Bull Eur Physiopathol Respir 8:1159–1172
10. Lonsdorfer J, Meunier-Carus J, Lamper-Benignus E et al (1972) Haemodynamic respiratory aspects of the Pickwickian syndrome. Bull Eur Physiopath Respir 8:1181–1192
11. Scharf SM (1984) Influence of sleep state and breathing on cardiovascular function. In: Saunders NA, Sullivan CE (eds) Sleep and breathing. Dekker, New York, pp 221–240
12. Schroeder JS, Motta J, Guilleminault C (1978) Hemodynamic studies in sleep apnea. In: Guilleminault C, Dement WC (eds) Sleep apnea syndromes. Liss, New York, pp 177–196
13. Shepard JW (1985) Gas exchange and hemodynamics during sleep. Med Clin North Am 69:1243–1264
14. Lugaresi E, Cirignotta F, Coccagna G et al (1980) Some epidemiological data on snoring and cardiocirculatory disturbances. Sleep 3:221–224
15. Bristow JD, Honour AJ, Pickering TG et al (1969) Cardiovascular and respiratory changes during sleep in normal and hypertensive subjects. Cardiovasc Res 3:476–485
16. Baust W, Bohnert B (1969) The regulation of heart rate during sleep. Exp Brain Res 7:169–180
17. Tilkian AG, Motta J, Guilleminault C (1978) Cardiac arrhythmias in sleep apnea. In: Guilleminault C, Dement W (eds) Sleep apnea syndromes. Liss, New York, pp 197–210
18. Martin RJ, Sanders MH, Gray BA et al (1982) Acute and long-term ventilatory effects of hyperoxia in the adult sleep apnea syndrome. Am Rev Respir Dis 125:175–180
19. Zwillich C, Devlin T, White D et al (1982) Bradycardia during sleep apnea: its characteristics and mechanisms. J Clin Invest 69:1286–1292
20. Miller JC, Horvath SM (1976) Cardiac output during human sleep. Aviat Space Environ Med 47:1046–1051
21. Boysen PG, Block AJ, Wynne JW et al (1979) Nocturnal pulmonary hypertension in patients with chronic obstructive pulmonary disease. Chest 76:536–542
22. Bradley TD, Rutherford R, Grossman RD et al (1985) Role of daytime hypoxemia in the pathogenesis of right heart failure in the obstructive sleep apnea syndrome. Am Rev Respir Dis 131:835–839
23. Coccagna G, Lugaresi E (1978) Arterial blood gases and pulmonary and systemic arterial pressures during sleep in chronic obstructive pulmonary disease. Sleep 1:117–124
24. Vogel JHK, Kelminson LL, Cotton EK (1967) Pulmonary hypertension during sleep. Am J Dis Child 113:576–580
25. Nowlin JB, Trogen WG Jr, Collins WS et al (1965) The association of nocturnal angina pectoris with dreaming. Ann Intern Med 63:1040–1046
26. King MJ, Zir LM, Kaltman AJ et al (1973) Variant angina associated with angiographically demonstrated coronary artery spasm and REM sleep. Am J Med Sci 265:419–422
27. Snyder F (1962) Autonomic nervous system manifestations during sleep and dreaming. Res Public Assoc Res Nerv Ment Dis 45:469–487
28. Lichstein E, Alosilla C, Chadda KD et al (1977) Significance and treatment of nocturnal angina preceding myocardial infarction. Am Heart J 93:723–726
29. Broughton R, Baron R (1978) Sleep patterns in the intensive care unit and on the ward after acute myocardial infarction. Electroencephalogr Clin Neurophysiol 45:348–360
30. Mohr R, Smolinsky A, Good D (1982) Treatment of nocturnal angina with 10° reverse Trendelenburg bed position. Lancet 1:1325–1327
31. Martin RJ (1984) Cardiorespiratory problems during sleep in the intensive care unit. In: Cardiorespiratory disorders during sleep. Futura, New York, pp 269–318
32. Kumazawa T, Baccella G, Guazzi M et al (1969) Haemodynamic patterns during desynchronised sleep in intact cats and in cats with sino-aortic deafferentation. Circ Res 24:923–937
33. Mancia G, Baccelli G, Adams DB et al (1971) Vasomotor regulation during sleep in the cat. Am J Physiol 220:1086–1093
34. Watson WE (1962) Distensibility of the capacitance blood vessels of the human hand during sleep. J Physiol 161:392–398
35. Parmeggiani PL, Zamboni G, Cianci T et al (1977) Absence of thermo-regulatory vasomotor response during fast-wave sleep in cats. Electroencephalogr Clin Neurophysiol 42:372–380

36. Seal JB, Zbrozyna AW (1977) Cardiovascular changes in various states of alertness and anxiety in dogs. XXVII International congress of physiology sciences. Paris, p 2022
37. Mancia G, Baccelli G, Zanchetti A (1974) Regulation of renal circulation during behavioural changes in the cat. Am J Physiol 227:536–549
38. Mullen PE, James VHT, Lightman SL et al (1980) A relationship between plasma renin activity and the rapid eye movement phase of sleep in man. J Clin Endocrinol Metab 50:466-469
39. Reivach M, Isaacs G, Evarts E et al (1968) The effect of slow-wave sleep and REM sleep on regional cerebral blood flow in cats. J Neurochem 15:301–306
40. Coote JH, Futuro-Neto HA (1980) Pattern of sympathetic activity to different vascular beds during paradoxical sleep. J Physiol (London) 312:29-30
41. Futuro-Neto HA, Coote JH (1982) Changes in sympathetic activity to heart and blood vessels during desynchronized sleep. Brain Res 252:259–268
42. Coote JH, Futuro-Neto HA (1981) A brainstem site producing the differential pattern of sympathetic activity characteristic of paradoxical sleep. J Physiol 317:38
43. Futuro-Neto HA, Coote JH (1982) Desynchronized sleep-like pattern of sympathetic activity elicited by electrical stimulation of sites in the brainstem. Brain Res 252:269–276
44. Coote JH (1982) Respiratory and circulatory control during sleep. J Exp Biol 100:223–244
45. Alexander JK, Dennis EW, Smith WE et al (1963) Blood volume, cardiac output and distribution of systemic blood flow in extreme obesity. Cardiovasc Res Cent Bull 1:39–48
46. Amad KH, Brennan JC, Alexander JK (1965) The cardiac pathology of chronic exogenous obesity. Circulation 32:740–749
47. Kaltman AJ, Goldring RM (1976) Role of circulatory congestion in the cardiorespiratory failure of obesity. Am J Med 60:645–653
48. Rochester, DF, Enson Y (1974) Current concepts in the pathogenesis of the obesity-hypoventilation syndrome. Am J Med. 57:402–420
49. Martin RJ (1985) Pulmonary artery pressure during sleep. Semin Respir Med 7:160–163

Part 7: Cardiovascular Risk and Sleep Apnea

Nocturnal Hemodynamics in Patients with Sleep Apnea

J. MAYER, H. GREB, B. HERRES, T. M. KLOSS, T. PENZEL, J. H. PETER, T. PODSZUS, and P. VON WICHERT

Introduction

Sleep apnea, a nocturnal disturbance of the respiratory regulation, has effects on the hemodynamics during sleep as well as during the day. The first systematic inquiries into these relationships were conducted as early as 1965 by Jung and Kuhlo [1]. In 1972, the research team of Coccagna and Lugaresi used direct measurements to document the blood pressure behavior during individual apnea episodes [2].

In the course of an apnea episode, the systemic arterial blood pressure (BP) shows a characteristic pattern. At the beginning of apnea, there is a rapid decline in BP values. As apnea continues, a plateau develops with a possible slight increase in mean BP, and with the onset of apnea-terminating respiration, BP swiftly increases, not only returning to baseline values, but reaching peak levels which are only normalized when undisturbed respiration continues. During obstructive apnea, the accompanying intrathoracic pressure changes correlate with a "saw tooth" pattern in the BP curve (see Fig. 1).

Recent epidemiological studies agree upon the point that there is a high degree of coincidence between sleep apnea and essential hypertension. Pronounced sleep apnea was found in 30%–50% of male hypertensive patients, and up to 90% of patients with marked sleep apnea suffered from hypertension [3–6]. But whereas a long-term connection between sleep apnea and hypertension has been established, and hemodynamic changes during individual apneas have been documented, little is known of the pathophysiological connection between acute blood pressure behavior in sleep apnea and its long-term effects. We therefore investigated the temporal course of BP behavior in sleep apnea patients during a whole night.

Methods

We conducted sleep laboratory long-term polysomnographic recordings in 14 patients (for data, see Table 1) suffering from severe sleep apnea with more than 200 episodes per night. Ten episodes per hour of sleep has come to be regarded as the threshold value for clinical relevance. Among the clinical diagnoses there were coronary heart disease in three, cardiac insufficiency (New York Heart Association - NYHA I-II) in nine, and systemic hypertension in 12 patients.

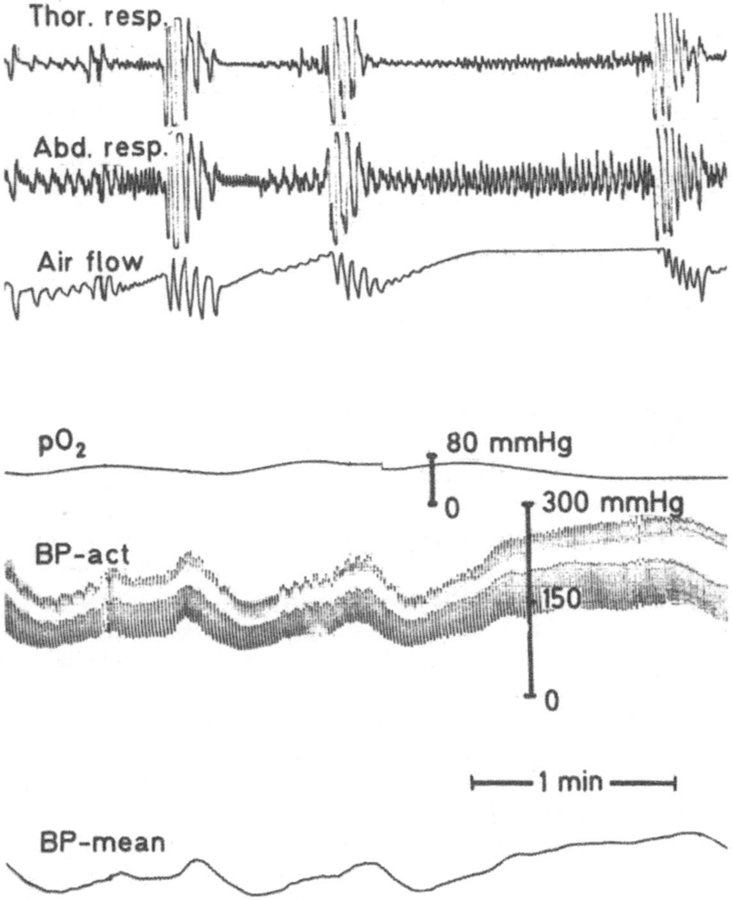

Fig. 1. Excerpt from a typical recording of blood pressure behavior during apnea, showing the recordings of thoracic *(Thor.)* and abdominal *(Abd.)* respiration (inductive plethysmography), nasal airflow (by thermistor), partial arterial oxygen tension (transcutaneously), continuous actual blood pressure, calculation of mean blood pressure

Respiratory activity was recorded by means of inductive plethysmography, using a thoracic and an abdominal belt, and additionally by means of a nasal thermistor. EEG, EMG, and EOG were used for sleep-wake classification. Systemic arterial BP was measured and recorded continuously by means of a catheter in the brachial artery.

For the evaluation of the recordings, we calculated the moving average of BP and of heart rate, by means of computed beat-to-beat analysis, for successive intervals of 10 min each over the whole run of the recordings. Within each interval, we determined the median value and excluded 5% of extreme values, considering only the range of values in which 95% of the recorded values were situated. For statistical evaluation we used the Wilcoxon test.

Table 1. Clinical data of the study population

Patient	Sex	Age (years)	Weight (kg)	Broca (%)	Number of apneas
1	m	49	115	164	758
2	m	35	97.5	135	363
3	m	61	82.5	112	324
4	f	67	70	140	630
5	m	40	87	106	482
6	m	59	118	144	340
7	m	62	102.5	155	621
8	m	63	105	125	460
9	m	55	120	170	310
10	m	46	79	100	205
11	m	47	82	111	314
12	m	35	90	95	632
13	m	51	105	130	513
14	m	55	108	130	753
Mean		51.8	97.3	129.8	478.9

Results

The systemic arterial mean BP reached its nocturnal minimum 1-4 h after the patients fell asleep. The BP was found to increase again 1-2 h before waking up. The difference between the BP reading during wakefulness and the nocturnal minimum averaged 5 mmHg.

Figures 2 and 3 show examples of the 10-min recordings and evaluations. The comparison of 10 min with high sleep apnea activity with interval characterized by normal respiration shows that the variability of the values (diastolic, systolic and mean BP, heart rate) is much greater during recurrent apnea. The individual results of the computerized evaluation of the distribution of values within the 10-min intervals have been summarized for the whole group in Fig. 4. The average variation of all parameters during wakefulness, and also during sleep with undisturbed respiration, is significantly different from the corresponding values during sleep with pronounced sleep apnea ($p < 0.01$).

Discussion

The present investigation shows that the nocturnal course of the BP curve in patients with marked sleep apnea is similar to the BP profile in healthy persons. As far as methodological differences permit a comparison with other studies, the decrease in BP after the onset of sleep and the corresponding increase in the morning seem to be less distinct [7, 8].

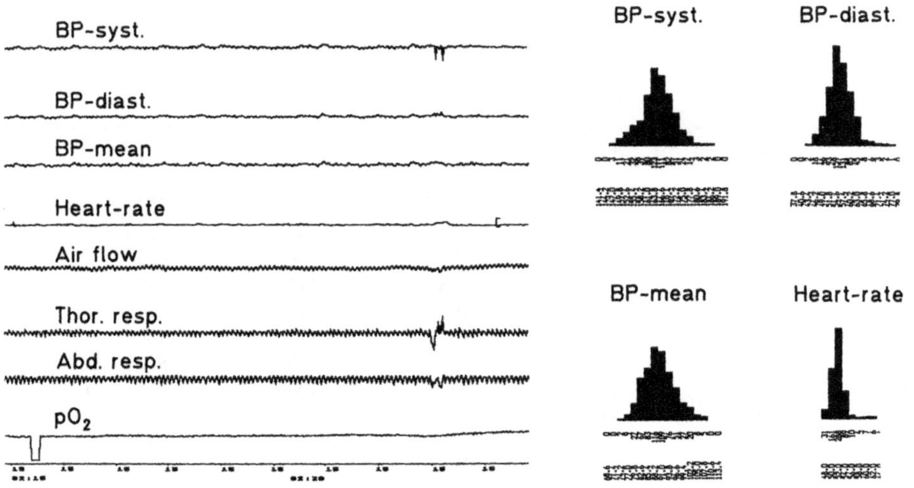

Fig. 2. Pattern of normopnea, recorded over 10 min: systolic, diastolic and mean blood pressure, heart rate, nasal, thoracic, and abdominal respiratory activities, partial arterial oxygen tension *(from the top). The histograms on the right* illustrate the distribution of individual values over the entirety of all beat-to-beat intervals during the 10 min of the recording. *The height of the bars* represents the absolute number of beat-to-beat intervals during which an individual value was measured, *the horizontal extension* of the histograms is an indication of the variability of the parameter values

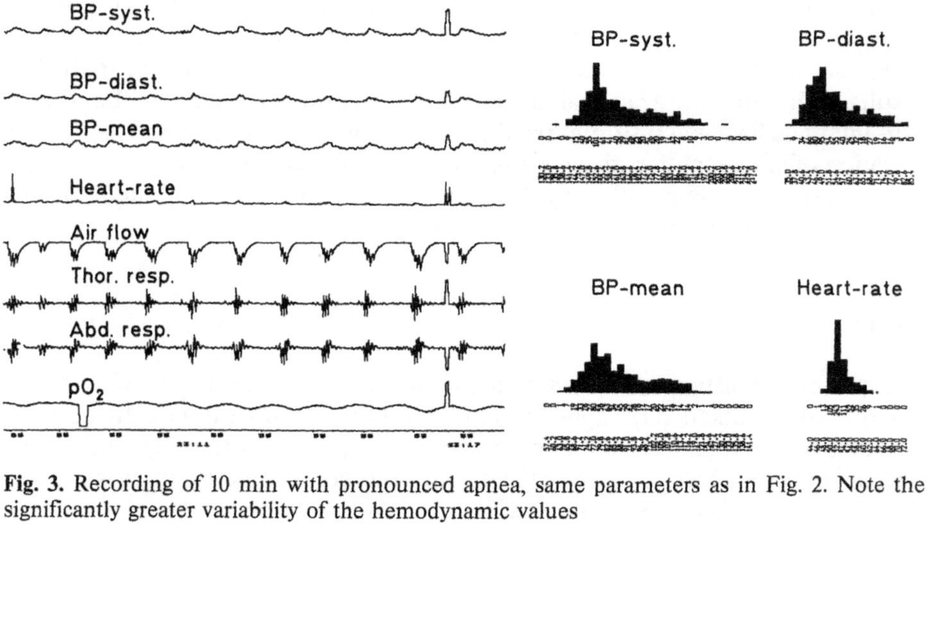

Fig. 3. Recording of 10 min with pronounced apnea, same parameters as in Fig. 2. Note the significantly greater variability of the hemodynamic values

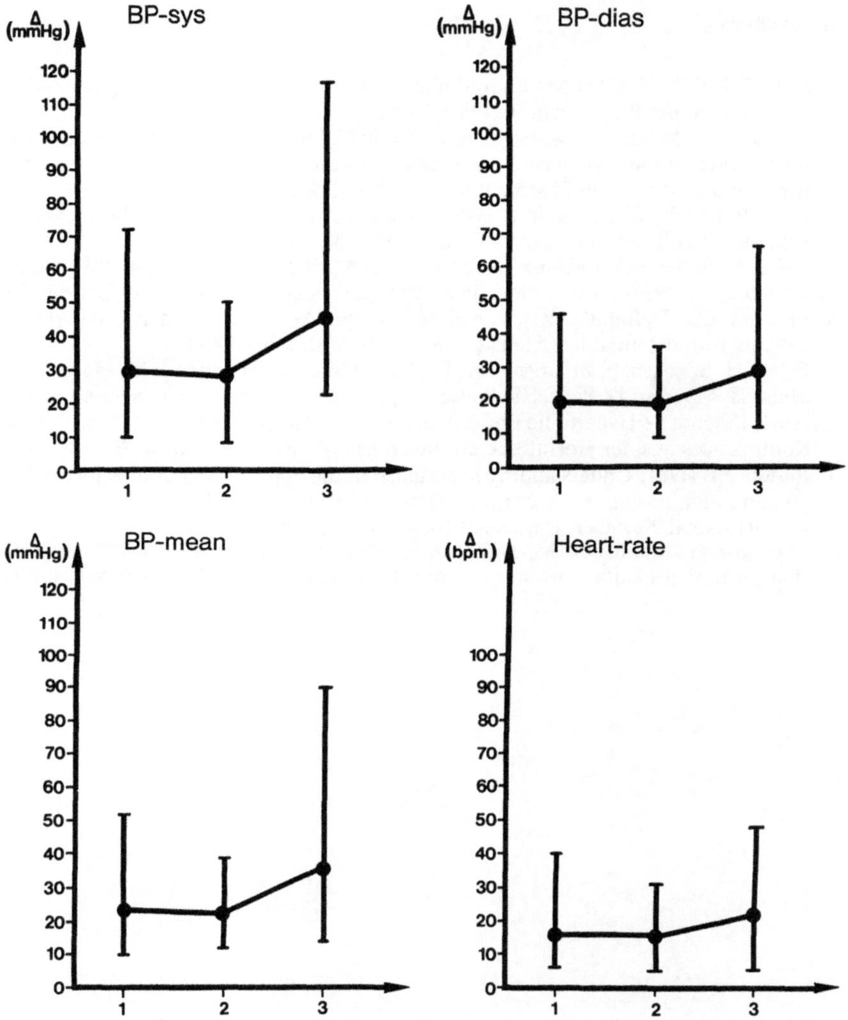

Fig. 4. Mean variability and range of three hemodynamic parameters and heart rate, distinguishing wakefulness *(1),* sleep with normopnea *(2),* and sleep with pronounced sleep apnea activity *(3).* The increases in variability in stage 3 are significant

The increase in variability of all recorded hemodynamic parameters in periods of high sleep apnea activity is highly significant. How this nocturnal increase in variability can induce hemodynamic changes even during the day, however, remains obscure. By way of speculation it may be suggested that it is either the disturbed structure of sleep itself via neural or hormonal mechanisms, or the stimulation of catecholamine due to hypoxia and mediated by peripheral and central chemoreceptors, which triggers mechanisms which, in turn, lead to persistent vasoconstriction, increased cardiac output, or chronic retention of water in the tissue.

References

1. Jung R, Kuhlo W (1965) Neurophysiological studies of abnormal night sleep and the pickwickian syndrome. Progr Brain Res 18:140–159
2. Coccagna G, Mantovani M, Brignani F, Parchi C, Lugaresi E (1972) Continuous recording of the pulmonary and systemic arterial pressure during sleep in syndromes of hypersomnia with periodic breathing. Bull Physiopathol Respir 8:1159–1172
3. Lavie P, Ben-Yosef R, Rubin A (1984) Prevalence of sleep apnea syndrome among patients with essential hypertension. Am Heart J 108:373–376
4. Kales A, Bixler EO, Cadieux RJ, Schneck DW, Shaw LC III, Locke TW, Vela-Bueno A, Soldatos CR (1984) Sleep apnoea in a hypertensive population. Lancet III:1005–1008
5. Fletcher EC, DeBehnke RD, Lovoi MS, Gorin AG (1985) Undiagnosed sleep apnea in patients with essential hypertension. Ann Intern Med 103:190–195
6. Peter JH, Bongartz F, Bräutigam W, Fuchs E, Gunawan H, Hügens M, Mayer J, Meinzer K, Meiss H, Motzkau D, Penzel T, Podszus T, Pusch O, Reinheimer V, Schnell H, v. Wichert P (1984) Essentielle Hypertonie und Schlafapnoe. In: Holzgreve H, Rost R (eds) Aktuelles und Kontroverses aus der Hochdruckforschung. MMV, München, pp 18–33
7. Raftery EB (1984) Understanding hypertension: the contribution of direct ambulatory blood pressure monitoring. In: Weber MA, Drayer JIM (eds) Ambulatory blood pressure monitoring. Steinkopff/Springer, Darmstadt New York, pp 105–116
8. Coccagna G, Mantovani M, Brignani E, Manzini A, Lugaresi E (1971) Arterial pressure changes during spontaneous sleep in man. Electroencephalogr Clin Neurophysiol 31:277–281

Plasma Levels of Catecholamines and Cardiovascular Parameters During Sleep in Patients with Sleep Apnea Syndrome

K. Ehlenz, U. Köhler, J. Mayer, J. H. Peter, P. von Wichert, and H. Kaffarnik

Patients with sleep apnea syndrome (SAS) have an increased incidence of cardiovascular diseases, e.g., arterial hypertension [1, 2]. Especially the physiological decrease in systemic blood pressure at night is often missing in patients with obstructive sleep apnea [2]. This is possibly produced by an increased sympathetic activity in response to hypoxemia during apnea. The urinary excretion of catecholamines is also increased in patients with SAS [2, 3] and the diurnal rhythm of excretion is lost [2]. Hitherto there have been no reports about the pattern of the plasma catecholamines in patients with SAS during sleep.

Methods

We studied nine male patients, eight with and one without sleep-related breathing disorders. Polysomnographic recordings were performed during sleep. In six patients, the arterial blood pressure was measured continuously. Blood samples were taken hourly via an indwelling catheter in a vein of the forearm. Norepinephrine (NE) and epinephrine (E) were determined by the HPLC technique with electrochemical detection (detection limit 5 pg/ml; interassay variability about 8%) [7].

Results

Shortly after puncture, we found elevated plasma levels of NE which decreased thereafter (Fig. 1). In three patients, the mean plasma NE level during sleep was below 100 pg/ml and three had values between 100 and 200 pg/ml. The other three persons had NE levels exceeding 300 pg/ml (Table 1), they had a history of pronounced hypertension. The patients of our study showed a great interindividual variation of plasma NE concentrations. The NE levels in the same patient, however, remained within a small range.

We calculated the correlation between NE plasma levels and arterial blood pressure or heart rate during sleep for every patient. There was no significant intraindividual correlation (data not shown). But patients with a history of hypertension and/or elevated nocturnal blood pressure had higher mean NE levels during sleep (Table 1). Only patient Plö had rather low NE levels in spite of a distinctly increased blood pressure at night.

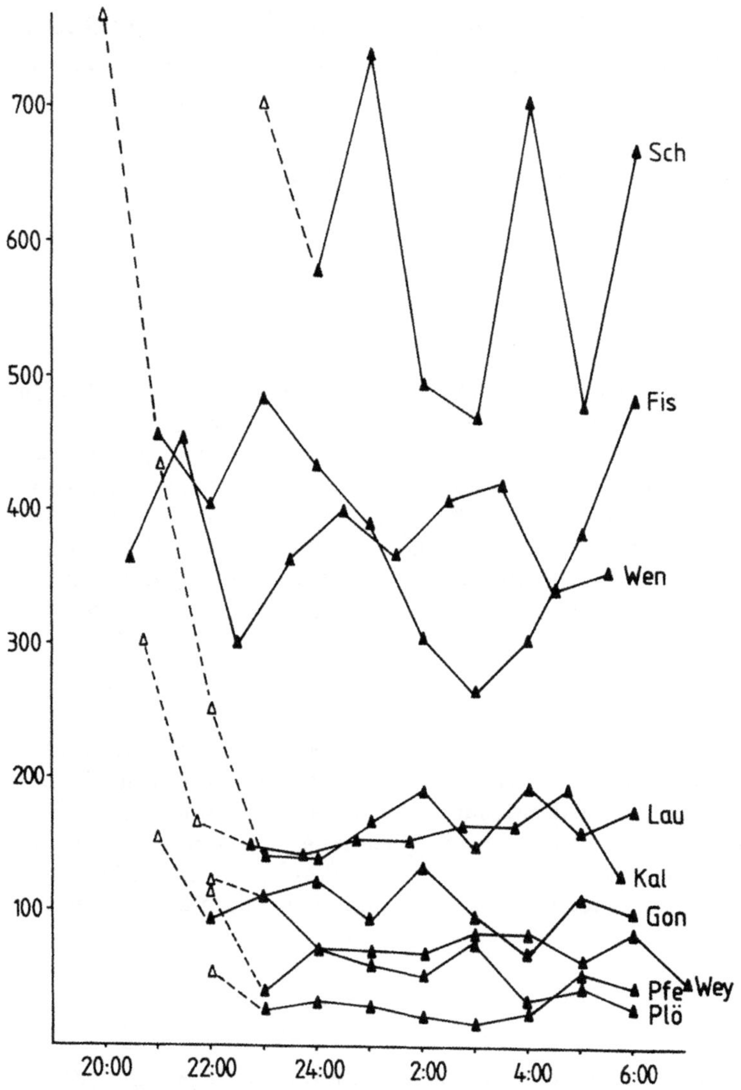

Fig. 1. Plasma levels of norepinephrine (pg/ml) shortly before sleep *(open triangles and broken lines)* and during sleep in nine patients (eight with sleep-related breathing disorders and one without)

There was no correlation between sleep apnea activity and mean NE levels. Patient Pfe, who suffers from severe sleep apnea, has very low concentrations of NE and low blood pressure during sleep. On the contrary, patient Wen, with a less severe SAS, reaches levels of NE which are ten times as high as those of patient Pfe (Fig. 2). The highest NE concentrations were found in patient Sch, who had only frequent hypopnoeic phases and no apnea.

Table 1. Cardiovascular parameters (mean arterial blood pressure and beats per minute) and plasma catecholamines in comparison to the history of hypertension and the apnea index during sleep in nine patients

Patient	History of hypertension	MAP (mmHg)	BPM	Ai (phases/h)	NE (pg/ml)	E (pg/ml)
Pfe	No	81.6 ± 5.2	67.4 ± 1.4	87	36 ± 12	8 ± 2
Plö	Moderate	105 ± 2.4	84.6 ± 1.1	18	53 ± 19	5 ± 3
Kal	No	84.7 ± 2.8	64.9 ± 2.6	64.4	159 ± 19	8 ± 4
Wen	Severe	135 ± 1.9	84 ± 2.7	27	378 ± 45	ND
Wey	Borderline	87 ± 5.3	51.8 ± 1.5	14.3	81 ± 21	5 ± 3
Fis	Severe	117 ± 2.5	56 ± 8	18.7	392 ± 78	13 ± 7
Gon	Moderate	103 ± 19	59 ± 6	10–4	103 ± 19	8 ± 3
Sch	Severe	ND	70 ± 8	Hypopnea	605 ± 114	8 ± 10
Lau	Moderate	ND	ND	1	162 ± 25	15 ± 6

Mean ± SE of the parameters which were measured howly. MAP, mean arterial blood pressure; ND, not determined; BPM, beats per minute; Ai, apnea index.

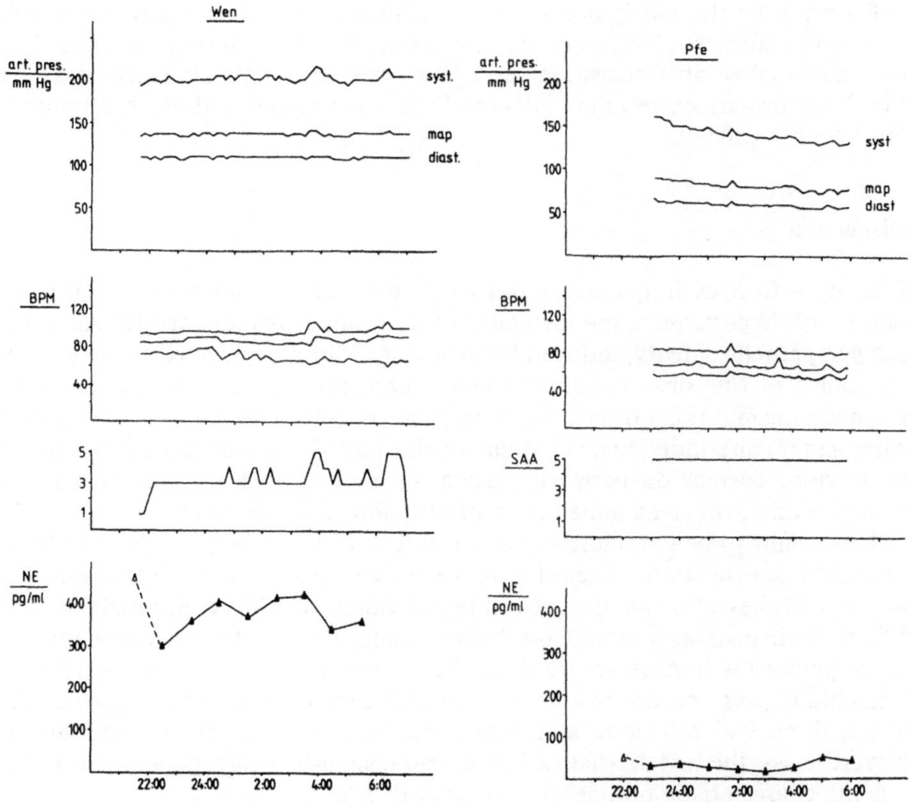

Fig. 2. Norepinephrine *(NE)* levels (pg/ml), sleep apnea activity *(SAA)*, heart rate *(BPM)*, and arterial blood pressure *(mmHg)* in two patients with SAS (*Wen* and *Pfe*)

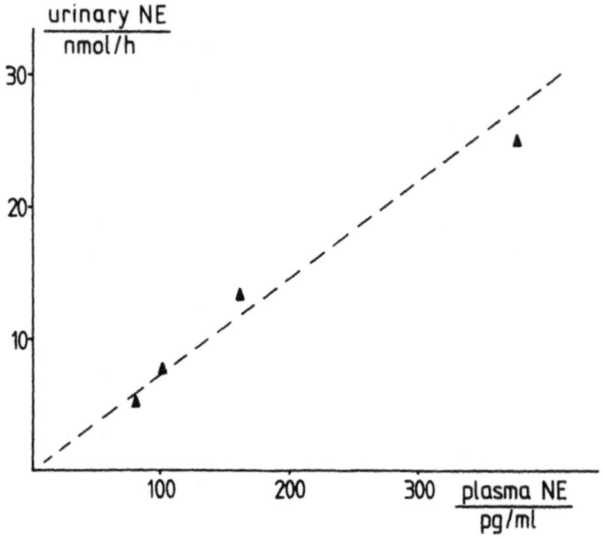

Fig. 3. Correlation between the mean norepinephrine *(NE)* plasma levels (pg/ml) and the urinary excretion rate of free norepinephrine (nmol/h) during sleep in four patients

Plasma E levels, which, according to Nishikara et al., show a positive correlation to wakefulness [4, 5], were very low as described for normal controls [4]. In four patients we also measured the urinary free catecholamines. As shown in Fig. 3, the urinary excretion of NE correlates very strongly with the mean plasma NE levels ($r = 0.99$).

Discussion

Patients with SAS frequently suffer from hypertension and, vice versa, in patients with hypertension the incidence of sleep apnea is increased [1]. As increased sympathetic activity, induced by hypoxemia during apnea, is supposed to be the cause of this observation, it seems interesting to measure the nocturnal plasma concentrations of NE and E in those people. The patients of our study show a great interindividual variability in plasma NE levels during sleep. There is no obvious correlation between plasma NE and severity of sleep apnea. One patient with grave sleep apnea even has the lowest levels of all.

This seems to be contradictory to the results of Fletcher et al. [2], who found increased catecholamine excretion in six patients with severe obstructive sleep apnea. But they also stated a great interindividual variability. Surprisingly, only 50% of their patients sufferd from hypertension, though the nocturnal apnea of those persons was more severe than of those studied by us. With regard to arterial blood pressure, our results were similar: two patients had no hypertension at all, three had moderate and only three patients had severe hypertension. Nevertheless, the lost diurnal variation - no decrease of catecholamines at night - is the characteristic finding in persons with SAS [2].

We found no intraindividual correlation between NE concentrations and blood pressure or heart rate during sleep. Stene et al. [6] found a significant correlation between blood pressure and NE levels when they studied the circadian rhythm of the two parameters in people who were normotensive. This correlation is most obvious at daytime when blood pressure and NE show a greater fluctuation than at night. It is possible that we did not find a significant correlation because our study was only performed at night. Considering the mean values of NE and arterial blood pressure, however, high plasma concentrations of NE correspond to a high arterial blood pressure. The three patients with marked hypertension had the highest mean NE levels.

It is noteworthy that one patient with very severe SAS had the lowest NE values. We suggest that some patients with severe SAS may not be, or are no longer, capable of developing an adequate sympathetic reaction to sleep apnea-induced hypoxemia.

Therefore our results might indicate that the primary cause of hypertension in patients with SAS is not the sleep apnea. But if a patient has pre-existing hypertension and sleep apnea, the hypertension may be aggravated by increased sympathetic activity following apnea-induced hypoxemia. This may be an explanation for the great variation in NE values. Therefore it seems important to us to divide patients with SAS into two groups, one with and one without a history of pronounced arterial hypertension.

Acknowledgements. I am indebted to my wife for revising the manuscript and to Mrs. U. Eisenack for skillful technical assistance.

References

1. Kales A, Cadieux RJ, Shaw LC, Vela-Bueno A, Bixler EO, Schneck DW, Locke TW, Soldatos CR (1984) Sleep apnoea in a hypertensive population. Lancet: 1005–1008
2. Fletcher E, Miller J, Schaaf J, Flectcher J (1985) Urinary catecholamines before and after tracheostomy in obstructive sleep apnea. Sleep Res 14:154
3. Clark RW, Boudoulas H, Schaal SF, Schmidt HS (1980) Adrenergic hyperactivity and cardiac abnormality in primary disorders of sleep. Neurology 30:113–119
4. Nishihara K, Mori K, Endo S (1985) Relationship between urinary excretion of epinephrine and wakefulness during sleep period in the daytime and nighttime. Sleep Res 14:26
5. Nishihara K, Mori K, Endo S, Ohta T, Ohara K (1985) Relationship between sleep efficiency and urinary excretion of catecholamines in bed-rested humans. Sleep 8:110–117
6. Stene M, Panagiotis N, Tuck ML, Sowers JR, Mayes D, Berg G (1980) Plasma norepinephrine levels are influenced by sodium intake, glucocorticoid administration, and circadian changes in normal man. J Clin Endoprinol Metab 51:1340–1345
7. Kremer R, Crawhall JC, Kolanitch R (1985) Rapid and reliable estimation of urinary free catecholamines in patients with pheochromocytoma: comparison with plasma catecholamines and vanillylmandelic acid excretion. J Chromatogr 344:313–318

Echocardiographic Findings in Sleep Apnea

W. Motz, C. Bethge, M. Klepzig, H. Blanke, and B. E. Strauer

Introduction

Sleep apnea is found in many patients with cardiovascular diseases such as coronary artery disease, congestive heart failure, and hypertensive heart disease. During long periods of sleep apnea, severe systemic hypoxemia occurs and pulmonary and systemic arterial pressures are markedly elevated.

Accordingly, the underlying cardiac disease which increases myocardial energy demand or reduces myocardial oxygen supply may be unfavorably aggravated by events of sleep apnea.

Moreover, it seems to be possible that sleep apnea is able to cause typical and specific cardiac lesions which are different from other underlying cardiac diseases. Consequently, it was the purpose of this study to determine:

1. Whether left ventricular global pumping function is impaired
2. Whether myocardial contractility, that is, myocardial function independently of influences exerted by pre- and afterload, is altered in sleep apnea syndrome
3. Whether in sleep apnea the prevalence of left ventricular hypertrophy is higher in comparison with patients without sleep apnea

We addressed these questions because it has been suggested that sleep apnea is the causative lesion for essential hypertension, and left ventricular hypertrophy represents the structural adaption of the heart in response to hypertension.

Methods

We studied 28 patients with proven sleep apnea syndrome. The minimum sleep apnea index had to be equal or greater than 10. The age range was 43–73 years.

Since arterial hypertension is known to cause severe and marked structural changes in the heart such as left ventricular hypertrophy, and, on the other hand, many patients with sleep apnea syndrome are hypertensive, it is impossible to differentiate between cardiac changes caused by sleep apnea as such and those caused by long-standing arterial hypertension.

Consequently, the 28 patients were divided into two groups:

a) patients with sleep apnea without arterial hypertension; and
b) patients with sleep apnea and arterial hypertension.

Echocardiography

One-(M mode) and two-dimensional echocardiograms were performed after a 30-min rest in the partial left lateral decubitus supine position with a Diasonics model 3400 imaging system and a 2.25 MHz transducer. M mode tracings were recorded in the short axis under simultaneous sector scanner monitoring in order to avoid projection errors. The tracings for left ventricular dimensions and septal and posterior wall thickness were recorded just beneath the mitral valve. The M mode tracings were evaluated according to the recommendations of the American Society of Echocardiography [1]. All readings were evaluated by two independent observers.

M mode echocardiograms were recorded at a paper speed of 50 mm/s. The two-dimensional echocardiographic examination comprised

a) the long axis view;
b) serial short axis view;
c) apical four-chamber view; and
d) the apical two-chamber view.

The long axis view was performed by positioning the image plane parallel to the left ventricular longitudinal axis. Serial short axis views were obtained by rotating the image plane at a 90° angle to the long axis plane and gradually angling the sector plane form aorta to apex. To record the apical four-chamber view, an image plane which is at a 90° angle to the ventricular and atrial septum was placed directly at the left ventricular apex. The apical two-chamber view was obtained by turning the transducer from the apical four-chamber view counterclockwise to visualize a sector plane being parallel to the ventricular septum and showing left ventricular atrium, aorta, mitral valve, and the left ventricle. All two-dimensional recordings were stored on a Sony-U-matic videotape.

Determination of Left Ventricular Hypertrophy and Geometry

The thickness of the ventricular septum (IVS), of the left ventricular posterior wall (LVPW), and the left ventricular diameter were measured at end-diastole at the beginning of QRS complex according to the recommendations of the American Society of Echocardiography [1]. The quotient of the IVS to LVPW-thickness was calculated to determine the extent of assymmetric wall hypertrophy. Left ventricular wall thickness–radius ratio th/r was calculated, where th was the mean left ventricular wall thickness and r the left ventricular radius at end-diastole.

Left ventricular muscle mass (LVMM) was determined by the established method of Devereux and Reichek [2]. Left ventricular end-diastolic volume (EDV) was determined by measuring the long and short axis of the left ventricle in the apical four-chamber view projection by two-dimensional echocardiography.

$$\mathrm{EDV} = \mathrm{m}^2 \times 1 \times \pi/6,$$

where m is the short, 1 the long axis of the left ventricle. Mass to volume ratio (M/V) was calculated as the quotient of left ventricular muscle mass and EDV.

Left ventricular systolic wall stress was calculated by using systolic arterial cuff pressure and left ventricular end-diastolic radius and end-diastolic mean wall thickness. Mean wall thickness was calculated as the arithmetical mean value oft left ventricular posterior wall thickness and interventricular septal thickness by M mode echocardiography.

$$SWS = \frac{Psyst \times r}{2\ d}$$

where SWS was systolic wall stress of left ventricle, Psyst the systolic arterial blood pressure, r the end-diastolic radius and d mean wall thickness of the left ventricle.

Results

The results are depicted in Table 1. Patients with sleep apnea without hypertension did not differ from normal persons in respect of left ventricular dimensions, hypertrophy and left ventricular function. However, patients with sleep apnea and hypertension showed an eccentric type of left ventricular hypertrophy. This is demonstrated by a significantly increased end-diastolic parameter with a slightly increased LVPW and IVS-thickness. Consequently, the LVMM was increased due to an increase in EDV. As a result of this the quotient of LVMM and EDV, the so-called MTV ratio, was decreased in patients with sleep apnea and hypertension. The hemodynamic consequence of these changes in left ventricular geometry was an increase in left ventricular systolic wall stress, which represents the ventricular afterload.

Table 1. Hemodynamic findings

	Sleep apnea without hypertension	Sleep apnea with hypertension
Psyst (mmHg)	142 ± 6.8	162 ± 7.4
Pdiast (mmHg)	88 ± 3.5	102 ± 3.3
Apnea index	29.5 ± 4.7	32.2 ± 5.7
Broca index	124.4 ± 5.7	126.2 ± 6.3
EDD (mm)	58 ± 2.8	66.3 ± 3.2
ESD (mm)	40.4 ± 2.5	46.8 ± 3.9
FS (%)	30.5 ± 1.8	30.7 ± 3.3
EF (%)	66 ± 2.5	63 ± 4.9
LA (mm)	33.9 ± 1.6	38.2 ± 1.9
LVPW (mm)	10.3 ± 0.42	11.4 ± 0.8
IVS (mm)	11.3 ± 1.7	12.1 ± 3.2
LVMM (g/m^2)	98 ± 6.4	168 ± 10.3
EDV (ml/m^2)	93 ± 0.25	158 ± 17.7
M/V (g/ml)	1.61 ± 0.36	1.06 ± 0.25
SWS (10^3 dyn/cm^2)	260 ± 22.2	327 ± 36.9

EDD, end-diastolic diameter; ESD, end-systolic diameter; FS, fraction of shortening of the left ventricle; EF, ejection fraction of the left ventricle; LA, left atrial diameter.

Nine of the patients were investigated invasively by cardiac catheterization. Six of the patients revealed severe coronary artery disease with stenoses of greater than 75% of at least one coronary artery. Two of the patients had a dilatative cardiomyopathy and two of the patients had no pathological findings.

Discussion

Sleep apnea frequently occurs in obese patients who are also frequently hypertensive. Since left ventricular hypertrophy is a structural consequence of the heart to a chronic sustained left ventricular pressure load [3], the prevalence of left ventricular hypertrophy in patients with sleep apnea is expected to be high. Consequently, one cannot differentiate between the specific lesions which are exerted by the so-called sleep apnea syndrome as such and hypertensive heart disease. Accordingly, we separated the patients with sleep apnea syndrome into two groups: those with and those without arterial hypertension. Since patients with sleep apnea without hypertension did not differ in respect of left ventricular dimensions and function from those without sleep apnea, it is concluded that sleep apnea as such does not cause specific lesions to the myocardium. On the other hand, patients with both sleep apnea syndrome and arterial hypertension demonstrated eccentric left ventricular hypertrophy. Eccentric hypertrophy is usually the end stage of concentric hypertrophy and indicates myocardial failure. Eccentric hypertrophy is associated with high SWS values, which means that an increased left ventricular afterload is imposed upon the left ventricle [3]. On the other hand, eccentric hypertrophy can also be caused by secondary diseases such as coronary artery disease. Since the duration of arterial hypertension is not known in these patients and also no systematic investigation of the coronary stages has been performed, it is just a matter of speculation whether this obviously high prevalence of eccentric hypertrophy in patients with sleep apnea is a consequence of the sleep apnea syndrome as such or whether the high prevalence of eccentric hypertrophy is caused by underlying secondary cardiac diseases. Further studies are necessary to clarify these very interesting points.

References

1. Sahn DJ, DeMaria A, Kisslo J, Weymann A (1978) Recommendations regarding quantitation in M mode echocardiography: results of a survey of echocardiographic measurements. Circulation 58:1072–1083
2. Devereux RB, Reichek N (1977) Echocardiographic determination of left ventricular hypertrophy in man. Circulation 55:613–618
3. Stauer BE (1983) Das Hochdruckherz, 2nd Edn. Springer, Berlin Heidelberg New York

Bradyarrhythmias in Patients with Sleep Apnea

U. Köhler, W. Rasbach, and J. H. Peter

Introduction

Sleep apnea activity (SAA) is, to some degree, a normal physiological finding in healthy subjects. Fewer than five apneic episodes per hour of sleep is generally regarded as a finding which does not demand clinical management or therapy, while results of more than ten episodes per hour are associated with severe risks such as a variety of cardiac findings, pathologically increased systemic and pulmonary artery blood pressure, as well as neurophysiological and psychological symptoms which constitute severe impairments of the patients' general well-being and their intellectual and physical powers.

Cardiac disturbances occupy a key role in the morbidity spectrum of sleep apnea. Sinus bradycardia $\leqq$ 30 bpm, heart blocks of higher degrees and asystoles $>$ 17 s have been reported in patients with SAA during the night [1–4]. Cyclical variation of the heart rate (CVHR) during the night seems to be the most specific finding in such patients [5]. This alteration of the sinus rhythm is characterized by decreases in heart rate down to extreme bradycardia during apnea and subsequent tachycardia accompanying the phases of apnea-terminating hyperventilation. Apart from a long-term detrimental effect on the cardiac function, extreme variation of heart rate during the night increases the risk of sudden nocturnal cardiac death.

We are therefore conducting a series of studies devoted to the prevalence of extreme cardiac findings, notably sinus bradycardia, among SAA patients, and to the pathomechanisms which connect severe apnea with specific cardiac results. One of the aims of this series is to find out if the long-term ECG is useful as an instrument in the early differential diagnosis of SAA.

Methods

We studied bradyarrhythmias in two groups of patients. Group I was a population of 18 patients with pathologically increased SAA (apnea index - Ai $>$ 10 episodes per hour), group II was a control group of 21 patients whith physiologically normal SAA (Ai $<$ 5). SAA was documented by means of overnight recordings of respiration (abdominal and thoracic by means of inductive plethysmography), partial arterial oxygen tension (transcutaneously), and ECG. Simultaneously with these recordings on our compact four-channel diagnostic unit, we recorded an additional two-channel long-term ECG (Oxford Medilog 4000).

Prior to the main investigation, all patients were clinically examined. There were no relevant cardiovascular diagnoses in either group. Mean overweight was 18.8% of normal weight according to Broca in the group of SAA patients, and 10.0% in the asymptomatic group. Both groups were comparable in terms of age. Mean age in group I was 51.5 (± 7.5, range 35–62), and 49.1 (± 8.8, range 32–60) in group II. The mean RR systolic blood pressure in group I was higher (141.1 ± 18.8 mmHg) than in the asymptomatic group (138.6 ± 2.4 mmHg). The same applies to the diastolic values (90.6 ± 12.7 versus 86.9 ± 6.8 mmHg).

Minimum, maximum, and mean heart rates were continuously calculated by computer on the basis of a window of four R-R intervals over the whole range of the recordings (17 h) as well as for three consecutive hours during the day (1600–1900) and at night (0100–0400). Heart rate minima during the night were determined by manual assessment of individual R-R intervals. The data of patients with minima < 35 bpm during the three nocturnal hours, according to this method, were subjected to a close analysis of frequencies < 35 bpm and < 45 bpm as well as asystoles. The apnea parameters used for statistical comparisons included the Ai, the proportion of apnea within the 10-min period of highest apnea activity, and the duration of each patient's 30 longest apnea episodes. Statistical significances were determined by means of the Wilcoxon test and Spearman's rank correlation.

Results

The results of the 17-h recording and the nocturnal apnea measurement are summarized in Table. 1. All patients in group I fulfilled the criterion of Ai > 10 (mean 25 ± 12.7). The highest Ai in group II was 4 (mean 1.4 ± 1.2). In the group

Table 1. Summary of results of the nocturnal apnea measurement and the ECG evaluations of the 17 h long-term recording and the recording during three nocturnal hours, as indicated

Number of patients	Group I (Ai > 10) 18	Group II (Ai < 5) 21
Ai (mean ± SD, range)	25.0 ± 12.7 (10.1–58.2)	1.4 ± 1.2 (0–4)
Longest apnea episode (s)	61 ± 25.7 (21–120)	16 ± 12.2 (0–45)
Heart rate maximum (17 h) (bpm)	128 ± 12 (104–150)	127 ± 13 (107–149)
Heart rate minimum (17 h) (bpm)	49 ± 10 (22–70)	50 ± 6 (36–63)
Mean heart rate (17 h) (bpm)	78 ± 9 (56–100)	74 ± 10 (56–93)
Bradycardia ≦ 30 bpm *(n)* (3 h)	1	0
Bradycardia ≦ 35 bpm *(n)* (3 h)	2[a]	1[b]
Asystole > 2.5 s *(n)* (3 h)	2 (3.2 s–3.4 s)	0
Second degree AV block *(n)* (3 h)	1[b]	0
Third degree SA block	2	0

[a] Occurred 20 times in one patient, nine times in the other
[b] Occurred only once

of apnea patients, there was a positive correlation between the frequency of apnea and age ($p < 0.05$).

The comparison of maximum, minimum, and mean heart rates did not show significant differences between the two groups. Within the group of apnea patients, the parameters of heart rate did not correlate with the apnea parameters or with bodyweight or age. In the control group, there was a significant connection between age and the minimum of heart rate: younger subjects had a lower minimum of heart rate during the night ($p < 0.05$).

There was one case of sinus bradycardia with a minimum of 35 bpm (based on the assessment of individual R-R intervals) in the control group (Fig. 1). Two patients exhibited bradycardia ≦ 35 bpm due to second degree atrioventricular

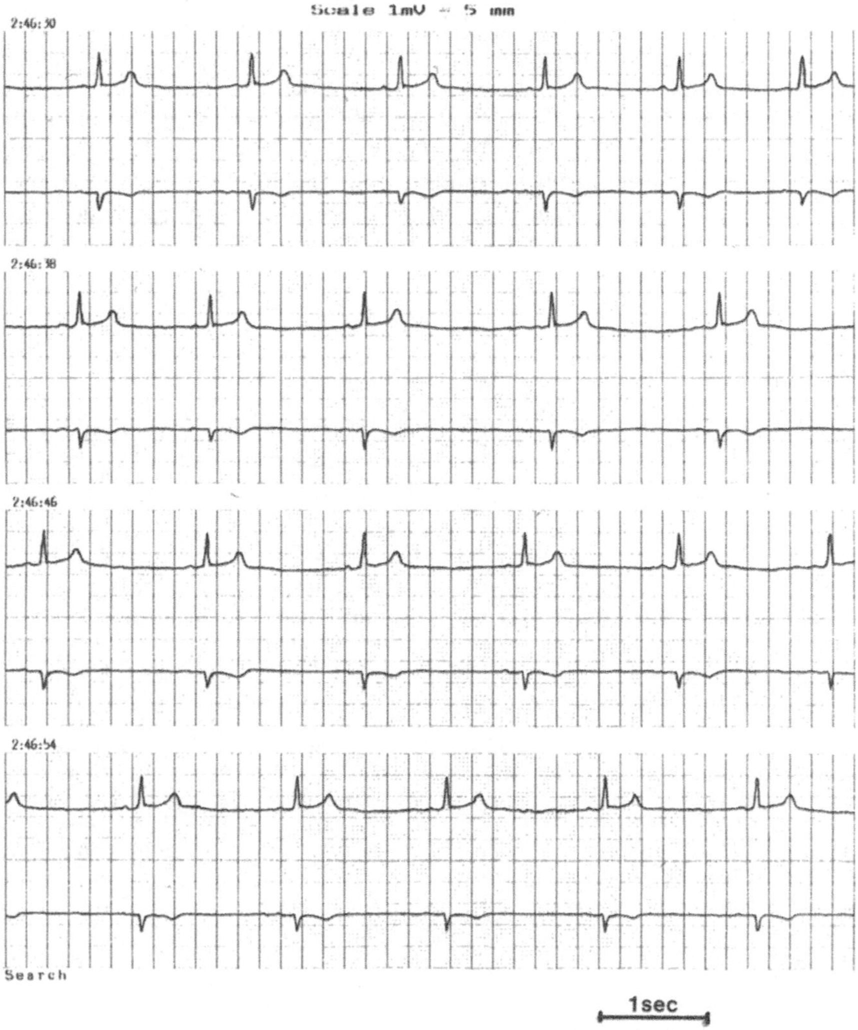

Fig. 1. Two-channel ECG recording of a patient without apnea: regular sinus rhythm of 40 bpm

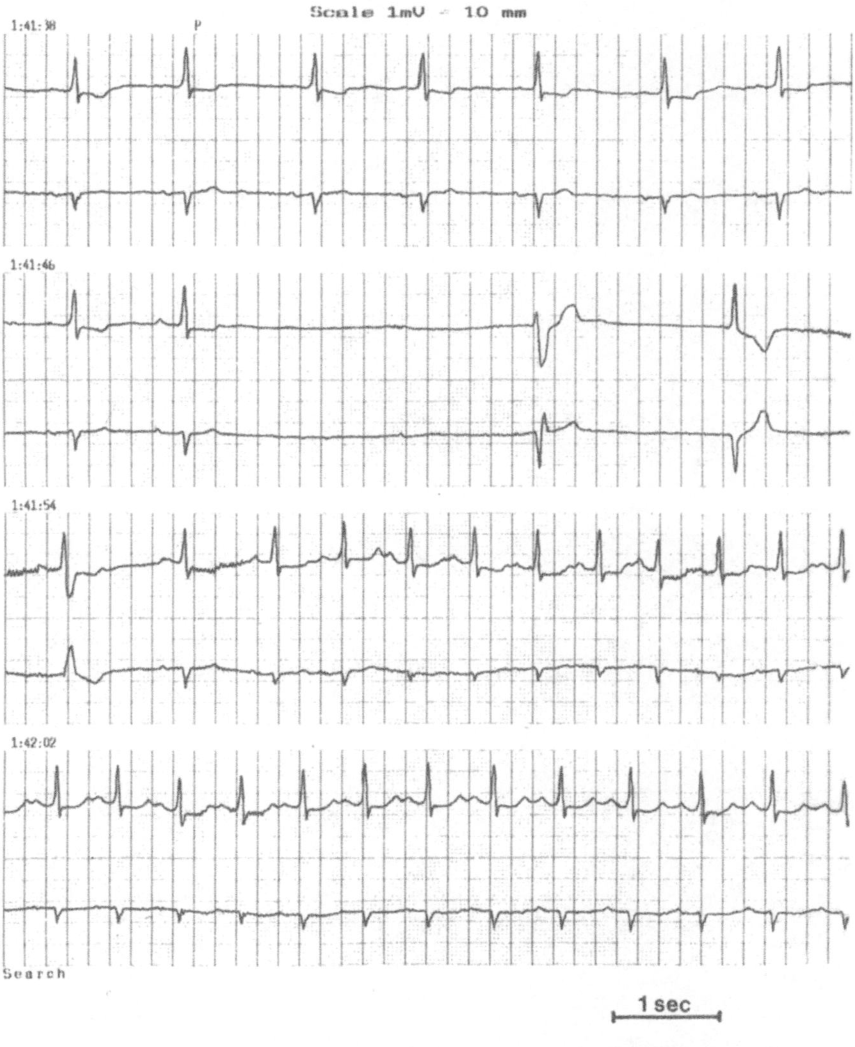

Fig. 2. Two-channel ECG recording showing instances of SA and AV conduction blocks with ventricular and nodal escape beats in a patient with sleep apnea

(AV) and third degree sinoauricular (SA) blocks in the group of sleep apnea patients (Figs. 2 and 3). The difference between the asymptomatic subject and the two patients with sleep apnea is illustrated by the fact that low heart rate > 35 < 45 bpm remained stable up to 24.8 min in the patient without apnea during the 3 h 0100–0400, whereas the two patients with sleep apnea exhibited recurrent short spells of low heart rate ($> 35 < 45$ bpm) lasting for up to 7.0 s in one, and 13.6 s in the other patient. In this patient, we observed 33 instances of second and third degree SA blocks within the three nocturnal hours singled out for close analysis.

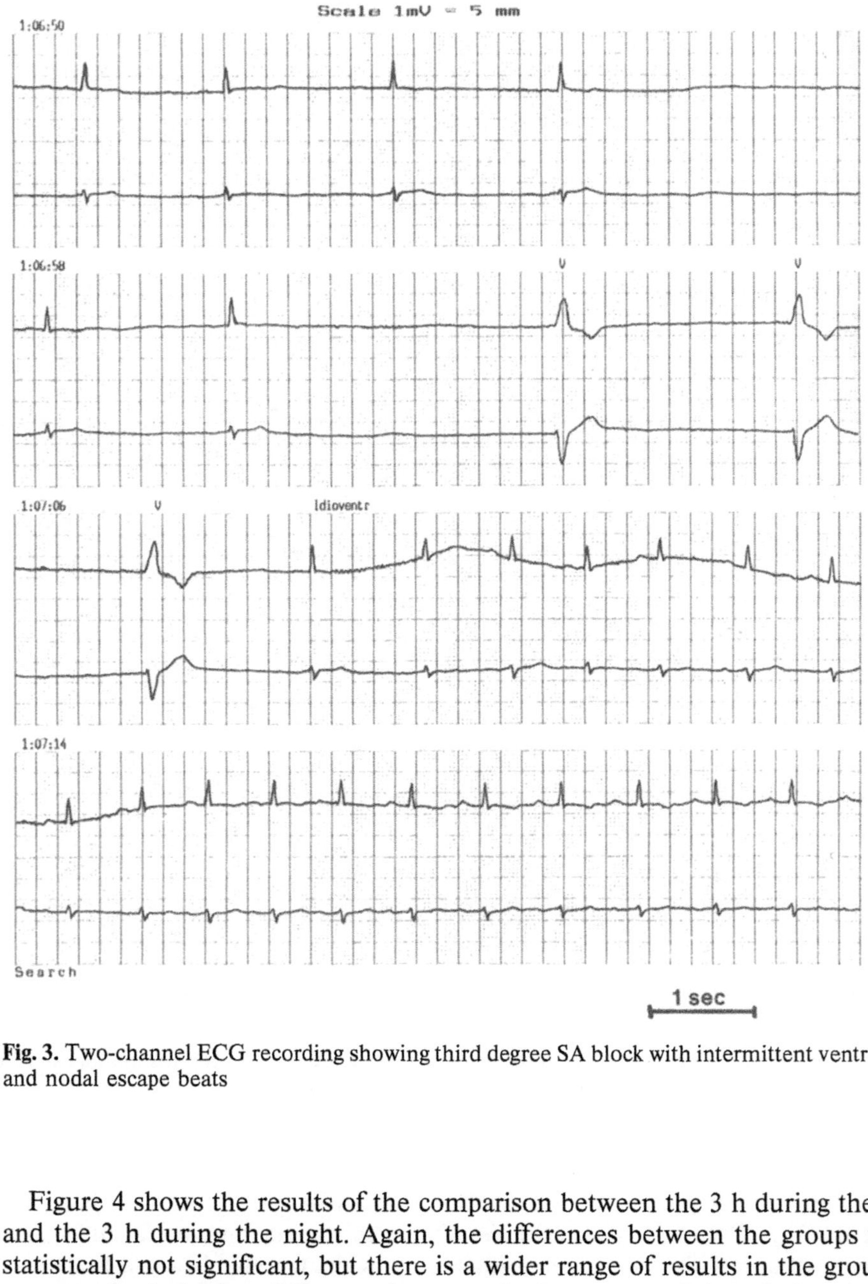

Fig. 3. Two-channel ECG recording showing third degree SA block with intermittent ventricular and nodal escape beats

Figure 4 shows the results of the comparison between the 3 h during the day and the 3 h during the night. Again, the differences between the groups were statistically not significant, but there is a wider range of results in the group of apnea patients (widest difference between the heart rate minima during the day 42 bpm, at night 52 bpm) than in the asymptomatic group (34 bpm during the day, 37 bpm at night). The difference between the daily and the nocturnal minima of heart rate is greater in the group with sleep apnea (mean 15 bpm) than in the control group (mean 9 bpm), but this difference was statistically not significant. The greatest difference between the diurnal and the noctural minima of

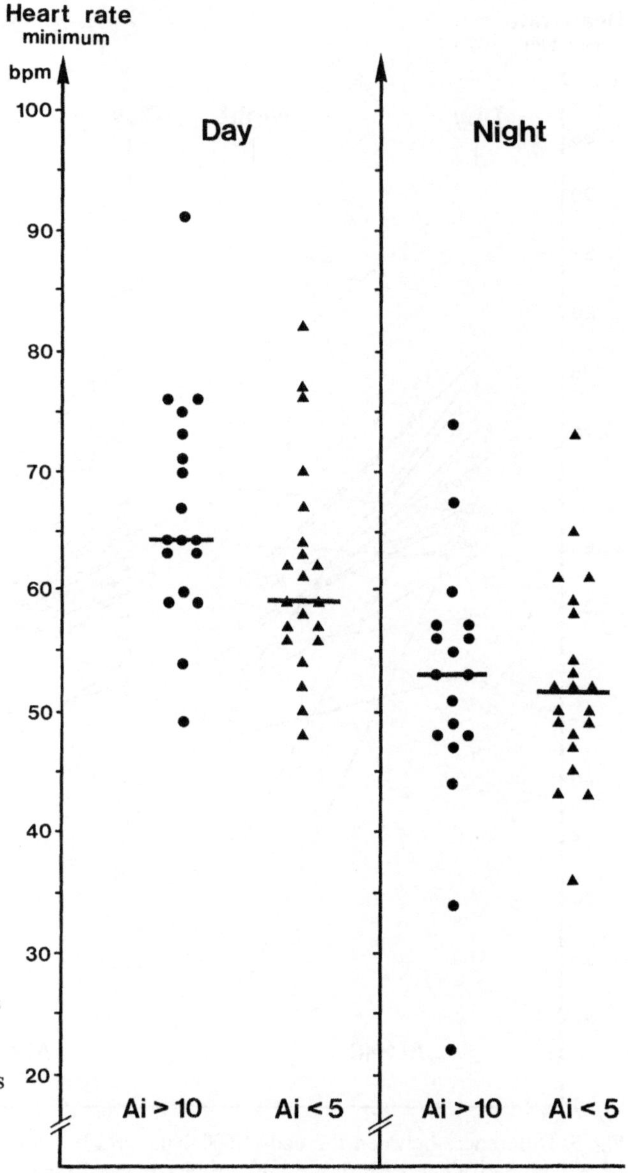

Fig. 4. Individual heart rate minima during the day and at night. Comparison of the hours 1600–1900 and 0100–0400. Median values are indicated. Differences between the groups with apnea (Ai > 10) and without apnea (Ai < 5) are not significant

heart rate was found in the two patients with second degree AV and second and third degree SA conduction blocks during the night (Figs. 4, 5).

Discussion

In our comparison of patients with pronounced sleep apnea and a control group of asymptomatic subjects, a significant relationship between cardiac parameters

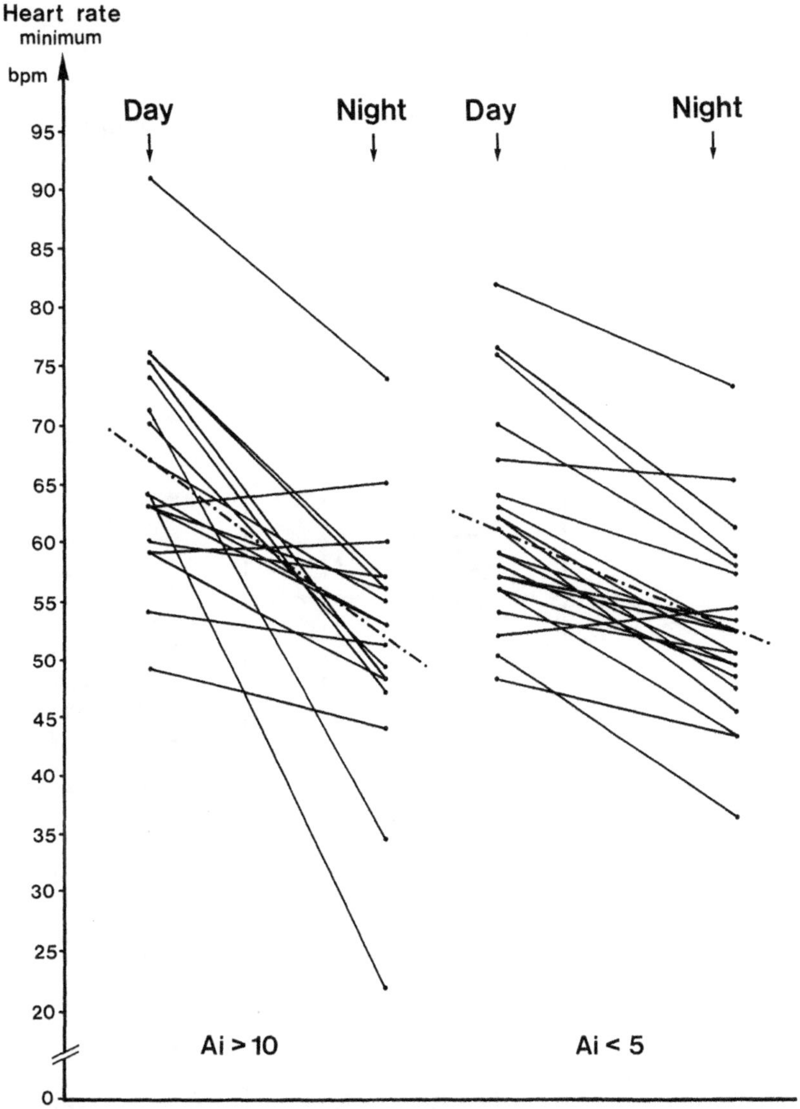

Fig. 5. Differences between the daily (1600–1900) and the nocturnal (0100–0400) minimum of heart rate, individual decreases in both groups, mean decrease inserted (–·–·–·–)

and apnea could not be established. There was a tendency toward a more distinct decrease from the heart rate minimum during the day to the nocturnal minimum in the apnea group. The average values of this comparison are influenced by extremely low minima in two patients with heart blocks during the night. Such heart blocks, on the other hand, as well as severe bradycardia and asystoles, were found to be less frequent than reported by other researchers. In two studies with 15 and 25 patients, Tilkian found extreme sinus bradycardia in 40% and 36%

respectively [2, 3]. Guilleminault studied a group of 50 patients with extremely severe apnea and reports asystoles $\geqq 2.5$ s in 30%, second degree AV blocks in 18%, and extreme bradycardia in 36% [1]. The rates reported by Miller [6] and by Shepard [7] are much lower: 4% (Shepard: 6%) second degree AV blocks, 9% (6%) asystoles, 9% (10%) of extreme sinus bradycardia. Judging from our own results, the frequency of asystoles (11%), bradycardia < 30 bpm (6%), or heart blocks (6%, 11%) is often overestimated as an indication in the differential diagnosis of sleep apnea. Nevertheless, these symptoms demand careful attention, and extreme findings should always warn the attending physician to consider sleep apnea as a possible cause.

Sinus bradycardia was also found in one subject in the control group. But whereas healthy, and especially younger, persons may exhibit a low heart rate during the night, the sinus rhythm is comparatively stable over long periods (compare Fig. 1). Our observations suggest that it is rather the degree of heart rate variation during the night which is the most typical ECG indication of sleep apnea. Short decreases in heart rate alternating with accelerations of the cardiac rhythm or a comparatively high mean heart rate during the night should alert to the possibility of sleep apnea with all the additional risks which have been reported. In a sequel to the present study we shall focus on the stability of the cardiac rhythm during the night, as we assume that heart rate variability is a better ECG-derived criterion for the recognition of sleep apnea than the occurrence of bradycardia.

References

1. Guilleminault C, Simmons F, Motta J, Cummiskey J, Rosekind M, Schroeder JS, Dement WC (1981) Obstructive sleep apnea syndrome and tracheostomy. Long-term follow-up experience. Arch Intern Med 141:985–988
2. Tilkian AG, Guilleminault C, Schroeder JS, Lehrman KL, Simmons FB, Dement WC (1977) Sleep-induced apnea syndrome. Prevalence of cardiac arrhythmias and their reversal after tracheostomy. Am J Med 63:348–358
3. Tilkian AG, Motta J, Guilleminault C (1978) Cardiac arrhythmias in sleep apnea. In: Guilleminault C, Dement WC (eds) Sleep apnea syndromes. Liss, New York, pp 197–210
4. Zwillich C, Devlin T, White D, Douglas N, Weil J, Martin R (1982) Bradycardia during sleep apnea: characteristics and mechanism. J Clin Invest 69:1286–1292
5. Guilleminault C, Connolly S, Winkle R, Melvin K, Tilkian A (1984) Cyclical variation of the heart rate in sleep apnoea syndrome. Mechanisms, and usefulness of 24 h electrocardiography as a screening technique. Lancet 1:126–131
6. Miller WP (1982) Cardiac arrhythmias and conduction disturbances in the sleep apnea syndrome. Prevalence and significance. Am J Med 73:317–321
7. Shepard JW (1985) Gas exchange and hemodynamics during sleep. Med Clin North Am 69:1243–1263

Part 8: Therapy

Treatment of Sleep Apnea by Prosthetic Mandibular Advancement

K. MEIER-EWERT, and B. BROSIG

Introduction

Obstructive sleep apnea in Western countries is a frequently encountered disease with a progressive course and serious sequelae. Its important aspects have been extensively reviewed [12]. Effective long-term therapy should combine high efficacy with minimal side effects and absence of risks. This ideal therapeutic method is still missing. Current methods of treatment and their published results are summarized in Table 1.

The cause of obstructive sleep apnea is an inspiratory occlusion of the oropharyngeal airway. It may be reduced or prevented by mandibular advancement which is produced surgically [2, 13] or by prosthetic treatment with a mandibular-protracting device [3, 11, 16, 17, 18, 19]. This prosthesis has to be built individually by a dentist [23]. It imitates the effect of the Esmarch maneuver and pulls the mandible 3–5 mm forward, opening the oropharynx by causing an artificial transitory progenia during sleep. Therefore it is called the Esmarch prosthesis.

Patients and Methods

A sample of 44 sequential, unselected patients was evaluated from 1982–1986. The group of patients consisted of 38 males and 6 females (mean age 52 years; range 34–74 years). All patients suffered from obstructive sleep apnea syndrome with an apnea index of at least 13 per h. The Apnea Index gives the number of apnea phases per hour. The mean apnea index of the patients sampled was 50.4 per h. Mean amount overweight was 18.1 kg. All patients had a diagnostic polysomnography which included EEG, EMG of musculus mentalis and both musculi tibialis anterior, noting horizontal eye movements, and recording of respiratory activity at the nose, mouth, thorax, and abdomen. Blood gas changes were monitored by recording O_2-hemoglobin saturation (Oximeter, Schuchardt, Wiesbaden) and O_2 and CO_2 partial tissue pressures (Oxycapnometer, Hellige, Freiburg/Bg). Sleep stages were scored visually according to the criteria of Rechtschaffen and Kales [21].

Once the diagnosis of obstructive sleep apnea had been established, all patients were seen by an ear, nose, and throat specialist. For prosthetic mandibular advancement an Esmarch prosthesis was built individually for each patient by one of three coworking dentists. To evaluate the effectiveness of the prosthesis,

Table 1. Effect of treatment in obstructive sleep apnea.

Reference	Type of treatment	No. of patients	Parameters	Improvement in percentage of baseline values
Surgical Interventions				
Guilleminault et al [9]	Tracheostomy	5 (severe cases)	Apnea index	97 (long-term)
Peiser et al. [21]	Weight reduction by gastric bypass	15 (selected of a total sample of about 100)	Apnea index	90
Caldarelli et al. [5]	(a) Submucous resection	23 (selected)	Apnea index	6
	(b) Palatopharyngo-plasty plus sub-mucous resection	17 (selected)	Apnea index	50.8
Dayal et al [8]	Nasal surgery	6 (selected)	Apnea index	39.8
Simmons et al [25]	Palatopharyngoplasty	20 (selected)	Apnea index	36.7
Drug treatment				
Rubin et al. [23]	Imipramine-HCl	13 (selected of a total sample of 31)	Apnea index	46.5
Brownell et al. [4]	Protriptyline	5 (double blind, crossover)	Apnea index	7
Mayer [15]	Theophylline	16	Apnea index	38.9
Hensley et al. [10]	Medroxyprogesterone	9	Apnea index	28 (n.s.)
Berry and Block [1]	CPAP	9 (selected)	Apnea index	85
McEvoy et al. [14]	CPAP	12 (sequential)	Apnea index	84
Sobers et al. [26]	Long-term CPAP	52 (unselected)	CPAP-compliance	63
Cambers et al. [7]	Long-term CPAP	52 (unselected)	CPAP-compliance	50
Cartwright et al. [6]	Tongue-retaining device	6 (unselected)	Apnea index	50
Meier-Ewert and Brosig [20]	Prosthetic treatment of Sleep Apnea Syndrome (in preparation)	58 (unselected)	Apnea time	53

CPAP = continuous positive airways pressure

each patient had polysomnographical, all-night recordings over 2 successive nights. Baseline values were taken from the 1st night recording (without Esmarch prosthesis) and compared to the values of polysomnography (with Esmarch prosthesis) during the following night. Of particular interest were the apnea index (number of apnea episodes per h) and apnea time, measured as a percentage of the total sleep time. As control parameters, total sleep time (TST) and time in bed (TIB) were used.

After each of the 2 nights, the patient's attentiveness was tested with a monotonous version of the "Mackworth clock" adapted from Quatember and Maly's vigilance test of the Vienna test system (G. Schuhfried, Mödling/Austria). For the 30 min test subjects sit in front of a screen, observing a light which moves around a circle of small quadrangles. Subjects are expected to press a button as fast as possible, when the light signal skips a quadrangle in a random fashion. As test parameters we used reaction time and number of missed signals. Pathological test results correlate with the severity of daytime sleepiness.

Results

In order to allow comparison with other publications in the field the sample of 44 patients was divided into two groups: group 1 showing more and group 2 showing less than 50% reduction of the apnea index during the night with the Esmarch prosthesis in place. Table 2 shows that 59% of our patients had their apnea index reduced by more than 50% in the night with the Esmarch prosthesis. This percentage is composed of patients from each of three coworking dentists with different success rates (range 42%–75%). If broken up into three groups with an apnea index reduction of 0%–30%, 31%–70% and 71%–100%, one third of our patients exhibited good to excellent improvements with an apnea index reduction of 71%–100%, a second third showed moderate to good improvement with an apnea index reduction of 31%–70% and the remainder (14 patients) showed unsatisfactory results with an improvement of 0%–30% (Table 3). To ensure that the reported percentage values of improvement are realistic, time in bed (TIB) and total sleep time (TST) were used as control parameters. Table 4 shows that neither changed significantly in the nights without and with the Esmarch prosthesis. In 19 patients with a reduction of apnea index of more than 50%, reaction time and number of mistakes were significantly decreased after the first night with the Esmarch prosthesis (Table 5). These vigilance test results correlate well with the patients' reports about feeling less sleepy.

Table 2. Treatment effect of Esmarch prosthesis in 44 unselected patients in two groups

Reduction of apnea index in percentage of baseline values	No. of patients	Percentage of total sample
more than 50	26	59
less than 50	18	41

Table 3. Treatment effect of Esmarch prosthesis in 44 unselected patients in three groups

Reduction of apnea index in percentage of baseline values	No. of patients	Percentage of total sample
71–100	15	34
31–70	15	34
0–30	14	32

Table 4. Apnea and sleep parameter without and with Esmarch prosthesis in 44 unselected patients. Time in bed (TIB) and Total Sleep Time (TST) did not change

Parameter	Esmarch prosthesis without	with	Improvement (in percentage) of baseline values	p*
Apnea time (in percentage of TST)	41.3 ± 23.8	18.6 ± 18.8	55	> 0.0005
Apnea index	50.4 ± 25	23.14 ± 19.6	54	> 0.0005
Control parameter				
TIB (min)	425.3 ± 48	429 ± 37	1	n.s.
TST (min)	378.3 ± 57	382.2 ± 58	1	n.s.

* t-test for correlated samples

Table 5. Vigilance parameter after nights without and with Esmarch prosthesis in 19 successfully treated patients (apnea index reduction > 50%)

Vigilance parameter	Esmarch prothesis without	with	p*
⌀ reaction time	0.46 ± 0.09	0.39 ± 0.08	> 0.05
No. of missed signals	8.9 ± 16.3	2.3 ± 6.9	>0.025

* t-test for correlated samples

Prosthetic mandibular advancement is more difficult in patients with artificial teeth. In such patients artificial dentures have always been removed and the prosthesis adapted to the upper and lower jaw.

Our results show that prosthetic mandibular advancement:
- is an effective treatment for sleep apnea, with immediate improvement in patients with and without retrogenia
- has few or no side effects
- shows higher success rates than drug treatment
- has lower risks than surgery
- is less expensive and less cumbersome than continuous positive airway pressure

Acknowledgements. We thank Dr. med. dent. Heinrich Schäfer who in collaboration with one of us (M-E) developed the Esmarch prosthesis and fabricated the prosthesis for 20 patients, our most difficult cases among them. The Esmarch prostheses for 12 patients were fabricated by Dr. Ulrich Handstein and for another 12 patients, by Dr. Lothar Grabs. We gratefully acknowledge their work and interest in this method. We thank Mrs. Hanna von Hessert and Mrs. Maria Kohl who performed all polygraphic recordings. Supported by Deutsche Forschungsgemeinschaft.

References

1. Berry RB, Block AJ (1984) Positive nasal airway pressure eliminates snoring as well as obstructive sleep apnea. Chest 85:15–20
2. Bear SE, Priest JH, Richmond DDS (1980) Sleep apnea syndrome correction with surgical advancement of the mandible. J Oral Surg 38:543–549
3. Brosig B, Meier-Ewert K (1986) Measuring treatment efficacy in obstructive sleep apnea syndrome. Eur Soc Pneumol Congress, Paris (abstract)
4. Brownell LG, West P, Sweatman P, Acres JC, Kryger MH (1982) Protriptyline in obstructive sleep apnea. A double-blind trial. N Engl J Med 307:1037–1042
5. Caldarelli DD, Cartwright RD, Lilie JK (1985) Obstructive sleep apnea: variations in surgical management. Larynogoscope 95:1070–1073
6. Cartwright R, Samelson C, Lilie J, Krawitz H, Knight S, Stefoski D, Caldarelli D (1986) Testing the tongue retaining device for control of sleep apnea. Sleep Res 15:III
7. Chambers GM, Birkemeier N, Walsh JK (1986) Nasal continuous positive airway pressure (CPAP) and home compliance. Sleep Res 15:112
8. Dayal V, Philipson EA (1985) Nasal surgery in the management of sleep apnea. Ann Otol Rhinol Laryngol 94:550–554
9. Guilleminault C, Cummiskey J (1982) Progressive improvement of apnea index and ventilatory response to CO_2 after tracheostomy in obstructive sleep apnea syndrome. Am Rev Respir Dis 126:14–20
10. Hensley MJ, Saunders NA, Strohl KP (1980) Medroxyprogesterone treatment of obstructive sleep apnea. Sleep 3:441–446
11. Kloss W, Meier-Ewert K, Schäfer M (1986) Zur Therapie des Obstruktiven Schlaf-Apnoe-Syndroms. Fortschr Neurol Psychiatry 54:267–271
12. Krieger J (1986) Les syndromes d'apnées du sommeil de l'adulte (sleep apnea syndromes in adults). Bull Eur Physiopathol Respir 22:147–189
13. Kuo PC, West RA, Bloomquist DS, McNeil RW (1979) The effect of mandibular osteotomy in 3 patients with hypersomnia sleep apnea. Oral Surg 48:392–395
14. McEvoy R, Thornton AT (1984) Treatment of obstructive sleep apnea syndrome with nasal continuous positive airway pressure. Sleep 7:313–325
15. Mayer J (1983) Untersuchung zur Wirkung von Theophyllin bei Patienten mit Schlaf-Apnoe-Syndrom. Thesis, University of Marburg, Marburg
16. Meier-Ewert K, Schäfer M, Kloß W (1984) Treatment of sleep apnea by a mandibula protracting device. In: Berichtsband 7th Eur congr sleep research München, p 217 (abstract)
17. Meier-Ewert K (1985) Neurologisch-polysomnographische Differentialdiagnostik hypersomnischer Syndrome. Prax Klin Pneumol 39:324–325
18. Meier-Ewert K, Schäfer H (1985) Behandlung des obstruktiven Schlaf-Apnoe-Syndroms mit einer mechanischen Bißklemme. Prax Klin Pneumol 39:327
19. Meier-Ewert K, Brosig B (1986) Prosthetic treatment of obstructive sleep apnea syndrome. Sleep Res 15:197
20. Meier-Ewert K, Brosig B (1987) Prosthetic Treatment of Sleep Apnea Syndrome (in preparation)
21. Peiser J, Lavie P, Ovnat A, Charuzi I (1984) Sleep apnea syndrome in the morbidly obese as an indication for weight reduction surgery. Ann Surg 199:112–115
22. Rechtschaffen A, Kales A (1968) A manual of standardized terminology, techniques and scoring system for sleep stages of human subjects. Public Health Service, US Government Printing Office, Washington DC
23. Rubin AE, Elroy GG, Peled R, Lavie P (1986) Preliminary clinical experience with imi pramine HCl in the treatment of sleep apnea syndrome. Eur Neurol 25:81–85
24. Schäfer H (1985) Das obstruktive Schlaf-Apnoe-Syndrom. Aufgabe für Neurologe und Zahnarzt. Zahnärztl Mitteil 75:1540–1541
25. Simmons BF, Guilleminault C, Miles LE (1984) A surgical treatment for snoring and obstructive sleep apnea. West Indian Med J 140:43–46
26. Sobers M, Mitler MM, Gutierrez F, Gaines S, Timms RM (1986) Acceptance of nasal CPAP and treatment compliance in patients with obstructive sleep apnea. Sleep Res 15:172

Review of the Therapeutic Approaches to Sleep Apnea

D. KURTZ, and J. KRIEGER

Since the first description in 1965 of the sleep apnea syndrome (SAS) by Gastaut et al. [29] and Jung and Kuhlo [41], many attempts have been made to define an efficient treatment for this syndrome. Unfortunately, most of the proposed methods, including weight loss and drug treatments, rapidly proved to be unsatisfactory; through their use only an inconstant improvement of daytime sleepiness or an insufficient reduction, if any, of the sleep-related apneas could be obtained. Only the tracheostomy, which was initially used by Kuhlo et al. [47], resulted in a complete reversal of the symptoms of obstructive sleep apneas (OSA); however, this technique, sometimes difficult to manage in obese patients, was often not well-tolerated by the patients.

A better knowledge of the pathophysiology of SAS has led to new therapeutic procedures: on the one hand, various surgical techniques whose aim is an enlargement of the upper airways; on the other hand, more or less mechanical devices whose application reduces or abolishes the sleep-associated inspiratory airway closure [40, 51, 60]. As will be shown later on, both techniques, though they may still be improved, represent a real therapeutic progress in comparison to the methods formerly proposed. However, before giving some insights into the management and the results of these new means of treatment, an overview of nonsurgical and nonmechanical treatments of sleep apneas will be presented.

Medical Treatment of Sleep Apneas

Weight loss

It is not actually surprising that weight loss had initially been considered as the major treatment for SAS; marked obesity was one of the main symptoms of the pickwickian syndrome described by Burwell et al. [10] and this syndrome was for a long time considered to be a cardiorespiratory consequence of obesity. Although the relationship between obesity and sleep apneas remains unclear, sleep apneas have been shown to increase with increased body weight. Among patients with SAS, Guilleminault et al. [36] noted that the majority of patients weighed more than 15% above ideal body weight. A reduction of the overweight has clearly been demonstrated as being followed by a decrease or a resolution of daytime sleepiness [37, 52, 59, 68, 87]. Moreover, this loss of weight was sometimes associated with a variable reduction of the sleep apneas and a lesser severity of O_2 desaturation associated with the apneic events [8, 37, 68], but only very rarely did the sleep apneas disappear completely after weight loss.

Though weight loss could be beneficial in a motivated patient, several problems remain: first, approximately 20% of the sleep apnea patients are not overweight; secondly, the deviation from ideal body weight varies in obese sleep apnea patients from 15% to 400% and no one knows the minimal amount of weight loss required before improvement is seen (9% of body weight according to Smith et al. [79]) or whether this minimal amount remains constant whatever the degree of obesity. Although in the extremely obese people reported by Harman et al. [37] a reduction of weight was effective on both daytime sleepiness and the apnea index, cases were reported where, despite a loss of more than 30 kg, either no clinical improvement could be noted or only daytime sleepiness improved, the sleep apnea index remaining unchaged [32, 52].

Finally, even in a motivated patient, a reduction of body weight is sometimes difficult to obtain or to maintain; diet therapy often fails and patients show a succession of weight loss and regain. Therefore, surgical interventions have been proposed and have been described as being successful: a reduction of gastric capacity by division [26, 86] or gastric bypass surgery [64] has been followed in a small number of extremely obese SAS patients by a dramatic reduction in the number of apneas per hour of sleep, which in Peiser's cases fell from 81.9 ± 43.5 to 15 ± 16.6 in the postoperative recording. However, one must be aware of the potential risk of severe postoperative complications (i.e., venous thrombosis, respiratory depression, infections, and massive atelectasis), so that, in the end, occasionally harmful gastrointestinal surgery should not be applied to SAS patients unless they present a morbid obesity.

Nervertheless, although the exact mechanism by which weight reduction improves daytime sleepiness and, to a lesser degree the sleep apnea index, remains unknown, and though weight loss often appears difficult to manage, a weight-reducing diet should be proposed to overweight sleep apnea patients as the first therapeutic procedure.

Drug treatment

The usefulness of drug treatments in SAS remains controversial, since, despite some positive results, most of the time the drugs employed failed to cure or even to improve patients showing sleep apneas, whatever their type.

Protriptyline

This tricyclic antidepressant with no respiratory depressant properties had been first tested in SAS patients by Clark et al. [16]; they reported a decrease in apnea frequency and duration after protriptyline treatment in 11 of 14 patients with OSA, but four patients nevertheless required tracheostomy, and the side-effects of the drug were often considerable.

In the study of Conway et al. [20, 21], four of the nine patients, who had OSA among various other symptoms, presented after protriptyline treatment a reduction in daytime drowsiness together with a fall in the number of apneas per hour of sleep. However, in severe SAS, the treatment appeared to be of low efficiency; even if efficient in mild SAS, its effectiveness decreased with time and uncomfortable side-effects led to the discontinuation of treatment.

Furthermore, two well-controlled studies [9, 77] clearly demonstrated that the major effect of protriptyline is a reduction in the amount of REM sleep, which obviously results in a decrease in REM sleep-related apneas. Since these apneas generally show the longest duration and, concomitantly, the lowest SaO_2 level, each reduction in REM sleep automatically results in a reduction of the total time spent during sleep in apnea and in an increase in nocturnal mean SaO_2. However, the apnea index remained unmodified in both studies, though in Smith's study during NREM sleep, apneas tended to become hypopneas. Whether this latter effect was due only to protriptyline remains questionable, since similar observations have been made in SAS patients recorded on several occasions without any drug treatment.

Finally, the beneficial effect of protriptyline treatment remains uncertain, though the two controlled studies mentioned above demonstrated an improvement in nocturnal SaO_2. If protriptyline treatment should nevertheless be undertaken, administration in a single dose (5–30 mg) 1 h before bedtime would appear to be useful only in mild OSA syndrome showing predominantly apneas during REM sleep. Even in these patients, anticholinergic side-effects or unpredictable cardiac arrhythmias may limit the use of the drug.

Chlorimipramine

This tricyclic antidepressant with sedative properties has been used in treating sleep apneas. However, the beneficial results indicated by Kumashiro [48] et al. and Schwartz and Rochemaure [72] could not be confirmed by Krieger et al. [44] in SAS patients with stable body weight.

Ventilatory Stimulants

Medroxyprogesterone Acetate (MPA). This oral synthetic progestin has been shown to improve blood gas values in normal subjects [76] and in pickwickians [85]. The efficiency of this drug in SAS patients has been contested by ORR et al. [62] in spite of data similar to those of Strohl et al. [81], who, in four of nine adult patients with OSA given 60–120 mg MPA per day, observed a resolution of daytime sleepiness and a decrease in the number of obstructive apneas during sleep. These responders had lower PaO_2 values and relatively higher $PaCO_2$ values before MPA administration than did nonresponders and they remained well during 6–8 months of MPA therapy, except for one patient who stopped the treatment because of alopecia. However, in a study of the effect of MPA on breathing and oxygenation in sleeping and awake chronic obstructive pulmonary disease (COPD) patients, Dolly and Block [23] noted increased mean PaO_2 and decreased $PaCO_2$ values during wakefulness, while, during sleep, no significant changes were observed in the number of sleep apneas and hypopneas or in the SaO_2.

These contradictory results indicate that further controlled trials of MPA in OSA seem warranted before the usefulness of this respiratory stimulant in treating sleep apnea patients can be assessed.

Acetazolamide. This carbonic anhydrase inhibitor has been reported to be beneficial in patients with predominant central apneas [89] but the study performed in six subjects was not a double-blind one and the long-term effect was variable.

Almitrine Bismesylate. A new ventilatory stimulant, which acts by increasing the ventilatory flow and by improving the $\dot{V}/\dot{Q}$ ratio, is supposed to decrease apneas during sleep by increasing the ventilatory drive, but this hypothesis has not been confirmed. In eight patients with SAS, who were given 200 mg per day almitrine bismesylate, no reduction in the number of apneas, either central or obstructive in type, could be observed [46]. The only significant effect was a reduction of the mean duration of respiratory events in NREM sleep but not in REM sleep, which perhaps resulted from the stimulation of peripheral chemoreceptors by the drug. This decrease was significant for hypopneas, both obstructive and mixed apneas, but surprisingly, not so for central apneas.

Doxapram. Given intravenously, doxapram also failed to reduce the number of sleep-related apneas, but according to Surrat et al. [84] improved SaO_2, probably by reducing the duration of the respiratory arrests.

Theophylline. Widely used in infants showing respiratory arrests or in adults with chronic obstructive lung diseases, theophylline has only recently been tried in adults with OSA [57]. According to Mayer et al. long-term treatment with theophylline resulted in marked decrease in pulmonary arterial pressure together with a significant reduction of apnea and hypopnea index. However, using the same drug in both acute and chronic administration, Guilleminault and Hayers [33] obtained clearly negative results.

Actually, all these ventilation-stimulating drugs act simultaneously on both the diaphragm and the upper airway muscles; consequently, they maintain the imbalance observed in OSA between the activity of the diaphragm and that of the upper airway muscles. Only a stimulant which would reinforce the upper airway muscles specifically could be effective in OSA. In animals, protriptyline, nicotine, and strychnine have been shown to act in such a way [5], but in man, their beneficial effect has not been established.

Miscellaneous Drugs

Besides ventilatory stimulants and antidepressant drugs, substances such as naloxone, bromocriptine, beta-blockers and tryptophan even nicotine [30] have been tried in SAS, but none of these drugs has appeared to be completely efficient [33]. The effectiveness of naloxone is still under discussion: no effect on sleep apnea has been noted by Guilleminault and Hayers [33] while Atkinson et al. [4] have observed, in a controlled study during naloxone infusion, a decrease in the average maximal oxyhemoglobin desaturation, though the number of desaturation episodes did not vary significantly. However, the 80% reduction in time spent in REM sleep could by itself explain the increase in mean SaO_2 during the night. By the use of 2500 mg of *L*-tryptophan at bedtime, Schmidt [70] observed a significant improvement in obstructive but not in central sleep apneas, especially during NREM sleep in patients with mild SAS.

Oxygen

The use of O_2 for the treatment of OSA repains controversial. Motta et al. [61], but also Martin et al. [56] and Alford et al. [2] reported a lengthening of the mean duration of the respiratory events while on O_2 therapy, which was not significant in Martin's study but highly significant in Alford's. Moreover, O_2 therapy was supposed to diminish the chemical stimulus for arousal, to worsen respiratory acidosis and to induce cardiac arrhythmias. However, Martin et al. noted in SAS patients (eight cases), who had received O_2 for 30 min (in comparison to room air breathing), a significant reduction in the total number of apneas and the percentage apnea time, as well as an attenuation of apnea-associated slowing of the heart rate. When given on a long-term basis, O_2 at a low flow during night-time decreased the number of OSA in three of five patients, but two of them lost weight concomitantly. In 20 patients with an overlap syndrome (i.e., sleep apneas and COPD), Alford et al. [2] noted that, when they were breathing O_2 instead of room air, there was a decrease in the disordered breathing events index, a reduction in SaO_2 during respiratory events and an increase in the mean nonapneic saturation. Furthermore, ventricular arrhythmias were not increased in 17 of 20 patients by supplemental O_2 and atrioventricular blocks were eliminated in two subjects.

However, though nocturnal O_2 supply could be beneficial in SAS patients, particularly in those with an associated COPD, nocturnal O_2 therapy should be administered only after close monitoring of respiration and cardiac rhythm during night sleep with and without supplemental O_2.

Finally, should one propose drug treatments for SAS? On the basis of the preceding review, the answer seems to be negative. Furthermore, it is certain that drugs could be harmful in sleep apnea patients, since several reports indicate an exacerbation of sleep apneas after the use of sedatives, hypnotics or alcohol: benzodiazepines particularly in aged people may exacerbate sleep-related apneas [12, 22, 45, 58]. Ingestion before bedtime of either vodka [24] or bourbon [31] may increase the number and duration of apneas [73]. Therefore, patients with SAS should discontinue the use of alcohol and sedatives, though further studies are necessary to establish the dose-dependent worsening of disordered breathing during sleep in patients taking alcohol or sleeping pills.

Surgical and Mechanical Treatments

Taking into account the low efficiency of drugs in the treatment of SAS, several surgical procedures and mechanical devices have been proposed since Kuhlo et al. demonstrated in 1969 the suppression of OSA by tracheostomy [47]. In the following chapter will be presented the different techniques, which, isolated or sometimes combined, have been applied to SAS patients. For each technique, the indications and effectiveness will be given on the basis of data from the literature.

Surgical Treatments

Tracheostomy

Bypassing the sleep-related upper airway obstruction, tracheostomy suppresses apneas and hypopneas which are obstructive in type. The disappearance of obstructive apneas is rapidly followed by a suppression in daytime sleepiness, and an improvement in sleep structure with a remarkable increase in deep slow-wave sleep. At the same time, most of the hypoxemic episodes vanish (except for the REM sleep-related hypoxemia), sinus arrhythmias or bradycardia are suppressed and pulmonary (and to a lesser degree systemic) arterial tension decreases. However, during the initial period following tracheostomy, an increase in central apneas and a persistent periodic breathing can be observed transitorily. All these findings have been confirmed by several authors, particularly by Lugaresi et al. [53], Coccagna et al. [17], Simmons et al. [75], and Weitzman et al. [88]. In a post-tracheostomy follow-up of 12–18 months, Guilleminault et al. [35] demonstrated an obstructive apnea index below five, together with a gradual decrease over time in the number of central apneas; however, plugging of the tracheostomy was followed in the 38 recorded patients by the recurrence of OSA, disturbances of night sleep and the reappearance of sinus arrhythmias. Therefore, it has been proposed that an uvulopalatopharyngoplasty (UPPP, see below) be performed in OSA at the same time as the tracheostomy or within a 6-week period. The hope was that after the patient's state had been stabilized by tracheostomy, the tracheostomy could be plugged, the UPPP alone being able to eliminate the obstruction of the upper airways. Only limited and unconvincing individual data are available [7].

Despite technical improvements, tracheostomy is often difficult to perform in SAS patients because of a short neck, altered oropharynx, and large amounts of fatty tissue that may interfere with the exposure of the trachea. Afterwards, granulation tissue may invade the tracheostomy site and lead to hemoptysis and tracheal obstruction; wound infections and recurrent purulent bronchitis may also occur despite the permanent skin flap proposed by Conway et al. [19].

Therefore, tracheostomy, though clearly effective in treating OSA, is physically and psychologically uncomfortable, and should be considered as an emergency treatment required only in case of severe cardiac arrhythmias or deep O_2 desaturation due to prolonged and repetitive obstructive apneas.

Nasal Surgery

It has been shown on one hand that nasal obstruction by either inflammation or allergic conditions favors the development of sleep apneas [54], and on the other hand, that increased respiratory airway resistance due to unilateral or bilateral mechanical occlusions of the nasal passages may cause an increase in respiratory events [50]. Therefore, the correction of nasal septal deformity has been used in the treatment of OSA [39, 67]. In nine out of 16 patients who underwent submucous resection of the nasal septum, the latter authors reported a reduction in diurnal somnolence, but the number of apneas decreased in four, remained stable in four, and increased in one patient [67]. With nasal surgery, an overall reduction of 50% in the apnea index has been noted in only eight of 23 patients reported by Calderelli et al. [11]. Therefore, nasal septoplasty does not appear to be a major treatment for OSA, but may be helpful and surely less invasive than UPPP.

Adenotonsillectomy

Adenotonsillar hypertrophy or tonsillar enlargement alone has been shown to favor the collapse of the upper airway muscles during sleep. Both in children [26, 55] and in adults [63, 67], the removal of tonsils has been reported to be followed by an improvement in daytime sleepiness, a reduction in snoring and a decrease, but not suppression, of the apneic events. In Rubin's five patients who underwent tonsillectomy, the apnea index, though reduced postoperatively, varied after tonsillectomy from 0.3 to 52.7. Therefore, adenotonsillectomy may be helpful for patients with OSA whatever their age; however, as far as the obstructive events are concerned, its effectiveness appears to be limited.

Reduction Plasty of the Tongue

This could also enlarge the upper airways and avoid inspiratory obstruction. Actually, as early as 1965, Gastaut et al. hypothesized that the projection of the tongue onto the posterior pharyngeal wall might cause upper airway obstruction [29]. More recently, this has been well-documented by Harper's study of genioglossal activity during sleep and sleep-related apneas. In a single patient with acromegaly, Afzelius et al. [1] noted a marked improvement after taking out a V-shaped wedge from anterior to posterior, parallel to the midline and extending posteriorly from the midportion of the mobile part of the tongue toward the base of the tongue.

Mandibular Surgery

The high frequency of OSA in children with Pierre Robin syndrome or in adults with retrognathia is well-known. Cephalometric studies have shown that most of these patients have an obtuse mentocervical angle, a chin deficiency, and usually a class II dental malocclusion. Therefore, the position of the tongue in the oropharynx is more posterior and hypotonia of the genioglossus seems more likely to produce an obstruction of the upper airways. These findings have led to new surgical techniques such as mandibular advancement and mandibular osteotomy with hyoid bone advancement.

Total Mandibular Advancement

This consists of advancing the lower mandibular segment with concomitant advancement of the tongue musculature so as to increase the hypopharyngeal space [65]. This rather complicated surgical procedure has only been performed on a few SAS patients (particularly on patients in whom the beneficial effect of UPPP was poor) and improvements in OSA have been poorly documented [65, 80]. Finally, this technique, which requires an intermaxillary fixation lasting 6 weeks and results in a change in dental occlusion, in the absence of concomitant maxillary advancement seems indicated only in highly selected patients, submitted to preoperative polygraphic monitoring with and without the use of a mandibular positioning device [3].

Mandibular Osteotomy and Hyoid Bone Advancement

This consists of an antero-inferior mandibular osteotomy [49]; this portion, which is the site of attachment of the genioglossus, is then pushed forward and secured to the maxilla with intraosseous wires. Concomitantly, the infrahyoid muscles are transected, allowing the hyoid bone to be pulled more anteriorly and superiorly; the fascia is placed around the hyoid body and the bone is suspended anteriorly [66]. The preliminary results in five patients appear promising, since in these cases the enlargement of the hypopharyngeal airways resulted in a drop in the obstructive apnea (OA) index.

At the same time, Kaya [42] suggested, based on three cases, that a medial sectioning of the body of an abnormally thickened hyoid bone along its vertical axis could suppress the OSA.

Uvulopalatopharyngoplasty (UPPP)

In the 15 years since Ikematsu's report on the effectiveness of excision of the pillar mucosa and partial resection of the uvula in suppressing snoring, Fujita et al. [27] have proposed uvulopharyngoplasty using a modified technique as a treatment for OSA. The widening of the oropharynx by a combination of tonsillectomy and removal of redundant mucosa and soft tissues of the uvula, soft palate, posterior pharyngeal walls and posterior pillars was thought to decrease upper airway resistance during sleep and thereby alleviate the obstructive respiratory arrests. Actually, eight of the 12 patients initially reported by Fujita et al. experienced a reduction in the apnea index together with an improvement in night sleep and a reduced tendency for daytime sleepiness. Later on, 33 out of 66 patients were considered by Fujita et al. [28] as responders to UPPP (i.e., showing a minimum of 50% reduction in the apnea index); in these patients, not only the number of apneas, but also their duration, the number of arousals associated with the resumption of respiration, the time during which SaO_2 was below 85% and the lowest SaO_2, were all significantly improved by about 50%. Nonresponders showed only less hypoxemia during sleep. After 1 year, polysomnographic evaluations were obtained for the 20 out of the 33 responders: the initial benefit, including a low apnea index, was maintained in those patients whose body weight remained stable [71]; each increase in weight was followed by an increase in OA [18]. Similar results after UPPP were reported by Guilleminault et al. [34] and Thawley [86], whereas in the study of De Berry-Borowiecki et al. [6] only 23% of patients with a moderate OSA syndrome had a significant reduction in the OA index after UPPP. In these studies the variables that distinguished responders from nonresponders had been: (a) body weight: only patients with more than 125% above ideal body weight were responders; (b) the site of obstruction: UPPP is only indicated in oropharyngeal obstruction without hypopharyngeal obstruction. The site of obstruction can be evaluated by cephalometrics and fiberoptic studies associated with the Müller maneuver [74]. By use of these selective criteria, a 72% reduction of the preoperative apnea index has been demonstrated after UPPP by Sher et al. [74].

Therefore, if a 50%–70% reduction in OSA would appear to be sufficient to prevent any complication due to the persisting 30%–50% of OSA, UPPP should be considered as useful. However, this technique modifies the palate, and complications due to changes in palatal function may occur (i.e., nasal regurgitation, nasal voice, dryness of the throat or even, in the case of an excessively extensive resection of the posterior pillars, naso-pharyngeal-palatal stenosis) [43].

Mechanical Treatments

Tongue-Retaining Device

A device which holds the tongue in a forward position has been used by Cartwright and Samelson [15]. This rather uncomfortable device reduced the number and duration of sleep-related apneas and improved the sleep architecture in 11 out of 16 patients. An increased severity of apneas associated with the supine sleep position [38] appeared to be the strongest indicator of the effectiveness of the tongue-retaining device. However, this device, given that it blocks the oral airway, cannot be used in OSA patients suffering from nasal disease.

Mandibular Positioning Appliance

This appliance has also been used successfully in children and adults with a hypoplastic mandible and moderate micrognathia.

Sleep Position Training

By wearing a gravity-activated position alarm on the chest, ten SAS patients have been trained to avoid the supine sleep position. According to Cartwright et al. [13, 14] number of sleep apneas and O_2 desaturation were significantly reduced in these patients.

Continuous Nasal Positive Airway Pressure (nCPAP)

This appears to be, since Sullivan et al. [83] first reported their results, the most promising and the most effective way of treating OSA. However, the following reports in this volume will provide further information concerning the technique used, the mostly positive results, as well as the inconveniences of this device.

Conclusions

During the past 20 years, weight loss, drugs, surgical procedures, and mechanical devices have been proposed for the treatment of SAS. Nevertheless, at present, it appears quite impossible to define clear-cut guideline for treating sleep apnea patients, since several questions remain without definite answers.

First, should all sleep apnea patients be submitted to treatment and should the same treatment be applied to severe, mild, or even asymptomatic SAS? Furthermore, on which basis should the classification according to graduated severity be based: number of apneas per hour of sleep; night-time or daytime hypoxemia; cardiac disturbances?

Secondly, which criteria should be used to evaluate improvement or curing of the SAS? Are all the SAS-related symptoms equally important: daytime sleepiness, overweight, number and duration of sleep apneas, hypoxemia, cardiac arrhythmias, pulmonary or systemic hypertension? To what degree is improvement in these symptoms required for the applied treatment to be considered as fully or partially effective [69]? If a decrease in daytime sleepiness associated with a variable decrease in the sleep apnea index is considered to be satisfactory, then weight loss, protriptyline treatment, nasal surgery, tongue-retaining devices or UPPP (though all only partially effective) could be chosen as therapeutic measures. If an increase in SaO_2 during the night, despite persistence of sleep apnea, could alone prevent complications due to respiratory arrests, then O_2 therapy or ventilatory stimulants could be helpful. However, if a suppression of all the obstructive apneas is required, tracheostomy, or better still nCPAP, would appear to be the most adequate treatment.

A clear answer to all these questions can only be possible if, in the near future, carefully designed, long-term studies using homogeneous groups of SAS patients become available. Therefore, until these answers can be obtained, the treatment of SAS should be as harmless as possible, thus, in our opinion, sophisticated surgical procedures are probably indicated in only a few, highly selected sleep apnea patients.

References

1. Afzelius L, Elmqvist D, Laurin S (1982) Sleep apnea syndrome caused by acromegalia and treatment with reduction plasty of the tongue. J Otorhinolaryngol Relat Spec 42:142–145
2. Alford NJ, Fletcher EC, Nickeson D (1986) Acute oxygen in patients with sleep apnea and COPD. Chest 89:30–38

3. Andrews JM, Guilleminault C, Holdaway RA (1983) Retaining devices and mandibular positioning appliances. Bull Eur Physiopathol Respir 19:611
4. Atkinson RL, Suratt PM, Wilhoit SC, Recant L (1985) Naloxone improves sleep apnea in obese humans. Int J Obes 9:233-239
5. Bonora M, St John WM, Bledsoe TA (1985) Differential elevation by protriptyline and depression by diazepam of upper airway respiratory motor activity. Am Rev Respir Dis 131:41-45
6. Borowiecki B, Kukwa AA, Blanks RHI (1985) Indications for palatopharyngoplasty. Arch Otolaryngol 111:659-663
7. Borowiecki B, Sassin JF (1983) Surgical treatment of sleep apnea. Arch Otolaryngol 109:508-512
8. Browman CP, Sampson MG, Yolles SF, Gujavarty KS, Weiler SJ, Walsleben JA, Hahn PM, Mitler MM (1984) Obstructive sleep apnea and body weight. Chest 85:435-463
9. Brownell LG, West P, Sweatman P, Acres JC, Kryger MH (1982) Protriptyline in obstructive sleep apnea. A double-blind trial. N Engl J Med 307:1037-1042
10. Burwell CS, Robin ED, Whaley RD, Bickelman AG (1956) Extreme obesity associated with alveolar hypoventilation. A pickwickian syndrome. Am J Med 21:811-818
11. Caldarelli DD, Cartwright RD, Lilie JK (1985) Obstructive sleep apnea: variations in surgical management. Laryngoscope 95:1070-1073
12. Carskadon MA; Dement WC (1981) Respiration during sleep in the aged human. J Gerontol 36:420-423
13. Cartwright RD (1984) Effect of sleep position on sleep apnea severity. Sleep 7:110-114
14. Cartwright RD, Lloyd S, Lilie J, Kravitz H (1985) Sleep position training as treatment for sleep apnea syndrome: a preliminary study. Sleep 8:87-94
15. Cartwright RD, Samelson CF (1982) The effect of a non surgical treatment for obstructive sleep apnea. JAMA 248:705-709
16. Clark RW, Schmidt HS, Schaal SF, Boudoulas M, Schuller DE (1979) Sleep apnea: treatment with protriptyline. Neurology 29:1287-1292
17. Coccagna G, Mantovani M, Brignani F, Parchi C, Lugaresi E (1972) Tracheostomy in hypersomnia with periodic breathing. Bull Physiopathol Respir 8:1217-1227
18. Conway WA, Fujita S, Zorick F, Sicklesteel J, Roehrs T, Wittig R, Roth T (1985) Uvulopalatopharyngoplasty. One year follow-up. Chest 88:385-387
19. Conway WA, Victor LD, Magilligan DJ, Fujita S, Zorick FJ, Roth T (1981) Adverse effects of tracheostomy for sleep apnea. JAMA 246:347-350
20. Conway WA, Zorick F, Hartse K, Piccione P, Roth T (1979) Protriptyline in the treatment of sleep apnea. Chest 76:349 (abstract)
21. Conway WA, Zorick F, Piccione P, Roth T (1982) Protriptyline in the treatment of sleep apnoea. Thorax 37:49-53
22. Dolly FR, Block AJ (1982) Effect of flurazepam on sleep disordered breathing and nocturnal oxygen desaturation in normal subjects. Am J Med 73:239-243
23. Dolly FR, Block AJ (1983) Medroxyprogesterone acetate and COPD. Effects on breathing and oxygenation in sleeping and awake patients. Chest 84:394-398
24. Dolly FR, Block AJ (1983) Increased ventricular ectopy and sleep apnea following ethanol ingestion in COPD patients. Chest 83:469-472
25. Eliaschar L, Lavie P, Halperin E, Gordon C, Elroy E (1980) Apneic episodes as indications for adenotonsillectomy. Arch Otolaryngol 8:492-496
26. Fairman RP, Sugerman HJ (1982) Gastroplasty for obstructive sleep apnea and morbid obesity. Am Rev Respir Dis 125:108 (abstract)
27. Fujita S, Conway WA, Zorick F, Roth T (1981) Surgical correction of anatomic abnormalities in obstructive sleep apnea: uvulopalatopharyngoplasty. Otolaryngol Head Neck Surg 89:923-934
28. Fujita S, Conway W, Zorick F, Sicklesteel J, Roehrs T, Wittig R, Roth T (1983) Evaluation of the effectiveness of uvulopalatopharyngoplasty. Sleep Res 12:248 (abstract)
29. Gastaut H, Tassinari CA, Duron B (1965) Etude polygraphique des manifestations épisodiques (hypniques et respiratoires) du syndrome de Pickwick. Rev Neurol 112:568-579
30. Gothe B, Strohl KP, Levin S, Cherniack NS (1985) Nicotine: a different approach to the treatment of obstructive sleep apnea. Chest 87:11-17

31. Guilleminault C (1980) Sleep apnea syndromes: impact of sleep and sleep states. Sleep 3:227-234
32. Guilleminault C, Eldridge FL, Tilkian A, Simmons FB, Dement WC (1977) Sleep apnea syndrome due to upper airway obstruction: a review of 25 cases. Arch Intern Med 137:296-300
33. Guilleminault C, Hayes B (1983) Naloxone, theophylline, bromocriptine and obstructive sleep apnea. Negative results. Bull Eur Physiopathol Respir 19:632-634
34. Guilleminault C, Hayes B, Smith L, Simmons FB (1983) Palatopharyngoplasty and obstructive sleep apnea syndrome. Bull Eur Physiopathol Respir 19:595-599
35. Guilleminault C, Simmons B, Motta J, Cummiskey J, Rosekind M, Schroeder JS, Dement WC (1981) Obstructive sleep apnea syndrome and tracheostomy. Long-term follow-up experience. Arch Intern Med 141:985-989
36. Guilleminault C, Van den Hoed J, Mittler MM (1978) Clinical overview of the sleep apnea syndromes. In: Guilleminault C, Dement WC (eds) Sleep apnea syndromes. Liss, New York, pp 1-12
37. Harman EM, Wynne JW, Block AJ (1982) The effect of weight loss on sleep disordered breathing and oxygen desaturation in morbidly obese men. Chest 82:291-294
38. Harper RM, Sauerland EK (1978) The role of the tongue in sleep apnea. In: Guilleminault C, Dement WC (eds) Sleep apnea syndrome. Liss, New York, pp 219-234
39. Heimer D, Scharf SM, Lieberman A, Lavie P (1983) Sleep apnea syndrome treated by repair of nasal septum deviation. Chest 84:184-185
40. Ingbar DH, Gee BE (1985) Pathophysiology and treatment of sleep apnea. Annu Rev Med 36:369-395
41. Jung R, Kuhlo W (1965) Neurophysiological studies of abnormal night sleep and the pickwickian syndrome. In: Abert K, Bally C, Stradé JP (eds) Sleep mechanisms. Progress in brain res, vol 18. Elsevier, pp 140-159
42. Kaya N (1984) Sectioning the hyoid bone as a therapeutic approach for obstructive sleep apnea. Sleep 7:77-78
43. Kramer M, Anand VK, Schoen L, Draper E (1985) Death associated with uvulopalatopharyngoplasty: a case report. Sleep Res 14:180 (abstract)
44. Krieger J, Mangin P, Kurtz D (1979) Syndrome d'apnées au cours du sommeil: effet de la chlorimipramine chez des sujets à poids stable. Rev Electroencephalogr Neurophysiol Clin 9:250-257
45. Krieger J, Mangin P, Kurtz D (1980) Les modifications respiratoires au cours du sommeil du sujet âgé normal. Rev Electroencephalogr Neurophysiol Clin 10:177-185
46. Krieger J, Mangin P, Kurtz D (1982) Effects of a ventilatory stimulant, almitrine bismesylate, in the sleep apnea syndrome. Curr Ther Res 32:697-705
47. Kuhlo W, Doll E, Franck MC (1969) Erfolgreiche Behandlung eines Pickwick-Syndroms durch eine Dauertrachealkanüle. Dtsch Med Wochenschr 94:1286-1290
48. Kumashiro H, Sato M, Hirata J, Baba O, Otsuki S (1971) Sleep apnoea and sleep regulating mechanisms. A case effectively treated with monochlorimipramine. Folia Psychiatr Neurol Jpn 25:41-49
49. Kuo PC, West RA, Bloomquist DS, McNeil RW (1979) The effect of mandibular osteotomy in three patients with hypersomnia sleep apnea. Oral Surg 48:385-392
50. Lavie P, Fischel N, Zomer J, Eliaschar I (1983) The effects of partial and complete mechanical occlusion of the nasal passages on sleep structure and breathing in sleep. Acta Otolaryngol 95:161-166
51. Lombard RM, Zwillich CW (1985) Medical therapy of obstructive sleep apnea. Med Clin North Am 69:1317-1355
52. Lugaresi E, Coccagna G, Mantovani M (1978) Hypersomnia with periodic apneas. In: Weitzman E (ed) Advances in sleep research, vol 4. Spectrum, New York
53. Lugaresi E, Coccagna E, Mantovani M, Brignani F (1970) Effets de la trachéotomie dans les hypersomnies avec respiration périodique. Rev Neurol 123:267-268
54. McNicholas WT, Tarlo S, Cole P, Zamel N, Rutherford R, Griffin D, Phillipson EA (1982) Obstructive apneas during sleep in patients with seasonal allergic rhinitis. Am Rev Respir Dis 126:625-628

55. Mangat D, Orr WC, Smith RO (1977) Sleep apnea, hypersomnolence and upper airway obstruction secondary to adenotonsillar enlargment. Arch Otolaryngol 103:383–386
56. Martin RJ, Sanders MH, Gray BA, Pennock BE (1982) Acute and long-term ventilatory effects of hyperoxia in the adult sleep apnea syndrome. Am Rev Respir Dis 125:175–180
57. Mayer J, Fuchs E, Hügens M (1984) Long term theophylline therapy of sleep apnea syndrome. Am Rev Respir Dis 129 [Suppl]: A252
58. Mendelson WB, Garnett D, Gillin JC (1981) Flurazepam induced sleep apnea syndrome in a patient with insomnia and mild sleep-related respiratory changes. J Nerv Ment Dis 169:261–264
59. Mitler MM, Weiler S, Walsleben J, Reitman MD, Hahn PM (1981) Obstructive sleep apnea: improvement with weight loss. Sleep Res 10:215
60. Moran WB, Orr WC (1985) Diagnostic and management of obstructive sleep apneas. Arch Otolaryngol 111:650–658
61. Motta J, Guilleminault C (1978) Effects of oxygen administration in sleep induced apneas. In: Guilleminault C, Dement WC (eds) Sleep apnea syndromes. Liss, New York, pp 137–144
62. Orr WC, Imes NK, Martin RJ (1979) Progesterone therapy in obese patients with sleep apnea. Arch Int Med 139:109–111
63. Orr WC, Martin RJ (1981) Obstructive sleep apnea associated with tonsillar hypertrophy in adults. Arch Int Med 141:990–992
64. Peiser J, Lavie P, Ovnat A, Charuzi I (1984) Sleep apnea syndrome in the morbidly obese as an indication for weight reduction surgery. Ann Surg 199:112–115
65. Powell N, Guilleminault C, Riley R, Smith L (1983) Mandibular advancement and obstructive sleep apnea syndrome. Bull Eur Physiopathol Respir 19:607–610
66. Riley R, Guilleminault C, Powell N, Derman J (1984) Mandibular osteotomy and hyoid bone advancement for obstructive sleep apnea: a case report. Sleep 7:79–82
67. Rubin AHE, Eliaschar I, Joachim Z, Alroy G, Lavie P (1983) Effects of nasal surgery and tonsillectomy on sleep apnea. Bull Eur Physiopathol Respir 19:612–615
68. Sampson MG, Wu CP, Gujavarty KS, Hahn PM (1984) Weight loss in obstructive sleep apnea. Sleep Res 13:162 (abstract)
69. Sanders MH, Rogers RM (1985) Sleep apnea: when does better become benefit? Chest 88:320–321
70. Schmidt HS (1983) *L*-Tryptophan in the treatment of impaired respiration in sleep. Bull Eur Physiopathol Respir 19:625–629
71. Schoen LS, Weisenberger S, Anand JK, Draper E, Kramer M (1985) Long term effectiveness of uvulopalatopharyngoplasty. Sleep Res 14:212 (abstract)
72. Schwartz BA, Rochemaure J (1973) Syndrome pickwickien. Traitement par la chlorimipramine. Nouv Presse Med 2:1520
73. Scrima L, Broudy M, Nay KN, Cohn MA (1982) Increased severity of obstructive sleep apnea after bedtime alcohol ingestion: diagnostic potential and proposed mechanism of action. Sleep 5:318–328
74. Sher AE, Thorpy MJ, Shprintzen RJ, Spielman AJ, Burack B, McGregor PA (1985) Predictive value of Müller maneuver in selection of patients for uvulopalatopharyngoplasty. Laryngoscope 95:1483–1497
75. Simmons FB, Guilleminault C, Dement WC, Tilkian AG, Hill M (1977) Surgical management of airway obstructions during sleep. Laryngoscope 87:326–338
76. Skatrud JB, Dempsey JA, Kaiser DG (1978) Ventilatory response to medroxyprogesterone acetate in normal subjects: time course and mechanism. J Appl Physiol 44:939–944
77. Smith PL, Haponik EF, Allen RP, Bleecker ER (1983) The effects of protriptyline in sleep disordered breathing. Am Rev Respir Dis 127:8–13
78. Smith PL, Haponik EF, Bleecker ER (1984) The effects of oxygen in patients with sleep apnea. Am Rev Respir Dis 130:958–963
79. Smith PL, Haponik EF, Gold AR (1984) The effect of weight loss on sleep disordered breathing. Am Rev Respir Dis 129 [Suppl]: A59
80. Spire JP, Kuo PC, Campbell N (1983) Maxillo-facial surgical approach: an introduction and review of mandibular advancement. Bull Eur Physiopathol Respir 19:604–606

81. Strohl KP, Hensley MJ, Saunders NA, Scharf SM, Brown R, Ingram RH (1981) Progesterone administration and progressive sleep apneas. JAMA 245:1230-1232
82. Sugerman HJ, Fairman RP, Lindenmann AK et al (1981) Gastroplasty for respiratory insufficiency of obesity. Ann Surg 193:677-685
83. Sullivan CE, Berthon-Jones M, Issa FG (1981) Nocturnal nasal airway pressure for sleep apnea. N Engl J Med 309:112
84. Suratt PM, Brown FD, Wilhoit SC, Findley LJ (1985) Treatment of obstructive sleep apnea with a respiratory stimulant. Sleep Res 14:220 (abstract)
85. Sutton FD, Zwillich CW, Creagh CE, Pierson DJ, Weil JV (1975) Progesterone for outpatient treatment of pickwickian syndrome. Ann Intern Med 83:476-479
86. Thawley SE (1985) Surgical treatment of obstructive sleep apnea. Med Clin North Am 69:1337-1358
87. Walsh RE, Michaelson ED, Harkleroad LE, Zighelboim A, Sackner MA (1982) Upper airway obstruction in obese patients with sleep disturbance and somnolence. Ann Intern Med 76:185-192
88. Weitzman ED, Kah E, Pollak C (1980) Quantitative analysis of sleep and sleep apnea before and after tracheostomy in patients with the hypersomnia-sleep apnea syndrome. Sleep 3:407-423
89. White DP, Zwillich CW, Pickett CK, Douglas NJ, Findley LJ, Weil JV (1982) Central sleep apnea. Improvement with acetazolamide therapy. Arch Intern Med 142:1816-1819

Five Years' Experience with Home Nasal Continuous Positive Airway Pressure Therapy for the Obstructive Sleep Apnea Syndrome*

F. Issa, R. Grunstein, J. Bruderer, L. Costas, V. McCauley, M. Berthon-Jones, and C. Sullivan

Introduction

Snoring sickness or obstructive sleep apnea (OSA) is now a well-recognized disorder which affects a relatively large percentage of the population [8]. Its two cardinal symptoms, excessive daytime sleepiness and chronic habitual snoring, should arouse the suspicion of the clinician to the presence of the disorder.

A number of approaches have been employed to treat OSA. Tracheostomy became the treatment of choice once upper airway obstruction was recognized as a key event [6]. Protriptyline and medroxyprogesterone are the two most commonly used drugs for the treatment of OSA [9, 11]. Surgical procedures aimed at enlarging the size of the upper airway [17] or reduction of body weight [12] have also been employed. We reported the successful management of OSA using nasal continuous positive airway pressure (nCPAP) in 1981 [14]. This form of treatment is based on the fact that collapse of the oropharyngeal airway is the underlying mechanism in OSA. Low levels of nCPAP physically support the collapsing structures (soft palate and tongue) and maintain the patency of the upper airway during sleep. Nasal CPAP is a simple, noninvasive method which can be used safely at home [16]. We report here our experience with home nCPAP therapy in 222 patients with the OSA syndrome over a 5-year period.

Methods and Protocol

Each patient was started on nCPAP following a full in-hospital assessment of the severity of the disease. This included measurement of lung volumes, daytime arterial blood gases, chest X-ray, ECG, thyroid function tests, full blood count, and biochemical profile. In selected patients a CT scan of the upper airway was performed. The severity of the disorder was assessed earlier through an all-night sleep study which provided the control data for sleep pattern and apnea indices.

In-hospital treatment with nCPAP was recommended for patients with moderate to severe OSA. The level of nCPAP required to induce quiet breathing was established in each patient using a circuit shown in Fig. 1. Patient education aimed at understanding the underlying mechanisms of the disorder and descrip-

* Supported by grants from the National Health and Medical Research Council of Australia.

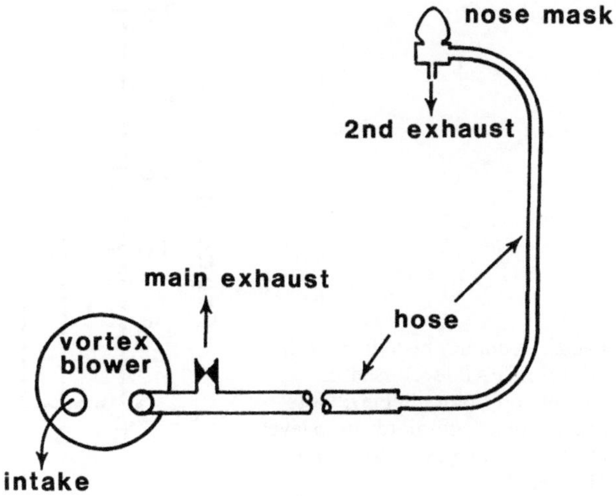

Fig. 1. Schematic diagram of home nCPAP system used to deliver a predetermined level of CPAP. A blower provides a high flow of room air. The main exhaust is placed near the blower, while the second exhaust could be placed anywhere within the connecting tubing system. A glue or nonglue nose mask is fitted to the nose

tion of the nCPAP system was carried out before discharge from the hospital. A large variety of prototype masks have been tried. In the first 3 years the basic mask consisted of an individually moulded nose mask which was glued to the nose with silastic (Elastomer 382, Dow Corning, USA). However, many patients were tried with nonglue varieties of this mask, and then in the last 2 years a variety of self-sealing masks has been in use.

The follow-up included frequent visits to the outpatient department. Repeat all-night sleep studies with and without nCPAP were performed at 6- and 12-month periods in order to examine the response to home treatment.

Results and Comments

The anthropometric data of OSA patients on home nCPAP are summarized in Table 1. The variability in nCPAP levels required to prevent upper airway obstruction is demonstrated in Fig. 2. Usually, 1–2 cmH_2O nCPAP higher than the level for NREM apneas was required for REM apneas. The intrasubject variability of nCPAP did not correlate with the severity of the disease. Patients were sent home with the nCPAP device set at 2–3 cmH_2O higher than the critical level of nCPAP. Two groups of patients required relatively higher levels of nCPAP

Table 1. Anthropometric data of patients on home nCPAP therapy

n	222
Male: female	10:1
Age (years)	13– 70
Weight (kg)	42–190
Height (cm)	152–197

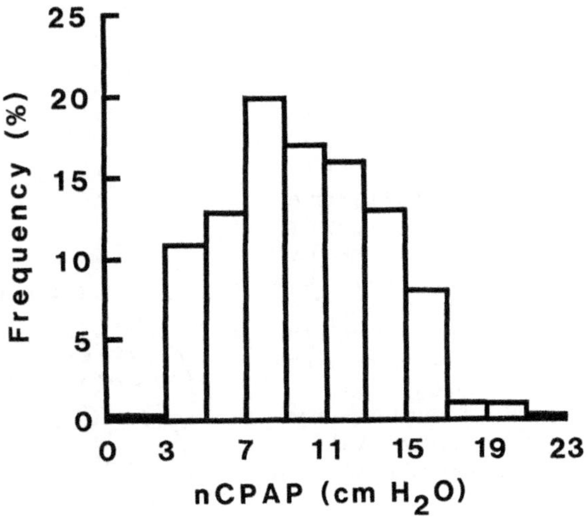

Fig. 2. Frequency histogram of the critical nCPAP level used in patients on home therapy. Note that the most commonly used level of pressure ranges between 7 and 13 cmH_2O

(range 15–20 cmH_2O). These were the patients with severe obesity-hypoventilation syndrome and patients with small nares. The level of CPAP measured at the nares in the latter group of patients does not represent the level at the oropharynx; much of the required pressure is dissipated at the nose.

Immediate Effects of nCPAP Therapy

Nasal CPAP prevented OSA in all patients, thus preventing sleep fragmentation and repetitive hypoxemia. Once apneas ceased to occur, the patient entered into long epochs of stage 3/4 NREM and REM sleep. The first noticeable effect immediately after the use of nCPAP is the disappearance of excessive daytime sleepiness; the patient stays awake for the entire day following the first night of treatment.

First Week of nCPAP Therapy

Continuous use of nCPAP leads to a further improvement in daytime alertness. Rebound of stage 3/4 NREM and REM sleep persists throughout the 1st week of treatment [4]. Discontinuation of nCPAP at this stage of treatment results in the reappearance of OSA within the first 10–15 min of sleep, and the re-emergence of excessive daytime sleep on the following day.

Of particular interest to the clinician is the treatment of patients with the severe obesity-hypoventilation syndrome. These patients are usually irritable and require special nursing care [15]. The upper airway is usually edematous in these patients, mainly due to repetitive trauma associated with the obstructive episodes. During the first few nights of nCPAP therapy, these patients develop rapid diuresis and an increase in hematocrit value. Since most of these patients are on diuretics for the associated congestive heart failure, a reduction or cessation of the drug is recommended. Continuation of nCPAP treatment reduces the edema of the soft palate and uvula thus increasing the size of the oropharyngeal airway. During the first 7–10 days of treatment this usually leads to a reduction of 3–5 cmH_2O in the nCPAP level required in these patients.

The rebound of deep sleep, particularly the long episodes of REM sleep, might impose a potentially dangerous situation in patients with severe obesity-hypoventilation syndrome. REM sleep is characterized by the depression of a variety of respiratory reflexes [2, 13] and an increase in arousal threshold to these stimuli [3]. In addition, the "abnormal" REM sleep recorded during a few nights of treatment is characterized by a depression of arousability for a variety of auditory, tactile, and other nonrespiratory stimuli in these patients. Selection of a subcritical level of nCPAP for treatment might result in partial upper airway obstruction during the abnormally long episodes of REM sleep. The defective response to loaded breathing in these patients [7], associated with the decrease in chemosensitivity and increased threshold to arousal, allows long periods of hypoventilation and dangerous hypoxemia to occur [5].

Long-Term Effects of Home nCPAP Therapy

Acceptance of home nCPAP is very high. The majority of patients use nCPAP for > 7 h/night, 7 nights per week. However, even though some patients may still use it less frequently, they do not report any daytime symptoms. In our experience, a minimum treatment of 3 nights per week is required before the reappearance of daytime symptoms. In those patients who elect not to use nCPAP frequently, the single most important motive to reuse nCPAP is the re-emergence of excessive daytime somnolence.

Long-term use of nCPAP does not lead to the total disappearance of OSA but it restores a normal sleep pattern. In a sample of six nonobese OSA patients, 2–3 years of home therapy resulted in a decrease in the group mean duration of apnea from 32.5 ± 2.0 to 27.0 ± 1.0 s ($p < 0.05$). This was associated with a concomitant decrease in apnea index (control: 55 ± 5, nCPAP: 18 ± 3 apneas per hour). There was also a significant improvement in the level of SaO_2 occurring during the obstructive episodes. The group mean lowest SaO_2 during apnea increased from $83\% \pm 1\%$ before treatment to $87\% \pm 1\%$ after treatment ($p < 0.05$). These changes were not associated with weight loss.

In our experience the most commonly reported side-effect of nCPAP therapy is nasal stuffiness. Nearly 50% of patients complain of nasal stuffiness, sometimes after the commencement of therapy. This side effect is either self-limited or disappears after a short period of using a nasal decongestant. However, in approximately 10% of patients, nasal stuffiness persists and requires continuous therapy (sympathomimetic or steroid nasal spray). Attempts to humidify the air may prevent this side-effect in some but not all patients.

Other possible side-effects may include irritation of the skin surrounding the nose due to the repeated use of silicone rubber or the long-term use of a mask made of irritating material. Stauffer et al. [10] have reported the occurrence of conjunctivitis from nCPAP. This side-effect is prone to occur with the use of nonglue masks. A nonfitting mask causes air to leak, usually at the junction of the cartilagenous and bony structures of the nose.

Our experience with long-term nCPAP therapy indicates that this form of therapy does not cause a deterioration in pulmonary function. Spirometry, lung volumes, and lung compliance did change in a group of patients 3–4 years after continuous use of nCPAP therapy. Nasal CPAP can also be used safely in patients with cardiac arrythmias. The improvement in the function of cardiovascular system is evident, particularly in patients with right-sided heart failure. Loss of edema in these patients is complete within the first 10 days of treatment. This improvement is partly due to a reduction in pulmonary artery pressure following the relief of nocturnal hypoxemia.

Conclusions

Nasal CPAP is a safe, noninvasive, and low-cost method for the treatment of OSA syndrome. Application of nCPAP should be started in hospital. A control all-night sleep study should first be performed in order to assess the severity of the disease. The exact level of nCPAP required to splint the upper airway should be determined rather than using a "guessed" level of nCPAP. In the majority of cases, patients' compliance depends on his/her understanding of the disorder, its symptoms, and the mechanism by which nCPAP prevents OSA. A detailed description of these facts to the patient and his/her bed partner encourages the continuous use of nCPAP.

References

1. Berthon-Jones M, Sullivan CE (1982) Ventilatory and arousal responses to hypoxia in sleeping humans. Am Rev Respir Dis 125:632–639
2. Berthon-Jones M, Sullivan CE (1984) Ventilation and arousal responses to hypercapnia in normal sleeping humans. J Appl Physiol 57:59–67
3. Bowes G, Phillipson EA (1984) Arousal responses to respiratory stimuli during sleep. In: Saunders NA, Sullivan CE (eds) Sleep and breathing. Dekker, New York, pp 137–161
4. Issa FG, Sullivan CE (1986) The immediate effects of nasal continuous positive airway pressure treatment on sleep pattern in patients with obstructive sleep apnea syndrome. Electroencephalogr Clin Neurophysiol 63:10–17
5. Krieger J, Weitzenblum E, Monassier JP, Stoeckel C, Kurtz D (1983) Dangerous hypoxemia during continuous positive airway pressure treatment of obstructive sleep apnea. Lancet II:1429–1430
6. Kuhlo W, Doll E, Frank MD (1969) Erfolgreiche Behandlung eines Pickwick-Syndroms durch eine Dauertrachealkanüle. Dtsch Med Wochenschr 94:1286–1290
7. Lopata M, Önal E (1982) Mass loading, sleep apnea, and the pathogenesis of obesity hypoventilation. Am Rev Respir Dis 126:640–645
8. Peter JH, Siegrist J, Podszus T, Mayer J, Selzer K, von Wichert P (1985) Prevalence of sleep apnea in healthy industrial workers. Klin Wochenschr 63:807–811

9. Smith PL, Haponik EF, Allen RP, Bleecker ER (1983) The effects of protriptyline in sleep-disordered breathing. Am Rev Respir Dis 127:8–13
10. Stauffer JL, Fayter NA, McLurg BJ (1984) Conjunctivitis from nasal CPAP apparatus. Chest 86:802
11. Strohl KP, Hensley MJ, Saunders NA, Scharf SM, Brown R, Ingram RH, Jr (1981) Progesterone administration and progressive sleep apneas. JAMA 245:1230–1232
12. Sugerman HJ, Fairman RP, Lindeman AK, Mathers JAL, Greenfield LJ (1981) Gastroplasty for respiratory insufficiency of obesity. Ann Surg 193:677–685
13. Sullivan CE, Kozar LF, Murphy E, Phillipson EA (1979) Arousal, ventilatory, and airway responses to bronchopulmonary stimulation in sleeping dogs. J Appl Physiol 47:17–25
14. Sullivan CE, Issa FG, Berthon-Jones M, Eves L (1981) Reversal of obstructive sleep apnea by continuous positive airway pressure applied through the nares. Lancet I:862–865
15. Sullivan CE, Berthon-Jones M, Issa FG (1983) Remission of severe obesity-hypoventilation syndrome after short-term treatment during sleep with nasal continuous positive airway pressure. Am Rev Respir Dis 128:177–181
16. Sullivan CE, Issa FG, Berthon-Jones M, McCauley VB, Costas LJV (1984) Home treatment of obstructive sleep apnea with continuous positive airway pressure applied through a nose-mask. Bull Eur Physiopathol Respir 20:49–54
17. Thawley SE (1985) Surgical treatment of obstructive sleep apnea. Med Clin North Am 69:1337–1358

Problems in the Application of Nasal Continuous Positive Airway Pressure for the Treatment of Obstructive Sleep Apnea. Hypoxemia During Sleep on Nasal Continuous Positive Airway Pressure Treatment

J. Krieger, and D. Kurtz

Introduction

Nasal continuous positive airway pressure (CPAP) as a treatment for obstructive sleep apneas (OSA) was first described 5 years ago by Sullivan et al. [15]; its efficacy has been confirmed by many authors [3, 6, 9, 10, 12–14], while others have stressed the problems they have encountered with this technique [16].

Our own experience with nasal CPAP is now 4 years old; this treatment has entered a period of routine use, especially since a commercial device reimbursed by the French health care system has become available. It seemed of interest to analyze the problems which we have encountered during this period of routine use of nasal CPAP; therefore we evaluated 35 consecutive patients over the past year. The problems we encountered were of three types: difficult acceptance, hypoxemia during sleep under nasal CPAP, and adverse effects. Because the first and the third have been largely developed elsewhere in this book, especially by Issa and Sullivan, we shall focus mainly on the problem of hypoxemia during sleep under nasal CPAP therapy.

Patients and Methods

The results reported here were obtained from 35 consecutive patients (4 women, 31 men) aged 17–75 years (mean : 52 ± SEM: 2) who were diagnosed as having an OSA syndrome on the basis of a polygraphic sleep recording (preceded by an adaptation night). The diagnostic recording was followed on the next night by a polygraphic recording while on CPAP therapy. CPAP was applied by means of a commercial device (SEFAM, Nancy, France). Both recordings included, in addition to standard EEG, EOG, and EMG of chin muscles [11], respiratory flow and volume (Fleisch No 2 pneumotachograph and Godart Statham pressure sensor and electronic integrator); thoracic and abdominal movements (mercury-filled silastic strain gauges); and ear oximetry (Hewlett Packard 47201 A). On the diagnostic night, the pneumotachograph was attached to a light airtight silicone nasobuccal mask. On the CPAP night, it was inserted in the expiratory line of the circuit, thus measuring the airflow of the CPAP device modulated by the patient's breathing; an off-set eliminated the airflow from the compressor; in addition, on the CPAP night, the applied pressure was measured in the nose mask and recorded, while a thermistor allowed one to be certain of the absence of airflow through the mouth. These polygraphic recordings were part of a set of routine examinations including, among others, pulmonary function evaluation (spirometry, body plethysmography, arterial blood gases in all patients, right heart catheterization in 20 patients).

Problems with Acceptance of Nasal CPAP Therapy

Two out of 35 patients were unable to sleep with nasal CPAP; these patients were aged 65 and 75 and were poorly motivated, which probably explains these failures.

Nasal CPAP is undoubtedly a constraining treatment with at least two components to this constraint: a physical component is related to the presence of a nasal mask, noise, and vibrations, all of which can be minimized by technical optimization of the CPAP device. A second component is a physiological one related to the changes in the mechanical conditions of breathing due to positive pressure breathing in itself; this may result in a feeling of choking. Therefore, it is important to allow the patient an adaptation period to CPAP while awake in a calm environment. Furthermore, it is of critical importance that the resistance of the expiratory line be minimal so as to avoid an increase in expiratory work which, added to the increased respiratory work due to positive pressure breathing in itself, could both impair the respiratory function and contribute to the discomfort of CPAP.

Among the 33 patients who tolerated nasal CPAP during the recorded night, 28 are presently on home treatment, the remaining five not being motivated enough to accept the constraint of nasal CPAP.

Furthermore, out of 15 other patients who had begun home treatment before the "routine period" described above, none has discontinued CPAP therapy (although some of them use it intermittently), this over a follow-up period of 1–4 years.

Hypoxemia During Sleep Under Nasal CPAP Therapy

We have previously described an OSA patient whose hypoxemia worsened while on CPAP treatment [7]. There are various reasons why OSA patients may remain hypoxemic during sleep under nasal CPAP therapy. We propose that these reasons be classified as: inadequate CPAP level, ineffective CPAP, and hypoxemia despite "effective" CPAP.

Inadequate CPAP Level

Once apneas are eliminated at a given CPAP level, patients often keep snoring. Snoring is not only an acoustic nuisance, but, as shown in Fig. 1, it may cause hypoxemia. A slight increase in the CPAP level generally results in the elimination of snoring and in an increase in SaO_2.

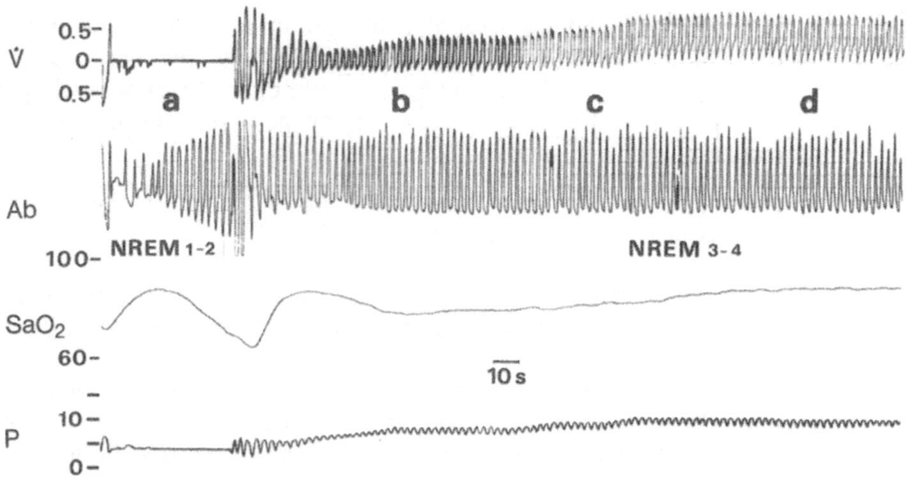

Fig. 1. Progressive achievement of an effective CPAP level. *On the left,* a pressure of 4 cmH_2O is ineffective in eliminating obstructive apneas *(a);* increasing the pressure to 8 cmH_2O eliminates apneas, but snoring persists, as indicated by vibrations on the inspiratory part of the flow curve *(b);* at 9 cmH_2O, snoring is eliminated, but the respiratory flow curve is still abnormal, with a sharp inspiratory peak followed by a plateau *(c);* only when a pressure of 10 cmH_2O is reached, does the respiratory flow curve have a normal shape *(d);* note that the elimination of snoring and the normalization of the flow curve are followed by an increase in oxyhemoglobin saturation. $\dot{V}$, respiratory flow ($l s^{-1}$; inspiration upwards); *Ab,* abdominal movements; SaO_2, oxyhemoglobin saturation (%); *P,* applied pressure (measured in the nasal mask; cmH_2O); *NREM,* non-rapid eye movement sleep; *1–2,* stage 1 or 2; *3–4,* stage 3 or 4

In addition to epidemiological studies showing an increased morbidity in snorers [5, 8], this observation further emphasizes the deleterious effects of snoring on oxygenation during sleep.

In some cases (Fig. 1), sleep is accompanied by hypoventilation and hypoxemia without snoring, which can be again corrected by an increase in CPAP, suggesting that the mechanism of hypoventilation is obstructed breathing.

In both cases, i. e. snoring and hypoventilation without snoring, the shape of the inspiratory part of the flow curve is abnormal, due to the presence of a plateau following a sharp inspiratory peak. Therefore, our criterion for an effective pressure is not only the elimination of apneas and snoring, but also the restoration of a normally shaped inspiratory flow curve (Fig. 1).

Once the effective pressure is reached, it is important to check that its efficacy is maintained throughout the night, since it very often occurs that a given pressure level, which is fully effective at the beginning of the night, becomes ineffective due to the resumption of snoring after several hours. For this reason, we consider that the minimal effective pressure cannot be established on the basis of a short recording, but requires a whole-night recording. In contrast to this intranight increase of the minimal effective pressure, there is no increase in the long term; if anything, the minimal effective pressure is decreased on the 6-month or 1-year repeat recordings, as compared to the initial recording.

Ineffective CPAP

In three patients we did not manage to reach a CPAP level which eliminated apneas. In fact, this problem overlaps with that of tolerance of nasal CPAP, since these patients (in whom pressures of 12-13 cmH_2O were ineffective) were awoken when higher pressures were applied. A detailed analysis of these three patients seems of interest: one, a 17-year-old, extremely obese girl, had hypertrophic rhinitis on the first CPAP trial; after medical treatment of her rhinitis, CPAP was efficient at a pressure of 10 cmH_2O one month later. The second patient was a 58-year-old man who was in a state of acute cardiorespiratory failure ($PaO_2 = 37$ mmHg; $PaCO_2 = 83$ mmHg) when CPAP was first applied; after 3 weeks of intensive care with tracheal intubation and respiratory assistance, a repeat recording showed that nasal CPAP eliminated sleep apneas; unfortunately, this patient did not accept home treatment and, since he lives in a remote area, we are unaware of his present condition. The third one was a 66-year-old man with an OSA syndrome associated with severe chronic obstructive pulmonary disease (COPD) [forced expiratory volume in one second over forced vital capacity ratio ($FEV_{1/FVC}$) = 0.57], and a history of several episodes of acute respiratory failure. In spite of repeated attempts, this patient was unable to tolerate pressures higher than 13 cmH_2O which failed to eliminate obstructive apneas, although it partially alleviated hypoxemia (Fig. 2).

Thus, CPAP was actually ineffective in only one out of 33 patients (3%).

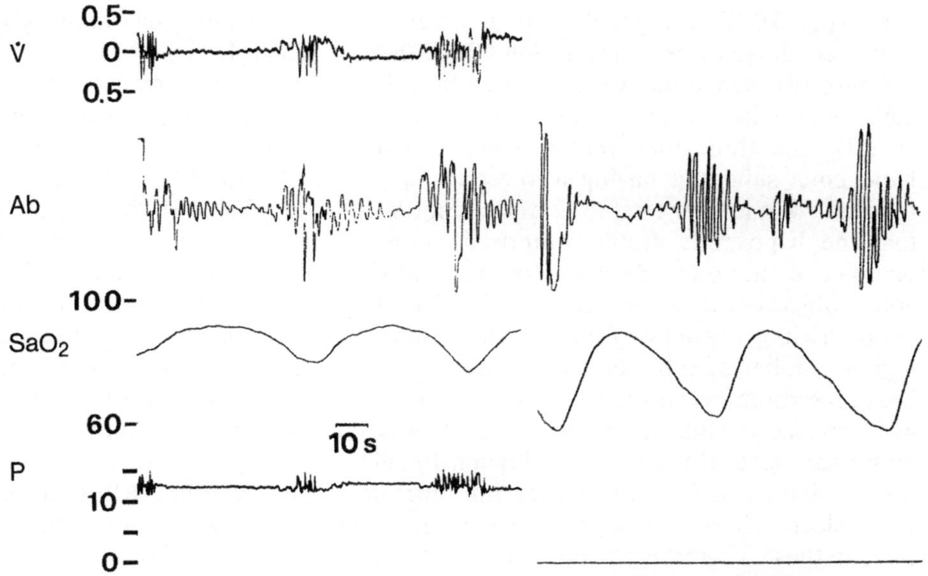

Fig. 2. Ineffective CPAP. In this patient, a pressure of 12.5 cmH_2O did not eliminate apneas *(left panel);* a higher pressure was not tolerated; note that when CPAP was discontinued, hypoxemia worsened considerably *(right panel,* respiratory flow not recorded). Abbreviations are the same as in Fig. 1

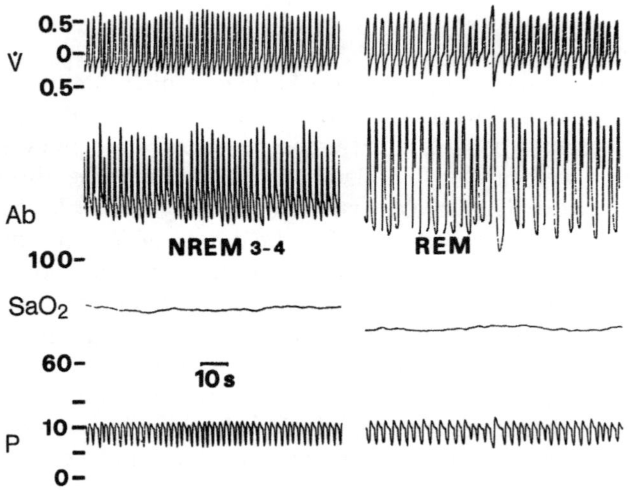

Fig. 3. Hypoxemia despite the elimination of apneas. Abbreviations are the same as in Fig. 1

Hypoxemia During Sleep Despite "Effective CPAP"

In ten patients, the minimal SaO_2 observed on nasal CPAP therapy was below 85% during NREM sleep and/or below 80% in REM sleep despite the elimination of apneas and snoring and the existence of a normally shaped inspiratory flow curve (Fig. 3). We compared these 10 patients to the 22 patients in whom SaO_2 remained above these levels during CPAP therapy (Table 1).

These two subgroups were not significantly different in age, overweight, or daytime sleepiness (as measured by their sleep latency on a multiple sleep latency test). As a whole, they were different in their respiratory parameters, the sleep hypoxemia subgroup having a lower FVC, a lower FEV_1/FVC and a higher residual volume over total lung capacity ratio (RV/TLC; Table 1); this indicates that the hypoxemic group comprised more subjects with restrictive and/or obstructive pulmonary disease. However, individual values overlapped considerably: subjects with an equally low FVC or FEV_1/FVC ratio or with equally "normal" lungs could be found in either subgroup. Probably, as a result of the higher number of subjects with pulmonary disease, the PaO_2 when awake and breathing room air was lower in the sleep hypoxemia patients as well as their presleep SaO_2, while their awake $PaCO_2$ was not different; in addition, their pulmonary arterial pressure was higher. Finally, sleep hypoxemia patients had lower minimal SaO_2 values during the untreated night, both in NREM and in REM sleep. These data suggest that the hypoxemic episodes observed during sleep in these patients are related to restrictive or obstructive pulmonary disease; however, the great overlap between individual values indicates that the factors analyzed are not the only determinants of the observed hypoxemia. This is in agreement with observations made in OSA patients after tracheostomy by Fletcher and Brown [2]. Out of 11 patients who had coexistent COPD and OSA,

Table 1. Comparison of the group of patients whose minimal oxyhemoglobin saturation (SaO_2 min) during sleep on CPAP therapy remained above 85% in NREM and above 80% in REM sleep (group A) with the group of patients whose SaO_2 min fell below either of these values (group B).

	SaO_2 min (%) NREM	SaO_2 min (%) REM	Age (years)	Over-weight (%)	Sleep latency (min)	FVC (% pre-dicted)	FEV_1/FVC (%)	RV/TLC (%)	PaO_2 (mmHg)	$PaCO_2$ (mmHg)	SaO_2w (%)	PAP (mmHg)	MEP (cmH_2O)
Group A $n = 22$	91.9 ± 0.4	89.2 ± 0.9	50.3 ± 2.1	40.8 ± 4.2	16.8 ± 1.8	96.0 ± 3.6	74.7 ± 1.9	32.8 ± 1.7	73.1 ± 1.7	40.6 ± 2.6	94.9 ± 1.6	14.2 ± 0.4 ($n = 16$)	8.7 ± 0.5
Group B $n = 10$	75.1 ± 3.3	63.5 ± 4.7 ($n = 8$)	52.3 ± 4.9	54.1 ± 10.0	15.8 ± 3.7	82.2 ± 3.8	65.5 ± 3.1	39.8 ± 2.4	60.6 ± 3.9	43.9 ± 2.4	90.4 ± 1.3 ($n = 9$)	20.5 ± 1.4 ($n = 4$)	10.2 ± 0.4
			NS	NS	NS	$p < 0.05$	$p < 0.02$	$p < 0.05$	$p < 0.01$	NS	$p < 0.001$	$p < 0.05$	$p < 0.05$

FVC, forced vital capacity; FEV_1, forced expiratory volume in one second; RV, residual volume; TLC, total lung capacity; PaO_2, $PaCO_2$, arterial oxygen and carbon dioxide tension while awake breathing room air; SaO_2w, oxyhemoglobin saturation before sleep onset on the diagnostic recording night; PAP, mean pulmonary arterial pressure; MEP, minimal effective pressure (i.e., level of CPAP which restored a normally shaped inspiratory flow curve); NS, not significant (data are presented as means ± SEM).

6 had hypoxemic episodes after tracheostomy, while 5 had none. The two groups were not different in terms of pulmonary function state. However, our results contradict the assumption made by Fletcher and Brown [2] that desaturation would not occur in apneic subjects free of intrinsic lung disease, since three of our sleep hypoxemia subjects had normal lungs. This demonstrates that lung disease is probably only one of several factors contributing to hypoxemia during sleep in CPAP-treated patients. One possible important factor, which was not explored in our study, nor in the aforementioned post-tracheostomy study [2], is an impaired chemosensitivity. If impaired chemosensitivity played a major role, one could expect a progressive improvement of chemosensitivity after elimination of sleep apneas with nasal CPAP, similar to the one described after treatment of OSA with tracheostomy [1, 4]; thus, hypoxemic episodes should disappear over time.

Nasal CPAP by itself cannot be considered to be a cause of the observed hypoxemia, since a comparison of the presleep values of SaO_2 on CPAP with the presleep values without CPAP shows that they were significantly lower in the non-sleep-hypoxemia group (93.9% vs. 94.9%, $p < 0.05$) but not different in the sleep hypoxemia group (90.0% vs. 90.4%, NS).

In those patients who experienced severe, prolonged hypoxemia during sleep, low-flow oxygen therapy, in association with nasal CPAP, has proved to be well-tolerated in our experience and helpful in maintaining a satisfactory oxygenation during sleep (Fig. 4) just as it was in tracheostomized OSA patients [2]. This associated treatment, which may be especially recommended for patients with pulmonary hypertension, warrants further investigation. Whether oxygen therapy may accelerate the restoration of normal chemosensitivity is not yet known. In this respect, ventilatory stimulants, especially those known to stimulate chemoreceptors, could theoretically be helpful in association with nasal CPAP, but they have not been systematically investigated in these patients.

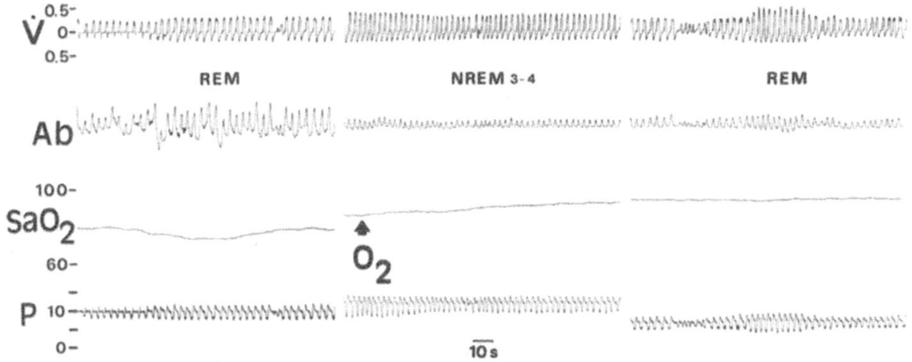

Fig. 4. Effects of additional low-flow oxygen therapy (2 liters per minute) in a patient who remained hypoxemic both in REM sleep (SaO_2 circa 75%) and in NREM sleep (SaO_2 circa 80%) before oxygen was started *(arrow)*. When low-flow oxygen is associated to CPAP, SaO_2 is maintained above 90% during NREM sleep and during REM sleep, despite irregular breathing typical of REM sleep

Adverse Effects

The only adverse effects we observed were skin irritation due to the nasal mask and complaints of a stuffy nose objectified by a hyperhemic nasal mucosa; this reaction, which we attribute to the heating of the air by the compressor, improved with local symptomatic therapy. It may be prevented in predisposed patients by humidification of the inspired air.

Of the 15 patients who underwent repeated follow-up examinations, none showed aggravation of either ventilatory performances or pulmonary hemodynamics after follow-up periods of 1–4 years.

In conclusion, nasal CPAP therapy is undoubtedly a constraining treatment. Nevertheless, the problems which arise with its use can be minimized when both the patient and physician are motivated and by optimizing the CPAP device and nasal mask, strictly defining the minimal effective pressure, and by associating low-flow oxygen therapy when the patients remain hypoxemic during sleep despite the elimination of sleep apneas. Under these conditions, nasal CPAP, as underlined by Kurtz in this volume, is clearly the most effective and safe treatment for OSA.

References

1. Aubert-Tulkens G, Willems B, Veritier C, Coche E, Stanescu DC (1980) Increase in ventilatory response to CO_2, following tracheostomy in obstructive sleep apnea. Bull Eur Physiopathol Respir 16:587–593
2. Fletcher EC, Brown DL (1985) Nocturnal oxyhemoglobin desaturation following tracheostomy for obstructive sleep apnea. Am J Med 79:35–42
3. Frith RW, Cant BR (1985) Severe obstructive sleep apnoea treated with long term nasal continuous positive airway pressure. Thorax 40:45–50
4. Guilleminault C, Cummiskey J (1982) Progressive improvement of apnea index and ventilatory response to CO_2, after tracheostomy in obstructive sleep apnea syndrome. Am Rev Respir Dis 126:14–20
5. Koskenvuo M, Kaprio J, Partinen M, Langinvainio H, Sarna S, Heikkila K (1985) Snoring as a risk factor for hypertension and angina pectoris. Lancet 1:893–896
6. Krieger J, Sautegeau A, Sauder P, Weitzenblum E, Kurtz D (1984) Syndromes d'apnées du sommeil. Traitement par la pression positive continue par voie nasale. Presse Med 13:2559–2562
7. Krieger J, Weitzenblum E, Monassier JP, Stoeckel C, Kurtz D (1983) Dangerous hypoxaemia during continuous positive airway pressure treatment of obstructive sleep apnoea. Lancet 2:1429–1430
8. Lugaresi E, Cirignotta F, Coccagna G, Piana C (1980) Some epidemiological data on snoring and cardiocirculatory disturbances. Sleep 3:221–224
9. McEvoy RD, Thornton AT (1984) Treatment of obstructive sleep apnea syndrome with nasal continuous positive airway pressure. Sleep 7:313–325
10. Rapoport DM, Sorkin B, Garay SM, Goldring RM (1982) Reversal of the "Pickwickian syndrome" by long-term use of nocturnal nasal-airway pressure. N Engl J Med 307:931–933
11. Rechtschaffen A, Kales A (1968) A manual of standardized terminology, technique and scoring system for sleep stages of human sleep. Brain Information Service, Brain Information Institute, University of California, Los Angeles
12. Remmers JE, Sterling JA, Thorarinsson B, Kuna ST (1984) Nasal airway positive pressure in patients with occlusive sleep apnea. Am Rev Respir Dis 130:1152–1155

13. Sanders MH (1984) The effect of nasal CPAP on patterns of sleep apnea. Chest 86:839–844
14. Sanders MH, Moore SE, Eveslage J (1983) CPAP via nasal mask: a treatment for occlusive sleep apnea. Chest 83:144–145
15. Sullivan CE, Issa FG, Berthon-Jones M, Eves L (1981) Reversal of obstructive sleep apnoea by continuous positive airway pressure applied through the nares. Lancet 1:862–865
16. Wagner DR, Pollak CP, Weitzman ED (1983) Nocturnal nasal-airway pressure for sleep apnea. N Engl J Med 308:461–462

Hemodynamics in Obstructive Sleep Apnea Syndrome Patients Treated by Coninuous Positive Airway Pressure

O. MARRONE, G. FERRARA, C. MACALUSO, F. MILONE, F. CIBELLA, V. BELLIA, and G. BONSIGNORE

Introduction

Heart failure has been considered as a possible consequence of obstructive sleep apnea syndrome (OSAS): it has been pointed out that the recurrence of obstructive apneas and of the related hypoxemic episodes cause recurrent increases in pulmonary artery pressure (P_{AP}) and that in the long run a sustained pulmonary hypertension and right heart failure (RHF) may result [4, 12]. This opinion has been recently challenged by Bradley et al., who demonstrated in a large sample of patients with OSAS that RHF occurred only in those patients who exhibited hypoxemia also during daytime [3]. In any case, the prevention of oxyhemoglobin desaturation and of hypertensive pulmonary levels during OSAS can be beneficial to the cardiocirculatory function.

Continuous positive airway pressure (CPAP) applied through the nares has been recognized as an effective way of preventing the onset of obstructive apneas and snoring and of the consequent oxyhemoglobin desaturations [11]. The aim of our investigation was to test whether the application of CPAP during sleep could ensure a constantly acceptable level of P_{AP}, preventing the pulmonary hypertensive peaks that possibly occur as consequence of the obstructive apneas.

Patients and Methods

We studied six patients, all obese, in whom OSAS had been diagnosed by means of polysomnography. The characteristics of the patients are shown in Table 1. Only

Table 1. Anthropometric and respiratory function characteristics of the sample

Patient	Age (years)	Sex	Weight (% ideal)	PaO_2 (mmHg)	$PaCO_2$ (mmHg)	FEV_1/VC
1	57	M	135	91	39	87
2	59	M	150	77	51	83
3	53	M	174	63	40	83
4	52	M	187	55	55	71
5	36	M	143	84	37	86
6	51	F	222	80	47	86

Table 2. Hemodynamic characteristics of the patients during wakefulness

Patient	Ps (mmHg)	Pd (mmHg)	$\overline{P}_{AP}$ (mmHg)	HR (beats/min)	Hb (g%)
1	35	15	19	72	16
2	25	6	14	74	16
3	29	10	20	90	16
4	55	20	33	78	18
5	25	12	19	75	17
6	35	8	22	74	16

one of the patients (no. 4) had an important alteration in arterial blood gas tensions during wakefulness; he was also the only one with a mild degree of airway obstruction, while all the other patients were normal in this respect. P_{AP} was measured during wakefulness (Table 2): patient no. 4 showed arterial pulmonary hypertension, while the other subjects had slightly increased or normal P_{AP} values.

All patients underwent a new nocturnal polysomnography after the introduction of a Swan-Ganz flow-directed catheter in the pulmonary artery. During the second half of the night, CPAP was applied at the level required to abolish apneas.

Since we did not measure the variation of the pleural pressure, we did not take into account the values of systolic pressure (Ps) and diastolic pressure (Pd) in the conditions when intrapleural pressures become more negative and more markedly influence their measurement, as happens during obstructive apneas. Therefore we considered only the values of Ps and of Pd before the onset of apneas. Heart rate (HR) was measured in the same periods, i.e., the ones when it reaches the highest values [13]. During CPAP application we repeated measurement of P_{AP}, which we compared with the previous ones, together with the relevant values of SaO_2 and HR. In two subjects (no. 4 and 5) P_{AP} measurements during CPAP application were not taken for technical reasons.

Results

The ventilatory and cardiocirculatory data (± SD) detected during sleep in our sample are presented on Tables 3 and 4. Before application of CPAP all the patients showed a high frequency of obstructive apneas (range 45–127 per hour), with a mean duration ranging between 18 and 40 s and a mean related desaturation ranging between 55% and 83%. In the intervals between the apneas, the P_{AP} values in all subjects were increased as compared to the wakefulness levels. In addition, in each subject some very high $\overline{P}_{AP}$ values were detected.

During CPAP application apneas disappeared, ventilation and HR became regular, SaO_2 remained constantly high, and the pulmonary hypertensive peaks were abolished, together with the tachycardias that precede the apneas. Only in patient no. 4 low SaO_2 values could still be observed during CPAP application,

Table 3. Respiratory and hemodynamic data during sleep without CPAP

Patient	Apneas/h	Mean apnea duration (s)	Mean lowest SaO_2 (%)	Ps (mmHg)	Pd (mmHg)	HR (beats/min)	Highest $\bar{P}_{AP}$ (mmHg)
1	60	40 15	75 11	55 17	25 6	82 7	41
2	75	37 8	83 4	32 2	10 1	79 1	37
3	45	23 15	81 8	26 4	16 4	80 6	46
4	127	18 9	68 12	61 13	32 7	85 5	59
5	81	38 8	55 3	41 8	31 7	85 3	57
6	50	20 6	70 7	37 4	16 3	81 11	34

Table 4. Respiratory and hemodynamic data during sleep with CPAP

Patient	CPAP (cmH_2O)	Mean SaO_2 (%)	Ps (mmHg)	Pd (mmHg)	HR (beats/min)	Highest $\bar{P}_{AP}$ (mmHg)
1	9	93	29 2	15 1	65 3	24
2	15	96	30 4	15 1	66 2	25
3	10	90	30 2	18 2	76 1	26
4	7	76			84 6	
5	11	95			79 2	
6	13	86	36 2	17 1	77 2	27

despite the abolition of apneas. That was probably due to hypoventilation especially during REM sleep, when values as low as 65% were detected, while during NREM SaO_2 remained around levels of 82%. Because of the fluctuation in SaO_2 values, HR was also variable and often high.

Discussion

CPAP was first described in 1981 as an effective method to prevent obstructive apneas during sleep [11]. It was then proposed that it acted by pushing forward the soft palate and tongue, sealing the oral cavity and keeping the nasopharyngeal airway patent. Later, other mechanisms of action were proposed, which could also play a role [8]. Since this first one, many reports have been published describing the acute and chronic effects of the use of CPAP on respiration during sleep, sleep structure and daytime symptoms of patients affected by OSAS [1, 3, 6, 7]. It has been shown that CPAP invariably abolishes obstructive apneas during sleep and, as a consequence, improves sleep structure, alertness, and sometimes also respiratory function during daytime [9, 10]. However, the effects of CPAP on pulmonary hemodynamics have not been described. The increase in P_{AP} during sleep in OSAS has been known for many years [4, 12], and there is no doubt that nocturnal hypoxemia plays an important role in determining it. CPAP prevents the desaturations, but may induce an increase in pulmonary vascular resistance as an effect of the pressure exerted upon the alveolar capillaries [5].

We found that CPAP prevents the peaks of pulmonary hypertension and usually stabilizes P_{AP} and HR at around values lower than those detected during the intervals between apneas. In the evaluation of these results we must take into account that the P_{AP} values reported are influenced by the pressure applied to the airway (9–15 cmH_2O in our sample) and therefore they are higher than those actually present in the pulmonary circulatory system. Nevertheless, they demonstrate the intervention of a therapeutic effect due to the correction of the apneas and of SaO_2.

Further studies are needed to assess the chronic effects of CPAP application on the P_{AP} detectable during wakefulness, as a consequence of a more prolonged correction of cardiorespiratory derangements due to OSAS.

References

1. Berry RB, Block AJ (1984) Positive nasal airway pressure eliminates snoring as well as obstructive sleep apnea. Chest 85:15–20
2. Bonsignore G, Marrone O, Milone F, Oddo S, Coppola P, Macaluso C, Bellia V, Ferrara G, Cibella F (1986) L'applicazione della pressione positiva continua per via nasale nel trattamento della sindrome dell'apnea ostruttiva nel sonno. Ann Ital Med Int 1:131–140
3. Bradley TD, Rutherford R, Grossman RF, Lue F, Zamel N, Moldofsky H, Phillipson EA (1985) Role of daytime hypoxemia in the pathogenesis of right heart failure in the obstructive sleep apnea syndrome. Am Rev Respir Dis 131:835–839
4. Coccagna G, Mantovani M, Brignani F, Parchi C, Lugaresi E (1972) Continuous recording of the pulmonary and systemic arterial pressure during sleep in syndromes of hypersomnia with periodic breathing. Bull Physiopathol Respir 8:1159–1172

5. Haynes JB (1982) Hemodynamic monitoring during supportive management. In: Petty LT (ed) Intensive and rehabilitative respiratory care, 3rd edn Lea and Febiger, Philadelphia, pp 114–131
6. Krieger J, Sautegeau A, Sauder P, Weitzenblum E, Kurtz D (1984) Syndromes d'apnées du sommeil. Traitement par la pression positive continue par voi nasale. Presse Med 13:2559–2562
7. McEvoy RD, Thornton AT (1984) Treatment of obstructive sleep apnea syndrome with nasal continuous positive airway pressure. Sleep 7:313–325
8. Rapoport DM, Garay SM, Goldring RM (1983): Nasal CPAP in obstructive sleep apnea: mechanisms of action. Bull Eur Physiopathol Respir 19:616–620
9. Rapoport DM, Sorkim B, Garay SM, Goldring RM (1982) Reversal of the "Pickwickian syndrome" by long-term use of nocturnal nasal-airway pressure. N Engl J Med 307:931–933
10. Sullivan CE, Berthon-Jones M, Issa FG (1983): Remission of severe obesity-hypoventilation syndrome after short-term treatment during sleep with nasal continuous positive airway pressure. Am Rev Respir Dis 126:177–181
11. Sullivan CE, Issa FG, Berthon-Jones M, Eves L (1981) Reversal of obstructive sleep apnoea by continuous positive airway pressure applied through the nares. Lancet I:862–865
12. Tilkian AG, Guilleminault C, Schroeder JS, Lehrman KL, Simmons FB, Dement WC (1976) Hemodynamics in sleep-induced apnea. Ann Intern Med 85:714–719
13. Tilkian AG, Guilleminault C, Schroeder JS, Lehrman KL, Simmons FB, Dement WC (1977) Sleep induced apnea syndrome. Prevalence of cardiac arrhythmias and their reversal after tracheostomy. Am J Med 63:348–358

Reversibility of Severe Cardiac Arrhythmias in Sleep Apnea Under Nasal Continuous Positive Airway Pressure Therapy

H. BECKER, M. FAUST, U. KÖHLER, and J. H. PETER

Introduction

While patients with sleep apnea (SA) do not exhibit significantly more cardiac arrhythmias during wakefulness than healthy subjects [1, 2], several investigators have been able to demonstrate an increase in arrhythmias during sleep in such patients as compared with patients not suffering from SA [1, 2, 6, 8]. These increases are closely associated with the apnea episodes.

The form of cardiac arrhythmia most characteristic for SA seems to be nocturnal sinus arrhythmia, which was found in 78%–100% of all patients who were studied [4, 8, 9]. Additional cardiac results include premature ventricular and atrial contractions (PVC/PAC), first to third degree atrioventricular (AV) conduction blocks, as well as sinus pauses. Frequency rates between 5% and 20% have been reported [1, 2, 8].

Nasal continuous positive airway pressure therapy (CPAP) could be shown to be an effective means of reversing apnea in a large proportion of patients with obstructive and mixed SA [3, 5, 7]. As apnea can be successfully treated with CPAP, and as disturbances of the cardiac rhythm are closely associated with this clinical picture, we asked what influence nasal CPAP therapy would have on the cardiac results in patients with sleep apnea. For a first study with this novel approach we selected five patients with severe apnea and cardiac arrhythmias.

Methods

Patient Selection

For the present study we selected five male patients who had been found to suffer from severe SA during screening investigations at our hospital in 1983–86 and who also suffered from characteristic cardiac arrhythmias. These patients were between 36 and 57 years old (mean 49.2). They all had extremely pronounced SA with an apnea index of 39–70 episodes per hour of sleep (mean 51.2). Patient no. 5 had central apnea, the others mixed or obstructive apnea. The clinical investigations showed systemic hypertension in four, two of whom also had pulmonary hypertension and myocardial insufficiency grade II (patient no. 2) and III (patient no. 1) according to the New York Heart Association (NYHA) classification.

Protocol

Recordings of respiration and long-term ECG were carried out on 3 consecutive nights. On the 1st night, control values were established, and no CPAP therapy was applied. On the 2nd night, the patients were given the opportunity to adjust to CPAP therapy, and we determined the individual amount of CPAP necessary for efficient apnea reversal (see Fig. 5). On the 3rd night, CPAP therapy was applied along with the recordings.

Measurements and Evaluation

Abdominal and thoracic respiration were measured by inductive plethysmography, and partial arterial oxygen tension transcutaneously. This method, in combination with the ECG, allows a clear assessment of apnea and has been successfully used by our research team for several years. A continuous long-term ECG (Oxford Medilog 4000) was recorded over 24 h and evaluated by visual analysis of the full disclosure records as well as by computerized evaluation routines. A second two-channel ECG (ELA Anatec) was applied just before the patients went to bed. This ECG permitted visual inspection on the screen as well as computerized beat-to-beat analysis over the whole sleeping period.

Results

On the 1st night of the recordings, when no therapy was applied, all cardiac arrhythmias, which had been demonstrated previously, could again be documented. All patients hat nocturnal sinus arrhythmia. Figure 1 shows a section of the long-term ECG recording in a patient without therapy. In addition, we found a second degree AV block in one patient and a third degree AV block and recurrent sinus pauses in another during sleep (Figs. 2–4). Nocturnal ectopies were found in four patients. Patients no. 2, 3, and 4 had PVCs class I, and patient no. 1 PVCs class VIa according to the Lown classification (Fig. 5).

Sleep apnea was efficiently reduced by nasal CPAP therapy in all patients. Figure 6 shows a sample recording illustrating the determination of efficient CPAP (for individual results, see Table 1).

CPAP therapy on the 3rd night of the investigation resulted in a reduction of sinus arrhythmia in four out of five patients. No significant reduction could be achieved in patient no. 5, who suffered from central SA. Heart rate variability in the other four patients was also distinctly reduced, as the automatically calculated histograms of the R-R beat-to-beat intervals analyzed during 3 h of sleep show (Fig. 7). Figure 8 shows that the difference between the maximum and the minimum heart rate during sleep, established by means of the Oxford Medilog

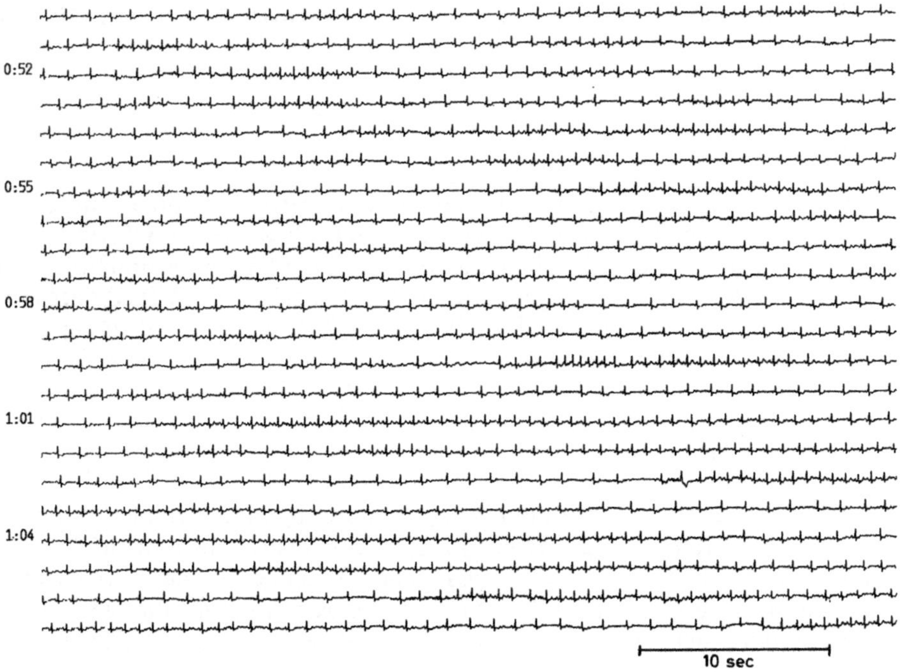

Fig. 1. Excerpt form the condensed long-term ECG (Oxford Medilog 4000, full disclosure) of patient no. 2 with severe SA before CPAP therapy, illustrating the cyclical variation in heart rate which is characteristic for the vast majority of SA patients

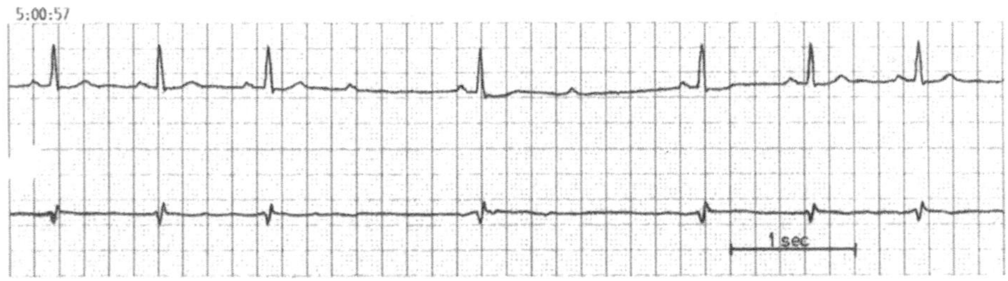

Fig. 2. Second degree AV conduction block in patient no. 1 before CPAP therapy

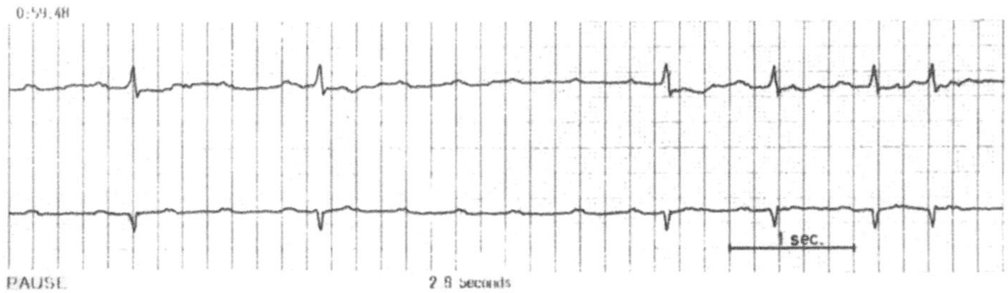

Fig. 3. Third degree AV conduction block in patient no. 2 before CPAP therapy

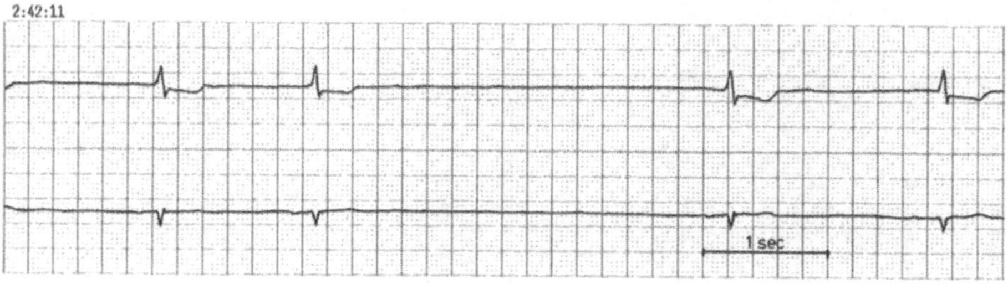

Fig. 4. Nocturnal sinus arrest in patient no. 2 before CPAP therapy

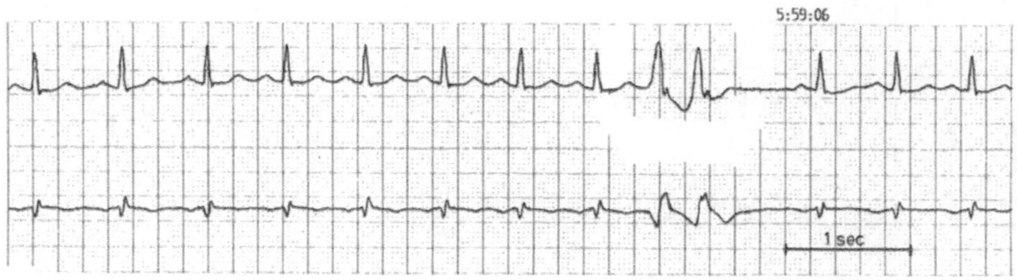

Fig. 5. Nocturnal couplet in patient no. 2 before CPAP therapy

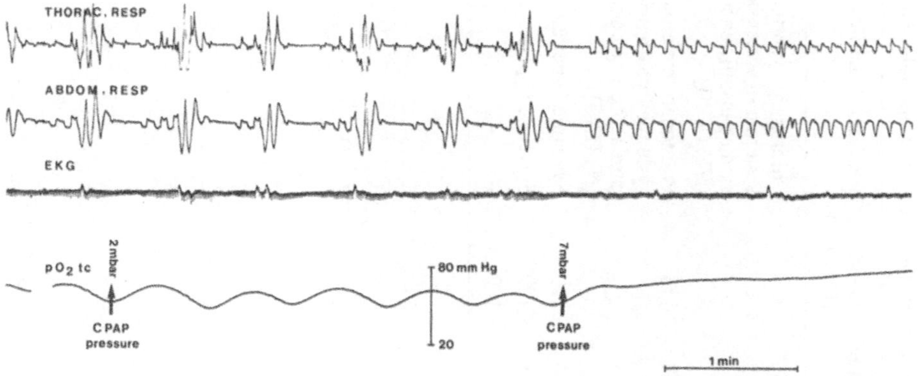

Fig. 6. Determination of efficient CPAP; recording showing successive apneas and their reversal after 7 mbar CPAP. *From the top:* thoracic and abdominal respiration (inductive plethysmography), ECG, partial arterial oxygen tension (transcutaneously). Insufficient (2 mbar) and sufficient (7 mbar) CPAP indicated

Table 1. Summary of the clinical data and relevant results before and after nasal CPAP therapy in five patients with pronounced SA

Patient No.	Age	Weight (Broca %)	Relevant diagnoses	CPAP (mbar)	Apnea index		Heart blocks		Ectopies	
					No CPAP	CPAP	No CPAP	CPAP	No CPAP	CPAP
1	56	186	Pulmonary hypertension, systemic hypertension, cardiac insufficiency (NYHA III)	12	39	6	Second degree AV	-	IVa	I
2	57	118	Pulmonary hypertension systemic hypertension cardiac insufficiency (NYHA II)	8	70	8	Third degree AV, sinus arrest	-	I	0
3	36	129	Systemic hypertension	8	47	3	-	-	I	0
4	48	129	Systemic hypertension	8	46	3	-	-	I	0
5	49	110	- - - -	8	54	10	-	-	0	0

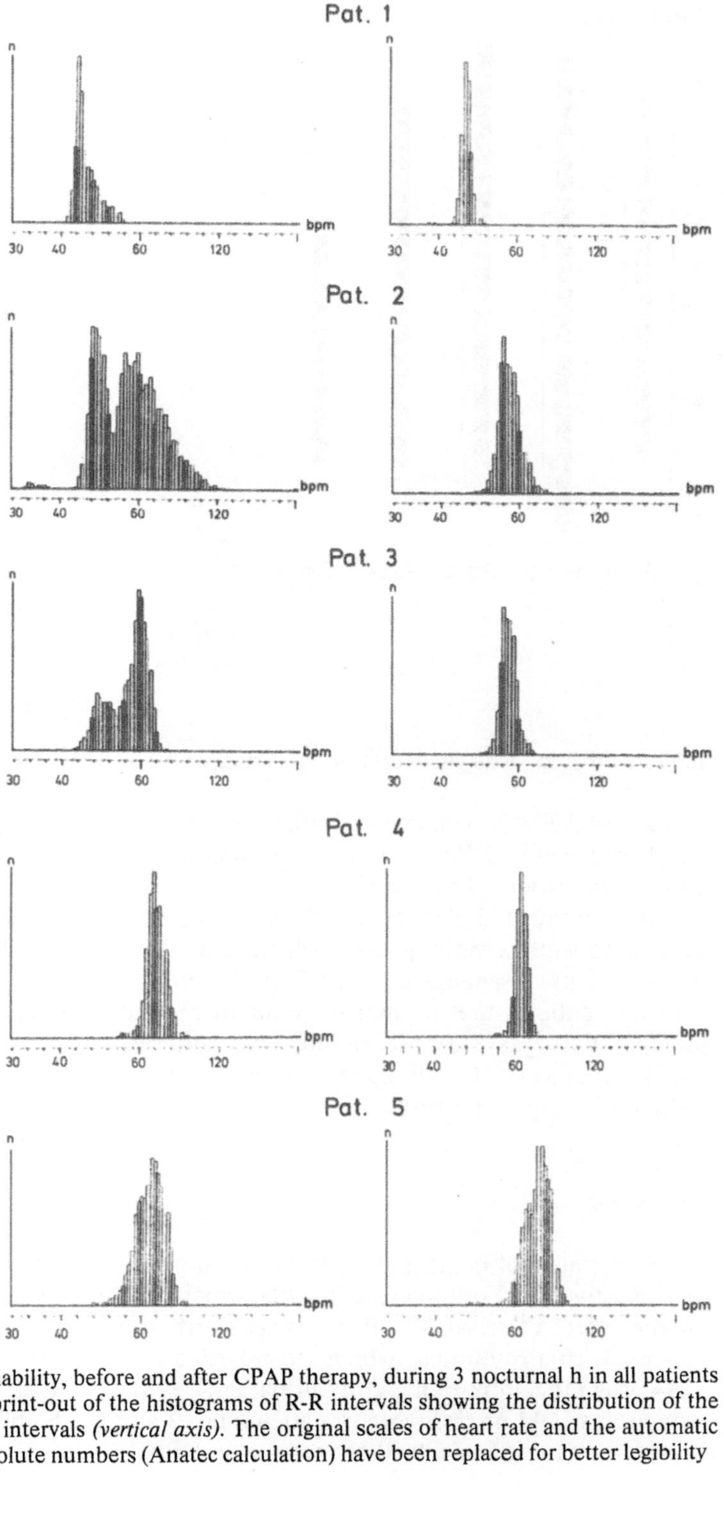

Fig. 7. Heart rate variability, before and after CPAP therapy, during 3 nocturnal h in all patients separately. Original print-out of the histograms of R-R intervals showing the distribution of the absolute numbers of intervals *(vertical axis)*. The original scales of heart rate and the automatic determination of absolute numbers (Anatec calculation) have been replaced for better legibility

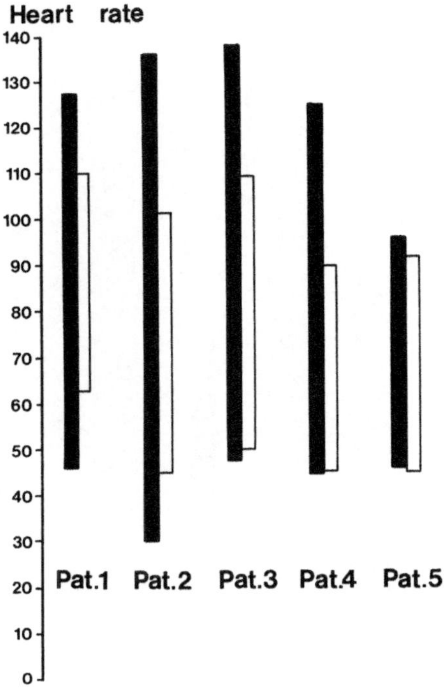

Fig. 8. Representation of the development of maximum and minimum heart rate during sleep, showing a distinctly smaller range after therapy. Based on the long-term Oxford Medilog 4000 ECG recordings. ■, without CPAP; □, with CPAP

4000 recording, was also distinctly reduced in four out of five patients after therapy.

Nocturnal PVCs, which had initially been found in four patients, were also clearly reduced by CPAP therapy. After therapy, occasional PVCs were observed only in one patient. The severity of the PVCs in terms of the Lown classification was also diminished. Second and third degree AV blocks, each occurring in one patient, as well as sinus pauses, which had additionally been found in one of these patients, disappeared after CPAP therapy.

In one patient, the number of premature atrial contractions increased after therapy. This was the only patient who suffered from central apnea (patient no. 5) and in whom CPAP therapy was also without demonstrable effect on sinus arrhythmia. The main results of this study have been summarized in Table 1.

Discussion

The occurrence of nocturnal cardiac arrhythmias has been described by numerous investigators. For the present study, which, to our knowledge, is the first ever on the effect of nasal CPAP on cardiac arrhythmias in SA, we selected five patients with arrhythmias, which are regarded as characteristic for SA.

SA was efficiently reduced in all patients by nasal CPAP therapy. A further reduction would be desirable in patients no. 2 and no. 5 and could possibly be achieved by means of a further increase in CPAP.

At the same time, CPAP therapy led to a massive reduction in nocturnal sinus arrhythmia as well as PVCs, and the complete suppression of AV conduction blocks, and sinus arrests. The sometimes severe cardiac arrhythmias which had been established before onset of the therapy could all be resolved.

The present results corroborate the results of an investigation by Guilleminault et al. [2], who found a far-reaching reversal of arrhythmias in 50 patients with SA and concomitant nocturnal arrhythmias after trachestomy therapy. Guilleminault, too, found that only PVCs, in a small number, were still present after therapy. Our own results show that severe nocturnal arrhythmias can also be prevented by an effective conservative therapy, that is by removing arrhythmogenic factors within the picture of SA, such as hypoxia, diminished pulmonary compliance, and intrathoracic pressure changes [10] by means of CPAP. In the light of these encouraging results, further studies which quantify and qualify the present findings should be undertaken in a greater number of unselected patients.

References

1. Bolm-Audorff U, Köhler U, Becker E, Fuchs E, Peter JH, Meinzer K, von Wichert P (1984) Nächtliche Herzrhythmusstörungen bei Schlafapnoe-Syndrom. Dtsch Med Wochenschr 109:853–856
2. Guilleminault C, Connolly SJ, Winkle RA (1983) Cardiac arrhythmia and conduction disturbances during sleep in 400 patients with sleep apnea syndrome. Am J Cardiol 52:490–494
3. McEnvoy RD, Thornton AT (1984) Treatment of obstructive sleep apnea syndrome with nasal continuous positive airway pressure. Sleep 7:313–325
4. Miller WP (1982) Cardiac arrhythmias and conduction disturbances in the sleep apnea syndrome. Am J Med 73:317–321
5. Remmers JE, Sterling JA, Thorarinsson B, Kuna ST (1984) Nasal airway positive pressure in patients with occlusive sleep apnea. Am Rev Respir Dis 130:1152–1155
6. Shepard JW Jr (1985) Gas exchange and hemodynamics during sleep. Med Clin North Am 69:1243–1264
7. Sullivan CE, Issa FG, Berthon-Jones M, McCauley VB, Costas LJV (1984) Home treatment of obstructive sleep apnoea with continuous positive airway pressure applied through a nose-mask. Bull Eur Physiopathol Respir 20:49–54
8. Tilkian AG, Guilleminault C, Schroeder JS, Lehrmann KL, Simmons FB, Dement WC (1977) Sleep apnea syndrome. Prevalence of cardiac arrhythmias and their reversal after tracheostomy. Am J Med 63:348–358
9. Tilkian AG, Motta J, Guilleminault C (1978) Cardiac arrhythmias in sleep apnea. In: Guilleminault C, Dement WC (eds) Sleep apnea syndromes. Liss, New York, pp 197–210
10. Zwillich C, Devlin T, White D, Douglas N, Weil J, Martin R (1982) Bradycardia during sleep apnea. Characteristics and mechanism. J Clin Invest 69:1286–1292

Current Research in Sleep-Related Breathing Disorders: Conclusions for Internal Diagnostics and Therapy

J. H. PETER

Internists and general physicians have been familiar with the relationship between sleep-wake disorders and internal diseases for quite some time. This connection is usually regarded from the point of view that a severe and/or consumptive primary disease interferes with the normal sleep-wake behavior, or that altered sleep-wake behavior is the result of certain medications, as is the case in antihypertensive therapy or steroid therapy.

Apart from general physicians, neuropsychiatrists customarily encounter sleep-wake disorders as a chief complaint. During the last 10 years, they have done much to accomplish an efficienct classification of sleep-wake disorders based on the patients' complaints and behavior [1]. In addition to epidemiological studies in the sleep-wake disorders thus classified, we are indebted to neuropsychiatry for epidemiological studies in other illnesses associated with disturbances of the sleep-wake behavior [2–4]. This approach led to the insight that not only insomnia, on which the main attention had been focused, but also hypersomnia and especially excessive daytime sleepiness (EDS) went along with increased general and internal morbidity as well as an elevated rate of mortality. Independently of the complaints associated with insomnia, these correlations were found to be based on the connection between nocturnal disturbances of the respiratory regulation, especially sleep apnea (SA), and cardiovascular, pulmonary, or cardiopulmonary diseases [5–7]. The connection between cardiorespiratory disorders and hypersomnia, on the other hand, had already been established in the classical studies in the pickwickian syndrome [8, 9]. Seventeen years ago, Jung and Kuhlo had also already described a parallel beneficial effect of tracheostomy on the cardiorespiratory and the psychophysical functional restriction in pickwickian patients [10]. Since the 1970s, a great number of studies have appeared wich – using clinical, pathophysiological, or epidemiological methods – elaborate on the relationship between nocturnal respiratory regulative disorders and cardiac arrhythmias, cardiac insufficiency, and arterial hypertension [11–15]. At the same time, epidemiological studies underscored the relevance of the nocturnal respiratory regulation, both within the context of sleep-wake disorders and of cardiovascular and cardiopulmonary risk factors and diseases [16–18].

The aim of the Marburg symposium documented in the present volume was the academic exchange of up-to-date information on sleep-related disorders and internal diseases. Among the participants were sleep physiologists, neuropsychiatrists, occupational physiologists, sociologists, epidemiologists, general practitioners, representatives of the pharmaceutical and technical instruments' industry, pneumologists, cardiologists, psychologists, engineers, technicians, physicists, and biochemists. The active contributors to the congress came from 11 countries in order to study and discuss the current international state of knowledge on sleep-wake disorders and internal diseases. Although it became evident that we are still in the early stages of understanding many relevant pathophysiological interrelationships, all presentations were unanimous in their recognition of the great significance of the problems under discussion. Snoring, sleep apnea, and desynchronized breathing, for instance, are beginning to receive the attention they deserve, as they impair both psychomental health and physical fitness, and reduce life expectancy. With the clinical importance of sleep-related breathing disorders now established, the general relevance and scope of the problem demands that we must immediately begin to draw practical conclusions for diagnostics and therapy in the fields of internal and general medicine, fully independently of the many questions which remain to be resolved in the future. Some of these conclusions will be discussed here.

The methods demonstrated for an early diagnosis of sleep-related respiratory regulative disorders lead us to believe that a significant decrease in general morbidity and mortality can be expected in the future. The symposium revealed that the significance of methods of early diagnosis has been underestimated up to now. In addition to the necessity for intensifying the efforts in the fields of clinical and therapeutic knowledge, important tasks in the education of the general population as well as the medical community challenge the researcher in this field.

Recent experience suggests that one well-equipped sleep laboratory is necessary for roughly 1 million inhabitants. We estimate that at least 2 million West German citizens exhibit a risk profile which urgently demands proper diagnostic management. As this risk profile is still largely unexplored, and the underestimation of the risks involved have prevented any safe quantitative assessment in the past, we can only judge from our present experience. On the basis of this experience, we estimate that at least 10% of those 2 million are in acute danger.

It is obvious that the large number of patients urgently in need of an apnea registration cannot be monitored with differential diagnostics under hospital ward conditions, not even in those countries where an adequate number of sleep laboratories exists. Biochemical screening methods with a sufficient degree of specificity and selectivity have not yet been developed. For these reasons, efficient ambulatory measuring techniques must be developed. As a prerequisite, detailed anamnestic reports are needed, and specific attention should be given to the following catalogue of indications:

a) Internal Medicine and General Medicine

- essential hypertension
- otherwise unexplained myocardial insufficiency, chest pains without evidence of coronary heart disease or other organic failure
- nocturnal cardiac arrhythmias
- obesity
- polycythemia
- otherwise unexplained recidivistic myogelosis in the neck and back

b) Neurology/Psychiatry and General Medicine
- reduced sleep latency and excessive daytime sleepiness, often in combination with difficulties in maintaining sleep
- permanent fatigue
- intellectual deterioration
- personality changes, depressions
- sexual dysfunction
- morning headaches

c) ENT and General Medicine
- loud and irregular snoring

There is a variety of parameters which lend themselves to ambulatory screening techniques. In the following we have drawn up a list of screening priorities which reflects our group's experience. As the individual measurements of separate parameters may prove cumbersome and only have limited reliability, our present combined solution intervenes on the way between preparatory ambulatory screening and comprehensive measurements in the sleep laboratory. During the past years, this portable unit has been found to be a reliable tool in the diagnosis of SA activity.

Rank order of separate analytic routines	Our present combined solution	Comprehensive stationary approach
1. Anamnestic questionnaire 2. Analysis of nocturnal heart rate (Holter ECG) —→ 3. Analysis of snoring 4. Analysis of respiration: inductive plethysmography, nasal thermistor 5. Continous blood gas monitoring (O_2 and CO_2 tensions)	1. ↓ 2 + 4 + 5: 4-Channel portable unit with ECG, inductive plethysmography, pO_2tc —→	Polysomnography in the sleep laboratory

Independently of the fact that, in view of the great number of persons in question, the amount of necessary recordings cannot be conducted under hospital ward conditions, there is still the problem of finding a standard of quantification for sleep-related breathing disorders (SRBD) which would permit a clear discrimination between what is still physiologically normal, and what is clearly pathological. The apnea index commonly used is based on the definition of apnea as a respiratory standstill exceeding 10 s, independently of their pattern. In addition to "central," "obstructive," and "mixed" apneas, hypopnea and desynchronized breathing must also be regarded as important SRBD. As the transition between physiological and pathological forms is somewhat fluid in all these varieties of SRBD, the diagnostical apparatus of the future will have to develop better evaluative guidelines than we have available today. We suggest that for any SRBD, a certain frequency and a certain duration of the individual occurren-

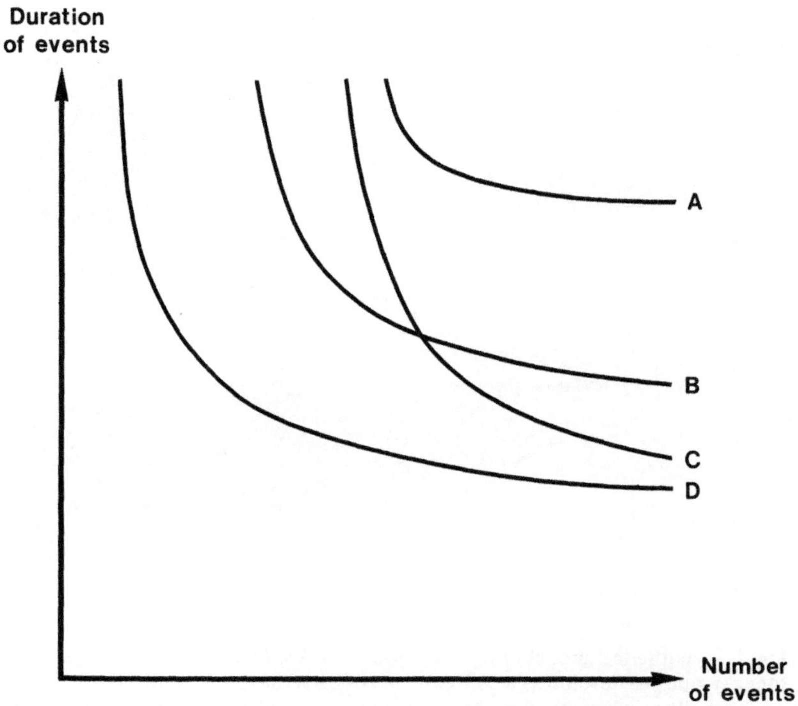

Fig. 1. Schematic illustration of the possible future determination of thresholds between physiological and pathological degrees of various sleep-related breathing disorders *A–D,* based on frequency and duration of individual occurrences. *A parallel to the horizonal axis* would imply that a disorder x is pathological as soon as its individual occurrence exceeds a certain duration, irrespective of its frequency; *a parallel to the vertical axis* would imply that the frequency of a disorder, independently of the duration of the individual instances, marks the transition into the pathological region. The determination of such curves for specific disorders would serve as guidelines for the clinical management of these diseases

ces will not be dangerous, but a high number of short individual instances or a small number of instances exceeding a critical duration will place the patient in a situation which demands clinical management (Fig. 1). It is imaginable that future research will be able to define borderlines between the physiological and the pathological region for each type of SRBD, depending on the duration and the frequency of its occurrence.

It cannot be stressed too often that early diagnostics are vital for the prevention of the composite clinical pictures which usually characterize SRBD in their advanced stages. Figure 2 shows a hypothetical model of the relationship between SA activity (SAA) and the findings which constitute the sleep apnea syndromes (SAS). The complete picture of the SAS does not fully develop until many years have elapsed. Usually SAA is detected when the patient seeks medical advice because of severe internal or psychophysiological complaints, but the

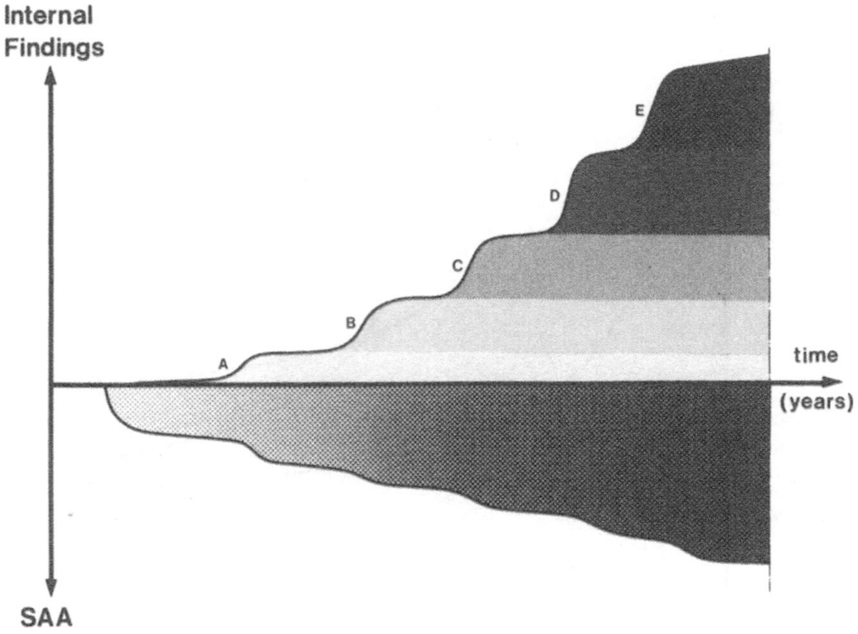

Fig. 2. Hypothetical model of the formation of SAS. Over the course of the years, internal and other symptoms develop as a consequence of SAA. Severe complications after a long history of SAA usually reinforce each other and cannot be completely reversed. Therapy must start before the multimorbid picture has formed

model makes plain that the diagnosis of SAA must take place before the entire picture of SAS has formed if there is to be a chance of intervening therapeutically and preventively in an effective way. Patients with high SAA are high-risk patients and must be identified as early as possible.

In terms of preventive and therapeutical measures, many questions remain to be solved. Weight loss in obese patients is essential. Tranquilizers, sedatives, anesthetics, alcohol, as well as other substances which have a depressant impact on the respiration must be avoided. Medications indicated in the treatment of a variety of diseases may interact with the mechanisms of SAA in a detrimental way. In the field of internal therapy we must train ourselves to ask the question: does any particular drug interact with vigilance, sleep, respiration during sleep, the cardiovascular system during sleep? This concerns sleeping pills and sedatives, but also many cardiocirculatory medications, antihypertensive agents, and antiarrhythmic drugs. The strong links within the triangle of sleep-wake regulation, respiratory control, and circulatory regulation should always be taken into account. Cardiovascular and cardiopulmonary disorders must be treated with special care and attention.

According to our experience, theophylline preparations have proved useful in the treatment of SAS, especially in its early stages. Should the relevant drug therapy attempts fail, we use nasal continuous positive airway pressure therapy.

The contributions to the symposium leave no doubt that the proper scope of the problems under discussion is now being recognized. Taken in their entirety, they express a growing concern and confidence in this field of research which leads us to expect that the problems which still await us are not insurmountable.

References

1. Association of Sleep Disorders Centers (1979) Diagnostic classification of sleep and arousal disorders. Sleep 2:1–122
2. Coleman RM, Roffwarg HP, Kennedy SJ (1980) Sleep-wake disorders based on a polysomnographic diagnosis. A national cooperative study. JAMA 247:997–1003
3. Lavie P (1983) Incidence of sleep apnea in a presumably healthy population: a significant relationship with excessive daytime sleepiness. Sleep 6:312–318
4. Guilleminault C, Dement WC (1978) Sleep apnea syndrome and related disorders. In: Williams RL, Koracan D (eds) Sleep disorders: diagnosis and treatment. Wiley, New York, pp 9–28
5. Guilleminault C, Eldridge EL, Simmon FB, Dement WC (1975) Sleep apnea syndrome - can it induce hemodynamic changes? West J Med 123:7–16
6. Coccagna F, Mantovani M, Brignani F, Parchi C, Lugaresi E (1972) Continuous recording of the pulmonary and systemic arterial pressure during sleep in syndromes of hypersomnia with periodic breathing. Bull Physiopathol Respir 8:1103–1113
7. Podszus T, Bauer W, Mayer J, Penzel T, Peter JH, von Wichert P (1986) Sleep apnea and pulmonary hypertension. Klin Wochenschr 64:131–134
8. Burwell CS, Robin ED, Whaley RD, Bickelmann AG (1956) Extreme obesity associated with alveolar hypoventilation. A pickwickian syndrome. Am J Med 21:811–818
9. Jung R, Kuhlo W (1965) Neurophysiological studies of abnormal night sleep and the pickwickian syndrome. Progr Brain Res 18:140–159
10. Kuhlo W, Doll E, Franck MC (1969) Erfolgreiche Behandlung eines Pickwick-Syndroms durch eine Dauertrachealkanüle. Dtsch Med Wochenschr 94:1286–1290
11. Bolm-Audorff U, Köhler U, Becker E, Fuchs E, Mainzer K, Peter JH, von Wichert P (1984) Nächtliche Herzrhythmusstörungen bei Schlafapnoe-Syndrom. Dtsch Med Wochenschr 109:853–856
12. Tilkian AG, Motta J, Guilleminault C (1978) Cardiac arrhythmias in sleep apnea. In: Guilleminault C, Dement WC (eds) Sleep apnea syndromes. Liss, New York, pp 197–210
13. Schroeder JS, Motta J, Guilleminault C (1978) Hemodynamic studies in sleep apnea. In: Guilleminault C, Dement WC (eds) Sleep apnea syndromes. Liss, New York, pp 177–196
14. Scharf SM (1984) Influence of sleep state and breathing on cardiovascular function. In: Saunders NA, Sullivan CE (eds) Sleep and breathing. Dekker, New York, pp 221–240
15. Podszus T, Bauer W, Mayer J, Peter JH, von Wichert P (1986) Sleep apnea and pulmonary hypertension. Klin Wochenschr 64:131–134
16. Siegrist J, Peter JH (1986) Schlafstörungen und kardiovaskuläres Risiko. Med Klin 81:429–432
17. Martin RJ (1984) Cardiorespiratory disorders during sleep. Futura, Mount Kisco
18. Köhler U, Mayer J, Peter JH, von Wichert P (1985) Cardiac arrhythmias accompanying sleep apnea activity (SAA) in patients with established sleep apnea and in general outpatients. Sleep Res 14:179

GPSR Compliance

The European Union's (EU) General Product Safety Regulation (GPSR) is a set of rules that requires consumer products to be safe and our obligations to ensure this.

If you have any concerns about our products, you can contact us on ProductSafety@springernature.com

In case Publisher is established outside the EU, the EU authorized representative is:

Springer Nature Customer Service Center GmbH
Europaplatz 3
69115 Heidelberg, Germany

Batch number: 10761697

Printed by Printforce, the Netherlands